# SELF HEAL

## THE COMPLETE HOME GUIDE TO NATURAL HEALING, HERBS AND NUTRITION

**Jill Rosemary Davies**

Newleaf

Newleaf
an imprint of
Gill & Macmillan Ltd
Hume Avenue
Park West
Dublin 12
with associated companies throughout the world
www.gillmacmillan.ie


© 2000 Jill Rosemary Davies
1 8586 00537
Print origination by Carole Lynch
Index by Susan Williams
Printed in Malaysia

A catalogue record is available for this book
from the British Library.

1  3  5  4  2

# ACKNOWLEDGEMENTS

I dedicate this book with love and gratitude to the memory of Dr. John Christopher for all his work and teaching and to Dr. Richard Schulze for keeping this herbal legacy alive and moving it on and into the 21st century. It is also dedicated to all herbalists worldwide for keeping and sharing the knowledge in the face of constant threats, legislation and land ravaging.

I may have written a book about natural healing and herbalism, but I am certainly not a natural writer and so, in effect, this book has been co-written by my friend Ruth Butterfield, whose patience, intelligence, organisational and editing skills have completed this work. Huge thanks also go to Alick and Kevin at Gateway Books for their gentle encouragement and support and to Deirdre Greenan and Michael Gill of Gill & Macmillan. For 'life' support during the writing of this book I would like to thank Dr. Shamim Daya, Professor Linda Fellows, Ray Hill from the BHMA, Anna Piper, Debs Chater, Andrea Stainsby, Jack Silverstone, Melanie and Abigail and also my wonderful family, Nityananda, Lorna and Jasmine.

My thanks go to all the practitioners, colleagues and students who have shaped the information in this book – in Britain, the USA and India. I wish I could list you all but I can't, so many thanks, even to those unmet, whose books have taught and inspired me.

Illustrators : Toby Driver (tree dressing, line drawings of plants), and Stephen Sturgess (culinary equipment).

# CONTENTS

CONTENTS

## Caution

*In general no doses have been given for the herbs, neither have the contra-indications of herbs been included as they are numerous and specific, those pregnant being in the highest category to avoid certain herbs. A list of contra-indications or more information and a dosage guide is available from:*

The Selfheal School for Herbalists and Natural Healers
The Cabins, Station Warehouse, Station Road, Pulham Market, Norfolk IP21 4XF; UK
Tel: 01379 608 082 & 01379 608 007, Fax & Tel: 01379 608 201 e-mail: Selfheal@aol.com
Herbs–Hands–Healing
Address as above
Tel.: 01379 608 201 e-mail: HerbsInfo@aol.com

# Introduction

## THE SELF HEAL WAY

The stars of this book are the plants, trees and flowers themselves. They are endearing, beautiful, mysterious, fundamental and primitive. The delight and use of their seeds, roots, bark, colour and form is phenomenal and, set amongst the rest of the intricate web of nature, they are truly miraculous. However, this book is not only about the plants, it is also about a combination of natural healing methods, healthy lifestyle and the use of herbs as potent tools for natural healing. Were this simply a book on herbal medicine, I feel that it would be dangerously easy to see plants as a direct substitute for conventional drugs. However, although it is often possible to gently and carefully substitute one for the other, on the whole it is best to use herbs as an integral part of life, combining them with the wealth of lifestyle choices we make and thus preventing and balancing dispositions.

Plant healing is deeply ingrained in our ancestry, yet the privilege of healing our own bodies has been increasingly taken away from us and put into the hands of doctors and conventional medicine. It is not surprising that night calls to doctors have doubled in the last few years, pill-taking has soared and the skills of home nursing have diminished. Many people tend to view ill-health as a 'supermarket affair', demanding quick answers with the cry, 'Give me a pill and make it go away, now!' However, for others, the yearning and desperation to know more about home natural healing skills, combined with herbs, is a pressing quest. So this book has been written in the understanding that herbalism and natural healing should be restored to the home as safely and effectively as possible.

All practitioners insist that, if there is any doubt as to the cause of a patient's condition, a doctor's diagnosis should be sought. From this you, and perhaps your local herbalist, can work on your body naturally until you regain full health. I will also be explaining the philosophy and ethos behind herbalism and natural healing. Perhaps you are not ill but just want to learn how to look after yourself. Knowing how to prevent ill-health, by understanding your body and having some practical insight in how to look after it, is all part of the ethos of natural healing. By gaining this knowledge, you will learn how to return some of the responsibility for your health back to where it should be, especially when one considers that 50% of Britain's 46,000 yearly patients dying from iatrogenic ailments (doctor involved) are associated with operations followed by diagnostic errors.

Many of the natural healing programmes in this book require the cleansing of the body via special foods. This is called detoxification and is fundamental to the natural healing process. Its basic importance rests upon the fact that the human body has the ability to regenerate itself, using its own genetic blueprint. Until recently it was believed that the time it took for the individual cells of the liver to regenerate, and thus create a new liver, was two years; now it is believed to be just a few months. This is phenomenally hopeful for so many people. Of course, the health of each new blood cell and thus each new organ reflects what it is created from – i.e. if we feed our bodies nutritionally deficient or toxic food we cannot expect to create healthy organs. However, with the correct directives and input, repairing our bodies is possible. Dr. John Christopher, Dr. Richard Schulze and Dr. Deepak Chopra – all of whom have been ground-breaking healers of the 20th and 21st centuries – have proven and continued to teach this inspiring thought for many years.

Other methods, which will be explained, include the use of water – to heat or cool the body in order to encourage circulation, to support and nurture, to de-stagnate, to cleanse and to provoke. As you read the chapter on diseases you will see how vigorous some of the programmes need to be in order to get results. You may be tempted to follow only part of a programme and to leave out some of the harder tasks but, if you are seriously ill, it is imperative that you carry out the treatment as directed. If your condition is not chronic then you may follow cleanses, such as a bowel or liver cleanse, specific to you, or simply as a preventative M.O.T. It is no coincidence that one of the most important health quests of the 21st century is the understanding of the immune and hormome systems, which is now being tested and punished in a myriad of ways. We must, therefore, ask more questions; and herbs are very good at providing some of the answers.

## WHY TRY HERBALISM?

Medical science took a big leap forward in Europe after the second world war with the development of a whole collection of drugs, including beta-blockers, anaesthetics, antidepressants, steroids and antibiotics, to name but a few. Some remain extremely useful, especially the anaesthetics, some painkillers and antibiotics when used in highly selective situations. Medical technology also took a big leap and, although some discoveries are now readily accepted as being useful and non-invasive, much new technology seems to have been designed simply to make lots of money for the manufacturers; while some is positively destructive, invasive and life-threatening.

Robert Mendelsohn M.D. in his book *Confessions of a Medical Heretic* says:

*I believe that modern medicine treatments for disease are seldom effective and that they are often more dangerous than the diseases they are designed to treat. I believe the dangers are compounded by the widespread use of dangerous procedures for non-diseases. I believe that more than 90% of modern medicine could disappear from the face of the earth – doctors, hospitals, drugs, equipment – and the effect on our health would be immediate and beneficial. I believe that modern medicine has gone too far, by using, in everyday situations, extreme treatments designed for critical conditions!*

We need to become more discerning about medical treatment and to ask for what we want instead of simply accepting whatever current medical development is thrust upon us.

Some natural healing methods may initially appear to be drastic, time-consuming, old-fashioned and crude. You may not have met anyone who has used them and be asking yourself whether they really work. A few of us, the recipients and facilitators of these methods, know that they do and, because of this, the knowledge has been kept alive. Now, more than ever, people need to be enlightened with the knowledge and ability to heal themselves. According to the World Health Organisation, the number of cancers is expected to double in most countries over the next 25 years. This is because we have an ever-increasing population which is living longer – but in a sicklier state. The Utopian ideals of the 1950s and 1960s enshrined in the National Health Service are visibly declining. With this in mind, it is important for every house-hold to have a clearer understanding of healthy daily living and self-help methods, and to be aware that little problems need not become large ones if they are dealt with early enough. Due to the over-use of antibiotics, vaccinations, poor nutrition and pollution, our children are becoming sicker and weaker with more persistent allergies than ever. We need to redress this widespread problem.

All too often we are scared away from herbs, regarding them as being the ex-clusive province of the professionals, but herbs naturally furnish us with our own healing laboratories in our own kitchens. Herbs are potent and their benefits are usually felt quite quickly.

In previous times, herbalists used only the plants in their own terrain, but personal territory has dwindled everywhere. As a means of sharing these resources and enrich-ing our knowledge, plants from luxuriant rainforests, spacious mountains and spartan deserts are now as easily available as those obtainable from a trip to the local garden centre. Yet, though we now have access to an incredible repertoire of healing plants, we actually have all we need on our doorstep, with everyday weeds capable of taking care of a host of viruses, bacteria, parasites and much more.

## THE 'ROOTS' OF HERBALISM

During his time as a hunter-gatherer, man, according to archaeological evidence, collected and consumed approximately 100 to 200 different plant species in any one year. This diversity of chemistry would have greatly protected the immune system and stimulated digestion more efficiently than does our modern diet. Not only did mankind flourish on this diet, but so did the animals that were subsequently con-sumed by man. Sadly, this cannot be said of the 'animal foods' of today.

Modern man's normal dietary range of plants is generally between only 20 and 40 species. These include carrots, cabbages, potatoes, parsnips, onions, apples, bananas, strawberries, peaches, lettuce, tomatoes, peas, broccoli, beans, wheat, blackberries, courgettes and marrows, oil made from sunflower (or in some cases olives), lemons, garlic, chillies and rice. If you look in the supermarkets, you will see that, on average, they stock 20–25 species. It is an unfortunate fact that many of these plants are also genetically engineered. Their original chemistry is far removed from the wild plants they once were, which is an important health consideration. Interestingly, a herbalist's materia medica is normally in the range of 100 to 200 plants, some of which are used frequently, some less so, while others are used very rarely; very much as the range of food species would have been used historically. Herbs give back the range of plants in our lives, their complex chemistries mixing to form patterns as individual and necessary as those taking place in every human being.

The Chinese, like many other cultures, spend a lot of time considering the correlation between our bodies and our entire existence, recognising that, in fact, we are cosmically part of the sun, stars, moon, earth and nature. Their diagnostic work also takes into consideration the effect of geographic location on our impressionable bodies – of heat, cold, damp, high or low altitude and the corresponding scale of temperatures of our own bodies, which consist mostly of water and minerals. Native American Indians, the Russians, the Aztecs and many other cultures have used these systems, which show a high degree of similarity in technique and wisdom. The Tibetans have similar, yet unique, forms of understanding disease, which have stemmed from their experience of day-to-day life on their harsh, barren mountainsides. The monks of these Tibetan mountains were often the primary healers of the outlying villages. Among other things, they were excellent at reading the eye; its colour, markings and its depths, with each area of the eye relating to particular parts of the body and giving clues about genetic tendencies, emotional predispositions and so on. We have our modern-day version of this therapy which we now call iridology and which remains a brilliant tool for assessing constitutional and genetic tendencies. Indian Ayurvedic medicine pays great attention to the clues of body structure, voice timbre and vital energy levels, right down to the colour of the saliva on the tongue.

In fact, all these old cultures have their own ways of tracking the roots of disease, but they overlap and arrive at the same destination via different routes. What they have in common is their attention to detail, the watching, feeling, seeing, remembering and experiencing; noticing the small alongside the large and the whole. These diagnostic and assessment methods are merely an extension of everyday life.

## MY INFLUENCES

As a natural healer, my aim is to empower and re-educate people within the home, using nature in all her forms, with her foods and herbs as allies, in order to remedy disease and rebalance the system. It is always very exciting to find 'like' spirits; I have met them in many countries including Britain, the USA, France and India. These people and places have all shaped and moulded me, but perhaps I was most greatly influenced by Dr. John Christopher, who for his time was a pioneer of modern herbalism and helped reshape and instigate the American herbal renaissance of the seventies, eighties and nineties. Not a week goes by without my thoughts and gratitude going out to him. I am especially grateful that I am legally allowed to practise as a herbalist in Britain as a direct legacy from Henry VIII and, more recently, through the work of the Medicines Control Agency (MCA), British Herbal Medicine

Association (BHMA) and European Herbal Practitioners Association (EHPA). Life for my American teachers (herbalists) has not been so easy. Dr. Richard Schulze, a colleague and main apprentice to Dr. Christopher has had to suffer the financial loss and indignity of having his herb stores smashed, spilled and confiscated. Dr. Christopher was similarly thrown into jail many times but he still healed many thousands of people and started up clinic after clinic – each after the last one had been shut down. Herbalism is illegal unless you are a qualified doctor in France, Spain, Belgium, Greece, Italy and other countries. However, plant usage is very much alive amongst the ordinary people in these countries and I have had the honour of learning a great deal from European herbalists, particularly those of the older generation who used only the herbs found growing around them, maybe 15 or 20 in total, to treat a wide range of diseases. Germany, Holland,

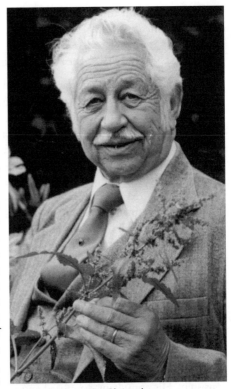

*Dr Christopher*

Sweden, Denmark and Britain remain among the few in Europe where herbalism can be practised solely as phytotherapy, whereas in developing countries, plants are still the main source of medicine. According to the World Health Organisation, as many as 80% of the world's people rely for their primary health care on traditional medicine, most types of which use remedies made from plants. The use of traditional medicine in developing countries is increasing. This is because populations are increasing, and governments want to encourage indigenous forms of medicine rather than relying on imported drugs, so there are strong moves to revive traditional cultures.

Dr. Christopher's style of herbalism is particularly useful for home use. This is partly because he was always working outside the law and, therefore, employed methods which could be safely used at home. His favourite saying was, *'There should be a herbalist in every home, a practitioner in every town.'* He often treated those who couldn't afford medical insurance, and used many revolutionary approaches for home health and first aid care that work simply, cheaply and efficiently. These methods have since been upgraded by his apprentice, Dr. Richard Schulze, to suit modern life and its contemporary diseases. Much of the style of natural healing and herbalism described in this book owes its origins to these two men. It has also been influenced by the teachings of Dr. Shyam Singha, an Ayurvedic practitioner, acupuncturist, osteopath and natural healer with whom I also served an apprenticeship. These people and others have been my inspiration and guides, both in my life and in my practice, which I first established in 1982.

## ILL HEALTH – THE GREATEST TEACHER

My teacher Dr. Christopher, was in and out of a wheelchair for most of his early life. His illnesses included serious spleen and liver disease and a crumbling spine, resulting from chronic arthritis and rheumatism, all of which became progressively worse. When he was thirty-five years old it was predicted that he would not reach his fortieth birthday, and it was probably this close brush with death that became a turning point in his life. He re-discovered herbs, food and water treatments, and finally examined his long-buried negative feelings about being abandoned by his original parents. Most of all he rebelled, went on to live to the age of eighty-two, married and had many children. He established flourishing clinics and taught herbalism, while continually learning himself from native American healers and inspiring many. He proved that a man who was once virtually a skeleton in a wheelchair could dramatically change the quality and direction of his life, transforming it through positive thought and action combined with natural healing methods. Read his book *A Herbal Legacy of Courage* for his full and spellbinding life story which was often beset with legal problems, fines and jail sentences, and his main text, *The School of Natural Healing*.

Another teacher, Dr. Richard Schulze, watched both his parents die of heart attacks, leaving him orphaned by the age of 14. By the time he was sixteen, he had himself begun to experience chest pains which became increasingly more painful and consistent. His consultant diagnosed angina and, as time went by, open heart surgery was recommended as his only hope; his combined parental gene package having now bequeathed him a life-threatening situation. Yet Richard felt there were many other methods and ways to treat his problem. At first he talked to a monk who suggested that he should not consume any meat or alcohol, and he felt a little better for these dietary restrictions. He went on to exclude fats (especially from cakes and pastries), fish and sugar. Someone else suggested that he should take plenty of exercise and, all in all, he began to feel a great deal better. Nevertheless, at the age of nineteen, he was scheduled for major open heart surgery. On discovering, however, that a friend of a similar age had died on the operating table undergoing the same surgery just the day before, he literally fled the hospital and continued his self-healing quest. To this day he remains healthy and more alive than almost anyone else I know, having used no drugs or surgery at any point in his life. His successful clinic, treating many thousands of terminally sick (and other) patients, was closed down by the Food and Drug Administration in 1994, but his work lives on ever stronger via his seminars, videos, teaching tapes and Herbal Medicine company.

My major personal experience of ill health started at the age of eighteen. It took the form of intense knife-like pains on my right side, sometimes lasting hours or days. I saw twelve bowel consultants, yet gained no insight or advice. When I was nineteen years old my stomach was cut open because it was suspected that I might have cancer. They found nothing, but removed my healthy appendix. I couldn't walk properly for months and I couldn't wear a bikini! But, after a while, I discovered yoga and the effects of its general balancing and internal massage, which started healing my problems. Eventually, I discovered healing foods, cleanses, herbs and colon health-care, through Dr. Christopher and other teachers.

## BOOK LIST

*Confessions of a Medical Heretic* by Robert Mendelsohn M.D. (Contemporary Books)
*Legacy of Courage* by Dr. J Christopher (Christopher Publications)
*The School of Natural Healing* by Dr. J Christopher (Christopher Publications)

# ONE

# Our Bodies, Our Health

## THE CLUES TO HEALTH AND SICKNESS

### WHY HAVE I BECOME ILL, AND WHAT IS WRONG WITH ME?

It is a great blessing if our body can transport us through life without too many recurring breakdowns. Being unaware of warnings, is part of the loss of many primal and gut instincts. When things do go wrong, we curse our body, treating it as something separate from ourselves – an entity that has failed in its service to us. What we fail to realise is that this reaction is the result of an ever-increasing disconnection with our body, and that the breakdown is the conclusion to a long series of unheeded warnings, which our body has been trying to communicate to us. These communications can be as simple as an awareness that we have not felt quite right for a while, that we have been unusually terse with our loved ones or simply the feeling that we can't cope any more. They can also take a more physical form, like a headache or indigestion – symptoms which we usually try to suppress with a pill rather than addressing the cause and questioning the reason for them. Sometimes, as with so many children nowadays, ill health becomes a way of life. Allergies, antibiotic usage, digestive disorders, they are all so common.

Listening to our body, observing and asking how and why we react to situations the way we do, can tell us an awful lot about ourselves. With physical symptoms, what is often required is a process of seeing the external signs and tracing them back to the inside. Initially, there may be just a jumble of clues and titbits of information, great and small. Every sensory ability has to be thrown into feeling more and gathering information, as in a great detective novel. This will invariably contain many false trails that must be patiently tracked by applying all available wisdom. Quick conclusions are as dangerous as over-complexity and tunnel vision. Simplicity and common sense should be your primary approach. A practitioner can often piece it all together for you and design a helpful route back to health, out of all the pieces.

In many cases of ill health, the disease progresses for some years before severe symptoms set in. The further on the disease is, the harder it is to find the source or to locate the actual moment, or moments, when the initial disharmony spawned the illness. So, seeing and being aware of ourselves is a lesson we can begin at any age and is one that it is never too early or too late to learn. In many ways it is a very natural process. Some may find comfort in knowing that it is their destiny. What is certain is that it is the course of action that follows that counts.

## THE BASICS THAT CAN BE ACHIEVED AT HOME

**Nutrition** – eat good foods, avoiding those that contain pesticides, hormones and any other additives or contaminants. Instead, concentrate on foods which are organic if possible and rich in vitamins, minerals and other desirable plant constituents. An occasional M.O.T. on the body through food cleanses is important. Today, digestive problems are rife and are at the bottom of much of our ill health. Weak digestive juices are often the cause.

**Medicinal Nutrition** – the use of healing plants to tone, support and stimulate.

**Herbalism** – make your own plant oils, tinctures, poultices, fomentations and decoctions.

**Hydrotherapy** – can be practised in the bathroom. Showering, soaking and steaming are just a few ways in which water can be used to circulate blood and massage internal organs and systems – giving them more oxygen and nourishment in order to avoid or dispel congestion and stagnation.

**Exercise** – which involves the body moving, flexing, circulating, pumping, inhaling, exhaling and detoxifying. Yoga and breathing exercises are especially good for all of these requirements, just as walking and running are for those mobile.

**Body Contact** – includes massage, yoga, reflexology, tai chi and other 'movement' therapies that help the body stay healthy and, if necessary, heal.

# TWO

# CELEBRATING NATURE'S ALCHEMY AND FRAGRANCE

*While the plant is growing, an enormous amount of electrical or vital energy is absorbed into the different parts of the plant. It is first generated by the sun, diffused through the atmosphere, the water and the earth; and the plants select what they need to build acids, alkalines, phosphates, carbonates, chlorides, glycerides, oils, fats, waxes and so forth.*

*In this profoundly wonderful vegetable kingdom that covers the earth with beauty, perfume and flavour, there is every conceivable requirement for every living creature, even to the breath of life. Plants arrange themselves into families, choose their own habitation and select their own food. Through long study of the chemistry of soil and plants we are able to predict what we shall find stored away in the leaves, roots, barks and fruits of particular plants for the purpose of supplying our own bodies with the specific material and specific energy we require.*

Excerpt taken from *The Advanced Treatise in Herbology* (early 1900s) by
Dr. Edward E. Shook.

There are many ways to make contact with nature. Anyone who has spent time communing with it will understand and feel its unseen gifts and potential as much as the more visible ones. The rocks, the earth, the many greens of foliage and the rainbow colours of the blossoms and flowers speak for themselves. A flower, when you stare into it, can heal by its colour and form alone, while its vibration and essence are something else.

Nature can respond like a true friend or lover, as events have shown time and again. Findhorn in northern Scotland continues to provide a wonderful experience and revelation of the power of love and tuning with nature, showing that plants are intelligent, responsive and emotional, lacking only, perhaps, the power of movement in an otherwise full spectrum of human abilities. On stony soil with windy aspects, unbelievable plants, fruits and vegetables have been produced, proving that really relating to nature can produce some surprising results – such as double-sized fruits and vegetables with no pests. This vibrational attunement with nature could produce even more wonderful benefits for world food production. Indeed we are going to need to assess our methods as time goes by. Perhaps we need to recall times when

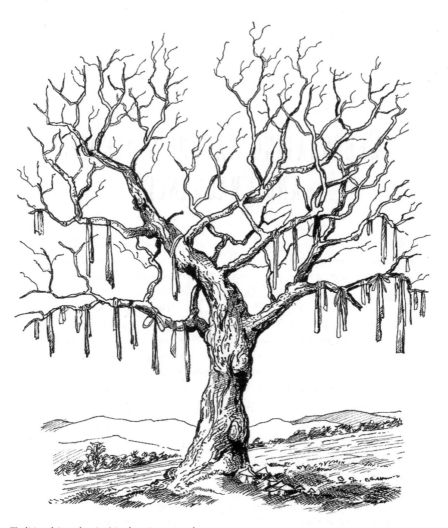

*Traditional 'tree dressing' in the winter months*

our relationship with growing things was founded on more simple gratitude and celebration.

All over the world trees were 'dressed' using ribbons or small toys tied on in the winter, in order to thank the tree for the splendour of its greenness and the joy of its blossom in spring and summer. In fact there were hundreds of ancient rituals for celebrating nature. 'Well dressing' was another, to thank the spring water for providing the basis for life.

Access to nature was, luckily, something I grew up with and it has affected my entire life ever since. My mother made home-made wine and I gathered for her the wild yellow broom flowers, nettle tops, blackberries, elderflowers, elderberries, dandelion flowers and birch sap required. Hours and hours over years and years spending time with these colourful plants gave me something that is very much a part of myself. Camping and travelling has given me an accumulative love of mountains, rivers, streams, woods and valleys; sun, rain, thunder, wind, cold and heat. Sometimes too tired to put a tent up, we have lain in powderdry ploughed fields, the odd ditch, or under a sheltering tree. Moonlight, darkness, firelight and stars have become familiar and friendly. It is there for us all to be touched with.

## THE SWEET SMELL OF NATURE

*The scent of plants on a wet early spring morning; the smell of newly-mown grass; the first roses of summer; the hot, dry, arid herbs on a scorched mountain.*

Smell is one of the most evocative memory joggers. Not only does it stop you at the time, helping you to extend and savour all that is present, but it also has a beautiful way of reviving memories to sweeten the present. When we remember someone, we very often remember their scent. We smell their individual pheromones ('pherein' meaning 'to carry' in Greek, and 'hormone' meaning 'to excite'). Pleasant smells make us feel happy, while noxious ones can irritate or depress. So, whether you like the smell of tar, bergamot essential oil, or the latest chemical perfume, is for you to decide, but the sensation will change your own body chemistry. It does this through a portion of the brain designated for emotional well-being, which is originally triggered by the nerves of the olfactory organ – i.e. the nose.

Essential oils come from all parts of plants and trees: barks, berries, seeds, leaves and flowers. They all basically work to balance our sympathetic and para-sympathetic nervous system, relaxing and bringing harmony and equilibrium and, at the same time, bringing clarity and awareness. This is why they were, and still are, burned in so many temples around the world in the form of incense: myrrh and frankincense from the East, sage from the West and lavender from the South.

## NATURE AND ITS HEALTH

Pollution has, to date, affected half of Britain's trees. Visible symptoms like sparse foliage, broken tops, bare branches or trees to which autumn seems to come early are the outward signs of complex internal problems. A survey done in 1991 showed that 56.7% of British trees had lost more than a quarter of their leaves. Britain ranks worst out of the whole of Europe: even heavily polluted Poland and the Czech Republic have relatively healthier trees. A combination of pollution and drought with ensuing infestations of insects and fungi seems to be the problem, resulting in the trees' natural defence systems becoming lower and lower. This mirrors our own alarming global rise in immune diseases and allergy problems.

Much land is being lost to development, it has become a victim to money and an increase in population. Historically, common land was often unlawfully sold off by the crown and church; more recently footpaths have been ploughed up by farmers and other landowners. Land has been given over to intensive farming, industry and housing. However, many people are now dedicated to reopening footpaths and pre-serving what little countryside we have left; some churchyards and cemeteries are now a haven for nature. Spending time out in nature will inspire us to save and create more. We should also remember that trees and plants are intelligent enough to adapt to changes in the environment, responding with new reactions in order to survive, to protect themselves from, or to transform, pollution. As major oxygenators, trees are very important. Thus replanting is essential in order to keep the atmosphere, and all who live within it, healthy.

Something that has increasingly struck me is that calcium-depleted soils produce sickly, weak trees which are prone to disease, while calcium-rich soils produce the opposite. Trees flourish in mineral and nutrient-rich soils, the much larger-leafed deciduous trees needing more nutrients than coniferous varieties. It is possible that we are in need of another ice age; where the rocks and earth are moved and crushed to re-feed the soil. Unfortunately, glaciers can take 900 centuries to re-mineralise the earth, and then a few more centuries would be needed to warm the ground up enough to grow anything again! But general loss of nutrient-rich undisturbed soils is certainly a huge factor in the loss of tree health. Interestingly enough, calcium is one of the most needed minerals for our own bodies; another similarity we have to plants. So, like all things, trees and humans are part of the same blueprint of nature.

## PLANT AID

Although some trees and plants are being killed off by mankind's pollution, this faith-ful flora continues to step in to help with the mess we have got ourselves into! In evolutionary terms, humans developed only because of the presence of the plant kingdom.

In the last fifty years, Britain has suffered the destruction of 97% of its wild flower meadows, 75% of its open heath, 96% of its lowland peat bogs and, 190,000 miles of hedgerow – enough to circle the earth seven times. Studies have shown that plants seem to provide the simplest and easiest way for combating the effects of airborne pollution – e.g. trees which have large areas of leaves with fairly rough or hairy surfaces are effective pollution traps. Hawthorn, with its open and branching shape, is a good 'trapper' using its canopy like a net. Dust that settles on the edge of a denser canopy, like that provided by lime or poplar, is much more likely to be blown away. Rough-fissured bark can also trap and trees planted in groups, with their increased ability to slow down passing air, help likewise. In effect, they are acting as air filters. There is also some research to show that trees 'lock up' in their tissues pollutants such as sulphur and nitrogen dioxide from car exhausts. A single mature beech can lock up two kilograms of carbon dioxide within one hour on a sunny day.

One problem close to my heart is that many playgrounds are unprotected by trees. Toddlers, infants and schoolchildren spend time playing in open suntraps, often at times of the day when the sun is at its most fierce. A few trees planted would give the vital shade needed to protect them from harmful ultraviolet radiation. An average six-foot eucalyptus costs very little; ten eucalyptus could pretty quickly make a huge difference to a playground, growing, as they do, three to four feet a season. As a species, they are naturally rich in ozone and anti-viral components which are then liberated into the air.

Plants and trees also provide noise barriers. Individual leaves absorb and reflect sound while the branches and general foliage 'scatter' the sound waves, making noises duller and softer.

## ALLOWING AND SUSTAINING NATURE AS MUCH AS POSSIBLE

Permaculture, or forest gardening, is something practised naturally by the native peoples of the rainforests, North American Indians and others. These old cultures simply made or found tiny clearings and worked with the forest canopy, dew, sun, earth, light, etc. to grow fruits, vegetables and other natural commodities, planting for their grandchildren and great-grandchildren as well as themselves. Forest gardening, as a system, works with nature and allows her to do the work wherever possible. One of its most important processes is 'maximum observation with minimum interference'. Permaculture takes into account the wind, sun, slope, climate, micro-climates and water-flow, and uses the minimum amount of machinery, so as to change or destroy as little as possible of this natural tapestry.

There is increasing interest in leaving nature alone and trying to learn from her instead of to master her. Such endeavours include the Permaculture Association based in Devon, a vegan community with similar interests in Cornwall, and organic farming schemes run in association with the highly successful 'box system' whereby organic fruits and vegetables are delivered to the doorstep weekly. The famous Alternative Technology Centre in Wales is another encouraging enterprise. 'Plantlife' is an organisation of paramount importance to herbalists in Britain because it addresses the issue of local herbs. Plantlife is Britain's only national plant conservation organisation working to protect and conserve Britain's wild flora in its natural habitat. It takes a strong lead on the quest for understanding and making changes in the 'how and why' of the symptoms of destruction and of the causes for the loss of wild plants. It actually conserves threatened species of plants (to include fungi) of which 232 are on the British government's 'danger list'. Some of the country's most respected botanists are involved. Plantlife now owns over 19 nature reserves which cover nearly 500 acres. In Spain and other European countries where nature reserves exist, herbs are gathered under strict supervision and care. This has a two-fold benefit: it provides an income for the reserve and provides much needed organic and wildcrafted herbs for herbalists and the general public. This could eventually be an interesting proposition for Britain.

Horticultural practices in general are trying to help our 'Green push' by using sustainable wood products for plant potting and packaging. Instead of using peat from disappearing peat bogs, moss (declining with the disappearance of boggy regions) or plastic pots which cause pollution, wood wool, root cloths, coconut fibre and more are coming into use. Key reasons for the use of certain materials are that they are sustainable, abundant or recyclable.

## PESTICIDES OR NOT

A problem arising from mono-farming concerns the use of chemical sprays. For years, because of the general gardening practices I employ, I have had no problem with slugs, white fly or other pests but, if I have had the odd greenfly, I have sprayed successfully using strong herbal teas or a minute dilution of lavender and other essential oils in water. In so doing, I use something the insects find off-putting to deter them. Another method, called companion planting, uses plant chemistry to keep pests at bay. For example, wormwood will produce a toxic chemistry which is effective at keeping invading nettles etc. away from other plants; this relationship between certain plants has often been applied to forest gardening. The idea of using essential oils and toxic plant chemistry is now being researched and is becoming more accepted, while the even more desirable technique of 'always keeping a balance' is being re-discovered by farmers and gardeners.

A few farmers now plant strips of wild flowers around fields of sweet corn or, in some cases, between batches of sweet corn and other vegetables. In time, perhaps, more trees will creep into the picture but, for now, the presence of a few more wild flowers and grasses have certainly been found to help maintain the balance between plant and insect predators and parasites. Even ICI has said that all gardens should have a small quantity of wild plant species and grasses near ornamental gardened areas, pointing out that these plants assist friends rather than foes. Lacewings and hoverflies, for example, lay their eggs on some of these weeds, and both destroy aphids. That's quite a quantum leap for a firm like ICI, but we need more leaps from them in many more positive directions.

Dr. Francis Brinker of the Eclectic Institute, Arizona, tells us that certain chemicals within the Prickly Ash species (American and Chinese varieties) act upon house flies, mosquito larvae, ticks and several leaf-eating insects, as well as being an ovicide for body lice and toxic to yellow meal worms. There is a great deal of research being carried out into natural insecticides. For instance, where eucalyptus grows not a single mosquito is to be seen!

Agricultural chemicals may be a problem to the West, but they have had even more serious consequences in the East. A ten million-strong peasants' revolt in 1994 tried to assuage some of the worst aspects of the GATT deal on world trade. Rural farmers in India and other developing nations want to let us know that their very survival is at stake. Their livelihood is being threatened and now a legacy of destruction can be seen, with farms, farmers and their families being forced into failure. These farmers are obliged to buy hybrid seeds from certain companies. Plants grown from these hybrid seeds do not set seed and therefore seed cannot be gathered from them for sowing the following year. Thus, the farmers have to buy more seeds from Western companies, at enormous expense. In addition, these genetically developed seeds actually depend upon chemicals for growth. This may be disgustingly brilliant for a monopoly on agribusiness, but is a threat to the very survival of small farmers, their families and indeed whole peoples. In fact, only a few very rich farmers will survive. These people will continue to starve, become

8

parted from their land, homes, lifestyle and, in short, everything they have or care for. Their own collected seeds have the excellence of centuries of improvement and adaptation to local conditions and are the best-suited for mixed sustainable agriculture. The imported 'miracle' hybrid versions are already reported to be giving lower yields and to require excessive water, which is simply not available.

## GET CLOSER TO NATURE AND MAKE A HERBAL PROFILE

Spending time in nature, where you can rediscover and hone gut instincts, can be given an extra purpose by making a herbal profile of your own. This will help you to appreciate that the trees and 'weeds' which grow around you are capable of feeding and healing you. You'll realise only too clearly that the whole body can be balanced and maintained with what is to be found commonly growing. See Appendix III for further instructions and guidance if you wish to make your own herbal profile. Be aware that some of these herbs do carry contra-indications.

## LET'S LOOK AT TWELVE HERBS

### BURDOCK (ARCTIUM LAPPA)

**Part Used:** Root

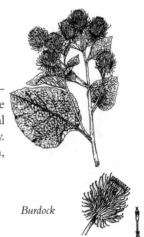

This is used as a root vegetable in Japan. Highly nutritious, it will sustain the pancreas and spleen while balancing blood sugar levels. It is a strong general immune herb, rich in tumour-inhibiting chemistry. As a prime blood cleanser it will clear the skin, bloodstream, lymph and colon of poisons.

*Burdock*

### DANDELION (TARAXACUM OFFICINALE)

**Parts Used:** Flowers, leaves and root

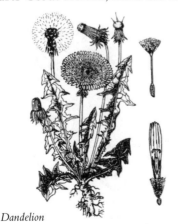

This is a wonderful herb for the liver, heart and kidneys. It helps stimulate liver function in general, aiding digestion as it does. It is also a prime kidney herb, helping to relieve water retention, but without exhausting the kidneys. In all, it treats gallbladder problems, oedema, high blood pressure, heart weakness, skin problems and many other conditions. Its yellow flower gives a clue to its work with the liver.

*Dandelion*

## ELDER (SAMBUCUS NIGRA)

**Parts Used:** Fruit, leaves and bark

The fruit is now recognised as a strong anti-viral, although this has long been part of ancient Native American Indian knowledge. The berries, leaves and flowers are useful for treating fevers and inflammation, due to their anti-inflammatory chemistry. All parts of the plant clean and clear the bloodstream and aid the clearing of mucus from the lungs. Externally, the flowers and bark are useful for sore eyes, minor injuries, skin problems e.g. eczema, psoriasis, warts, inflammation and irritations.

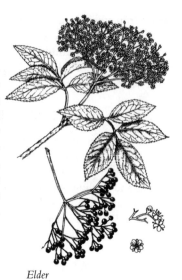

*Elder*

## HAWTHORN (CRATAEGUS OXYACANTHA)

**Parts Used:** Flowers, leaves and berries

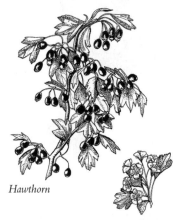

All parts of the hawthorn are very safe for use on the heart, and many heart patients regularly pick the leaves, berries and flowers and make tea from them. It acts like a beta-blocker, blocking heart receptor cells and unblocking again as needed by the individual. It is a very clever herb, ideal for improving circulation, coronary blood flow, regulating heart rate and blood pressure. It also has antibacterial qualities. Its red berries give us a clue to its work with the circulatory system.

*Hawthorn*

## LIME TREE (TILIA EUROPAEA OR CORDATA)

**Part Used:** Flowers

A wonderful musty and heady aromatic fragrance issues from these summer blossoms. It is a good herb for the nervous system, sedating, calming and relaxing. It relaxes spasms, improves digestion and often helps migraine and high blood pressure. It is also used for circulatory problems like hardening of the arteries, and for urinary infections and catarrh.

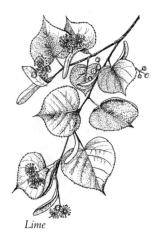

*Lime*

## MAHONIA (MAHONIA AQUIFOLIUM)

**Parts Used:** Roots, root bark and occasionally the fruit

This is a very common hedgerow plant found all over Britain. It also grows prolifically in America where Native American Indians used it to treat the liver and skin. It has the ability to inhibit the over-production of skin cells associated with psoriasis and is used frequently in Germany because of this with great success. Whenever you see Berberis mentioned in a formula, Mahonia will often do just as well. It is

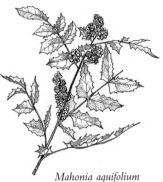

*Mahonia aquifolium*

a very useful plant and a prime liver tonic. It also has a beneficial effect on the bowel because, by stimulating bile flow, it helps stimulate peristalsis, which is vital because this in turn helps release toxins. If you don't want to dig the roots up, then just collect an autumn bunch of the grape-looking fruits. The yellow spring flowers bring attention to its use as a liver herb.

## NETTLES (URTICA DIOICA)

**Part Used:** Herb

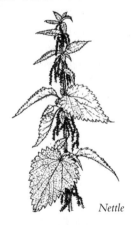

*Nettle*

Nettles are rich in many vitamins, minerals and trace elements, and are particularly high in available calcium, magnesium and iron. Nettle is a wonderful blood cleanser and will greatly help anaemia (and any excess menstruation or haemorrhage). It is an old European rheumatism and arthritis remedy and was originally brought to Britain by the Romans.

## OAK (QUERCUS ROBUR)

**Parts Used:** Bark, leaves, galls and acorns

This is a bitter, astringent plant, rich in anti-viral and antibacterial chemistry. Due to its strongly astringent (tannin) qualities only small amounts can be taken internally. It is ideal for treating some types of diarrhoea. It is also a wonderful herb for the immune system. However, it is mainly used for

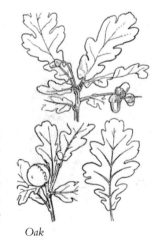

*Oak*

mouth washes and as a gargle for sore throats, gum and mouth problems. This tree was a staple source for many Native Indian tribes around California where the white oak still grows in profusion. It really sustained these people who often left the acorns in water for days to wash away the tannin and then crushed them. The resultant 'flour' was very nutritious and good for boosting immunity.

## Plantain (Plantago major)

**Part Used:** Herb

This is a wonderful antibacterial herb and can be taken internally for bacterial infection or put directly as a fresh poultice on wounds. It also has antihistamine properties, which makes it useful for allergies, insect bites, etc. It cools, helps reduce inflammation and acts as an efficient blood and lymph cleanser.

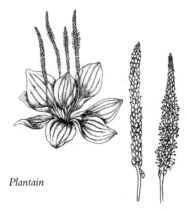

*Plantain*

## Red Clover (Trifolium pratense)

**Part Used:** Herb

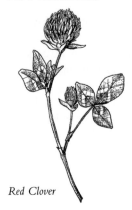

Red Clover is an unequalled blood cleanser which is always used for degenerative disease and specifically for cancers of the lymph system and bloodstream. It is also capable of relaxing spasms and will help release water retention and induce sweating when needed. Its red flower gives a huge clue to its blood cleansing capabilities.

*Red Clover*

## St. John's Wort (Hypericum perforatum)

**Part Used:** Flowers and top leaves

This summer solstice yellow flower has been used for 100 years in Europe for a wide variety of diseases both internally and externally. The list is impressive and modern research is now able to support its older uses – externally for wounds, bruises, burns, nerve pain (dental, etc.), internally for liver and gall-bladder complaints, bladder and lung problems, dysentery,

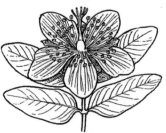

*St. John's Wort*

worms, diarrhoea, hysteria and nerve complaints. It outstrips the sale of Prozac in Germany because it has the ability to heighten serotonin levels in the brain. (St. John's wort should not be taken with drugs containing serotonin; it can also cause light sensitivity in some individuals; It is advisable to seek professional advice before taking this herb.)

## YARROW (ARCHILLEA MILLIFOLIUM)

**Part Used:** Herb

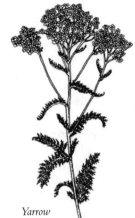

This is a commonly found herb along road and field verges. Aromatic and bitter, it affects digestion favourably and lowers blood pressure. As a strong astringent it can staunch heavy blood loss. Traditionally in Europe and North America it has long been used for fevers, colds, flu and other viral diseases.

*Yarrow*

*If you own a garden, I'd like to share with you a small list of trees that can help you enlarge your existing repertoire and herbs to add to those that you may already possess, e.g. culinary ones, plus lemon balm, etc.*

## EUCALYPTUS (EUCALYPTUS SPECIES)

Rich in rutin, this tree's leaves will not only help strengthen the walls of the vascular system but, as a strong anti-viral, it will make a wonderful tea – for flu, colds, coughs, etc. (It is used for the treatment of malaria all over the word.)

## JUNIPER (JUNIPERUS SPECIES)

This is another anti-microbial plant with a particular affinity to the urinary tract. The leaves of this shrub are used; make them up as a tea. A few juniper berries can also be used over a short term.

## PINE (PINUS SPECIES)

As a prime antioxidant, a cup a day made from the needles will keep your body literally 'alive'. Pine is also a strong anti-viral and anti-infection aid.

## GINKGO (GINGKO BILOBA)

Favoured for its abilities with the brain and memory, it also has prime immunosupportive chemistry as well as vascular maintenance properties. A simple tea can be made at any time of year from the leaves, but late summer yellow-green ones are the best.

## BOOK LIST

*Advanced Treatise in Herbology* by Dr. Edward E. Shook (Christopher Publications)
*Forest Gardening* by Robert A de Hart (Green Books)
*Herbal Medicine Makers Handbook* by James Green (Wildlife and Green)
*Plant Spirit Medicine* by Tom Brown (Swan Raven and Company)
*Rolling Thunder* by Doug Boyd (Dell Publishing)
*Secret Life of Plants* by Peter Thompkins and Chris Bird (Perennial Library)

## RESOURCES

For details of local Organic Box Systems contact:
**Friends of the Earth**, 26-28 Underwood Street, London N1 7JQ. Tel: 0171 490 1555
or, **The Soil Association**, Bristol House, 40-56 Victoria Street, Bristol, BS1 6BY. Tel: 0117 929 0661
**Royal Botanic Gardens**, 47 Kew Green, Richmond, Surrey, TW9 3AB. Tel: 0181 332 5000
**For a list of Suppliers of Essential Oils contact**: Aromatherapy Trade Council, PO Box 38, Romford, Essex, RM1 2DN
**Plantlife**, The Wild Plant Conservation Charity, 21 Elizabeth Street, London SW1W 9RP.

# THREE

# THE PLANTS THEMSELVES

## BEST QUALITY HERBS

The best herbs to use for medicinal or culinary purposes are those collected from the wild, in areas where the plant is found growing naturally, away from contaminants. However, the colossal increase in demand for herbs has meant that, some of the time, they are being collected from unsuitable wild sources, such as roadside verges, or that wild sources are being over-plundered. Efforts are more recently being made to collect with permission from National Parks.

This huge increase in demand and a belated desire for quality have led to an upsurge in organically grown herbs. Hundreds upon hundreds of acres of herbs are now being grown in parts of Europe (in particular Germany and in some parts of Britain), the USA and Canada. Some herbalists and herb chemists see benefits in this, in that it becomes easier to standardise the chemical constituents in the plants and harvesting can become 'controlled'. This is done by using gas chromatography and other techniques to test plants for their optimum or peak harvesting time. These harvested plants can consequently be more rapidly and carefully stored, dried or processed, with a minimum of delay and spoilage. However, botanical herbalists know that plants growing in the wild will produce more 'primitive' and original chemistry as they fight to survive selective pressure, producing some aggressive chemistry. For instance, with the herb cascara sagrada (Rhamnus purshiana), which is heavily harvested in the temperate rainforests of North America, demand instigated its cultivated growing in an area where it grows wild! This turned out to be unsuccessful, as the laxative chemistry in the cultivated variety was shown to be much less active than that found in the wild harvested barks. Monoculturally grown herbs will increase over time and, in the long term, could alter the chemistry of plants and eventually may even genetically change them forever. I have no personal answer to this because we need a great deal of herbs, we have diminished land and we do not want to defoliate our wild areas.

The question of good quality herbs was always a vital one to herbalist Dr. Christopher and it was a treat to find his standard of excellence in times when many people paid little attention to such details. He insisted on sourcing only clean, wild-crafted or organic herbs, processing them in a way that retained their vibrancy and quality, much as the older herbalists had done. Pesticides are a fact of modern farming methods and 'poisoned herbs' could be found in his day just as they are now. Dr. Christopher taught his students to carefully choose the sources from which they bought their herbs and to check how they were stored and then later prepared. For this reason, he liked herbalists to prepare and even pick their own herbs in order to make their own tinctures, ointments and other preparations to a high standard. He even went as far as insisting that anything for external use should be of the same quality as that for internal use. His legacy of high standards lives on with many of his students, now excellent herbalists in their own right. To this day, herbal preparations vary in their quality and, sadly, I have met people who have not had beneficial experiences from some preparations. This is very likely due to the poor quality of the original herb and then how it was prepared.

Twenty years ago it was hard to find organically grown herbs, so my personal choice was to grow my own as far as possible, to seek out organic herb growers in Britain and to import from American wild-crafters as and when I needed to. Nowadays, needs and trends have changed dramatically and access to good quality herbs has become relatively easy. However, my own experiences do not necessarily reflect the 'norm' so, let's take a close look at the whole issue.

There is a recognised need for greater control on herb quality. As a result, rules and regulations have been put into place by the Medicines Control Agency (MCA) which is addressing the quality, origins, storage and preparation of herbs grown in or imported into Britain. The problem of quality has become larger during the last few years because herbalism has become increasingly popular, with demand pushing up the need for greater amounts of herbs. To this end, a few importers have become less fussy in order to meet the ever-growing demand, with some herbs having been substituted or adulterated – as has been proved by laboratory testing.

Toxic metals have been found among some imported herbs. Faecal matter has been found amongst some crude herbs – where human faeces have been used to fertilise fields. Radioactive waste has also been found, as some herbs are still collected from places in and around disaster areas, often by poor people who are anxious to make a living and for whom herb collecting is still a way of life. Medical and other toxic wastes are buried or burnt, and the fumes and leakages from these can contaminate the herbs in the area. Since the 1940s, there has been a thirty-three-fold increase in the use of pesticides, including insecticides, herbicides, fungicides and other agents, with a ten-fold increase in potency. Used on herbs, this is disastrous. According to the American National Cancer Institute, cancer rates increase by seven or eight times through ingestion of pesticide-contaminated foods – not something that sits comfortably with herbs which are going to be used for medicine.

Sulfured herbs are now available; apricots and peaches are sulfured to keep their colour and for storage, but do we want sulfured herbs as well? Rodents and insects are sometimes found among herbs. Microbes – for example fungi and bacteria – need to be kept to a minimum, but herbs are often sprayed in transit with noxious chemicals like ethylene oxide, thus causing them to become toxic. Bacteria, such as E-coli and those causing typhoid, have been found in herbs, particularly low-growing plants, in monsoon seasons.

Some herbs are sprayed with antibiotics because this bypasses the need for expensive laboratory testing to determine toxicity and microbial levels (which are often unacceptably high). The resulting products are called 'pre-treated' and passed as 'clean'. Another way in which herb companies have sought to 'clean up' herbs is by using autoclaving, a cleaning process that utilises steam. Originally used solely for surgical tools, this sterilisation technique is now used on herbs in an attempt to severely lessen the risk of contamination. Yet another method is to irradiate herbs, a very worrying method recently used on some foods.

The bottom line is that organic (or clean, wild collected) herbs have to become the only type of herb acceptable to the industry. The public needs to demand only these. This needs to be coupled with procedures to analyse each plant's authenticity of species and correct storage facilities, including that of fresh tinctures or freeze dried herbs, to ensure minimum spoilage and maximum potency.

## PLANTS AS INVESTMENTS AND MONEY-MAKERS

Plants are becoming an increasingly profitable investment. Europe and the USA, Japan, China, Brazil and Mexico have been swept by a huge demand for herbs, which has led to an enormous increase in profits. In China, sales of traditional medicines have more than doubled in the last five years, while India's booming export trade in medicinal plants has risen almost three-fold during the last decade. In Germany, over 80% of all physicians regularly use herbal products. In the USA, herbs and natural supplements were worth $12 billion in 1998, which was double that of 1994. Britain, like everywhere else, is being swept along on the herb revival boom.

On the other hand, pharmaceutical companies were not doing so well financially and a lot of companies have swallowed each other up in a bid to survive. In 1990, the pharmaceutical market profit was 15%; by 1994 it had fallen to 9%. In the West, this drop in revenue has halted research programmes, as the money to fund them simply hasn't been available. Consequently, scientists were asked to be more creative! One idea which they have developed is to focus on the older generation and its 'ageing' problems. With the World Health Organisation predicting that the incidence of cancer will double or triple, due to the increase in the number of older people, this would seem a likely target. Another trend, already being developed in some areas of alternative medicine, is the move to bypass the doctor and sell more products directly to the public, either over the counter or through mail order. Pharmaceutical companies have begun 'copying' herbs and we'll see more of this trend in the years to come. Several pharmaceutical companies are investigating methods to standardise medicines from plants. In the past, only single-molecule botanicals could be identi-fied. Without proper identification, researchers cannot prove the safety and efficacy of these agents because there are batch-to-batch inconsistencies. Previously, pharma-ceutical companies have not submitted applications for herbal medicines because companies could not receive patents for these substances. However, recently a phar-maceutical company developed the first pharmaceutical versions of multi-molecule herbal medicines by standardising the active molecules and their interactions. Meanwhile, other herbal concoctions can now be seen for sale by other pharma-ceutical companies.

Cuts have been made to research programmes looking at single herbs and trying to isolate their 'magic bullet' components. For years, pharmaceutical companies were in the habit of throwing away the 'best bits' while looking for the 'magic bullet'. This was reflected in a lesson learned in 1995. Flavonoids are a component of many plants, but this particular plant chemical had been constantly discarded for twenty years. In hindsight this lesson was indeed a bitter and costly one, because flavonoids are known to be antioxidants – a new 'buzz' word among the more nutritionally aware. Antioxidants are known to inhibit and treat a wide range of illnesses and conditions including cancer, strokes, heart disease, emphysema, late-onset diabetes, rheumatism, arthritis, ulcers, cataracts, Chron's disease, senility, arterio/athero sclerosis and old age; flavonoids do this by preventing our cells from 'rusting' or 'ageing'.

Now, pharmaceutical companies are looking at multi-species herbal formulae, using many herbs in mixtures that are then tested. This is how herbalists have always worked! Looking back into history, our ancestors grazed plants in the days of hunting and gathering, ingesting a broad range of plant species, which kept them well. Now science is beginning to look down this avenue, in the hope that their next billion lies at the end of it. It may well do, but I feel we can graze for ourselves. When some drugs come to the end of their patents and therefore their value as incomes expire (which will be soon, in some cases), the pharmaceutical industry will, no doubt, make an even greater investment in 'natural' Green pills.

## PLANT COLLECTION

Plant chemistry varies according to the time of day and season. Traditionally, some plants were always collected prior to sunrise and others were never collected after sunset. In all, plant collection contained many important 'quirks', which are now being proved to be of value through scientific evaluation. It is possible, however, to figure out some basic factors:

**Leaves** – spring leaves are best because they have new sap in them. Their energy has not yet been drawn away to produce flowers or seeds.

**Bark** – spring is best, just as the sap rises. This is also when the newly-formed bark is most easily cut off.

**Flowers** – these are at their peak just after they have opened.

**Seeds** – these are at their peak in late summer and early autumn.

**Berries** – usually autumn is the best time to collect these. Look for good, deep colour and tight, glowing skin.

**Roots, rhizomes, root bark, and tubers** – collect in late autumn when all the top foliage has died down, but before the 'stores' are used during the winter and spring. However, spring time is an option and will produce slightly different chemistry, but do it before major foliage and stem production has begun.

## DRYING

Once harvested, the way in which herbs are dried and stored is of paramount importance. When a herb is picked it immediately starts to decay, bacteria and fungi increase and the plant chemistry ebbs with its colour, smell and texture. It is vital to arrest this process as quickly as possible. The water content and type of fibrous material to be dried out varies in each plant and some plants need to have their readily lost oils conserved very efficiently. Still others are more affected by the climate; for example, if it is constantly damp and rainy, fungal spores can completely destroy the plant. General rules for drying are to keep the plant out of direct sunlight and in constant aerated heat.

## BASIC PREPARATION OF HERBS

A herb is sometimes used on its own or as part of a formula that contains several herbs. The latter, termed polypharmacy, employs a teamwork effect which is appropriate when the power of a single herb needs assistance. Very often the formula consists of one main herb with others acting as support. The support team can be made up of one or two herbs, or even ten or twelve. The main herb may, for example, be required to soothe the impaired tissue, while the others assist in nourishment, or to help eliminate toxins, assist in nerve or blood supply and/or to calm and sedate. These single or multiple herb choices can be used as tinctures, teas (infusions), decoctions, ointments, syrups, poultices, pessaries, capsules, salves and ointments.

Differing forms of administering a herb or herbs are chosen for whether external or internal uses are needed. Also a choice has to be made as to which method and by what means the specific beneficial chemistries are to be extracted – for instance the main chemical constituents in ginkgo leaf are best extracted using water and therefore a tea or decoction is ideal, whereas for Echinacea root, alcohol is best and therefore a tincture is ideal. Sometimes these methods can be mixed, thus gaining all available chemistries.

All plants used in the basic preparation of herbs should be organic or wildcrafted.

### HERBAL TEAS – INFUSIONS

These can be made using a specialised tea-pot. If using the latter or indeed a mug or cup, then a tea-sock is ideal, as this simple cotton sock on a wire rim can be set into the mug, cup or pot and left to infuse with the herbs and boiling water.

Use 12–25g of dried herb or 25–50g of fresh herb to 750ml of distilled water. Infuse the herbs in a mug or teapot for 5 to 25 minutes. Chamomile is the only exception – use 12g of this herb to 750ml of water and infuse for only five minutes.

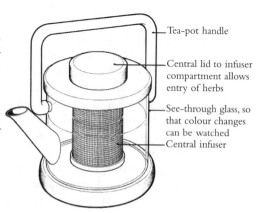

Tea-pot handle

Central lid to infuser compartment allows entry of herbs

See-through glass, so that colour changes can be watched

Central infuser

*The tea-pot infuser*

## Dosage Guide for Seven-Minute Infusion:-

| | | | |
|---|---|---|---|
| Adults: | 3 cups a day | Children (under 12): | 1¹/₂ cups a day |
| Children (under 3): | ³/₄ cup a day | Adults (over 70): | 1¹/₂ cups a day |
| Adults (over 75): | ³/₄ cup a day | | |

You can mix many herbs together. In fact it's better to do so, because, that way, you get a range of chemical properties and effects, and no one herb can dominate in either flavour or effect. Change your herb mixes regularly.

## DECOCTIONS

A decoction is similar to a herbal tea but is designed for using the harder parts of herbs, such as nuts and hard seeds, barks, rhizomes and roots. With these harder parts of plants, an infusion may not extract all the medicinal properties that are locked into them. Therefore, you need to heat them for a longer period of time.

A basic decoction is made by adding 12g–25g (depending on how bulky they are) of dried herb to 750ml of cold spring water (250ml may evaporate during boiling). It is best to let the herbs soak and re-hydrate in the water for up to 12 hours, if you have the time, and then slowly bring the mixture up to a boil. Let it simmer for between 10 and 30 minutes.

Divide resultant liquid (approx. 500ml) into 3 cups and drink at intervals through-out the day.

## TINCTURES

These are mixtures in which the medicinal components of the herbs have been extracted, ideally into grain alcohol or vinegar. Alcohol or vinegar tinctures should be made as follows:

## To Make Tinctures at Home – Standard Quantity

Use 230g (8oz) of dried roots, berries, leaves or flowers, or 460g (16oz) of fresh material, with enough vodka to cover it. This will be a minimum of 900ml (32floz).

1.  Place the chosen material in a liquidiser or food processor and cover with vodka; standard 45% proof is effective, but 70-80% proof is even better. Blend the ingredients. The mixture will be particularly stiff and hard if using berries, making it difficult for the blades to turn and requiring more vodka to get these to break down. Once the mixture is well blended, pour the tincture into a dark, airtight container – a dark glass jar or a kilner jar is ideal.
2.  Shake well, label your jar carefully, then store it in a cool place out of direct sunlight.
3.  After two days, measure the contents and add water. For dried berries, leaves and flowers add 20 per cent of the volume if using 45% proof vodka, and 50–60% if using 70–80% proof vodka. Leave for 2–4 weeks, shaking at least twice a day.

4.  Strain through a jelly bag, preferably overnight, until you have strained the last drop. For the best result, use a wine press.
5.  Pour the resultant liquid into dark jars, label and store in a cool, dark place. For personal use, decant into a 50ml (2floz) tincture bottle.

Some herbalists like to plan the making of tinctures around the moon phases, using the gravitational waxing and waning of the moon to add power and energy as the old herb alchemists did. To do this, start the process when the moon is new, then strain and bottle at the full moon.

To keep tinctures over a long period of time, wax the stopper and store in a dark place. When administering a tincture internally if you wish to avoid the alcohol, you may evaporate 98–99% of the alcohol from the solution by putting it into a little boiling water. Otherwise, simply add your tincture to a little cold or warm water, or fruit juice.

## Average Recommended Dosage for Tinctures

The average recommended dosage for tinctures made from berries, leaves, flowers, barks, root barks, rhizomes and seeds varies from herb to herb, so consult a herbal practitioner for guidance.

## Dosage for Everyday and Long-term Use:

Adults: 1tsp (5ml) of tincture diluted in 5tsp (25ml) of water (or fruit juice), 2–3 times daily, e.g. a total intake of approximately 15ml per day
Children aged 7–12 years: 1/2 adult dose
Children aged 3–7 years: 1/4 adult dose
Children aged 3 years: 2–5 drops twice a day
Dose varies from individual to individual and depending on whether or not a single herb or formula is being used.

Commercially produced tinctures of a professional standard can be used. Some are of a very high quality, but always choose those that are organic or wildcrafted. Some combine tinctures with infusions and decoctions for extra benefit.

## HERBAL SYRUPS

A herbal syrup is basically a maceration, an infusion, a decoction or occasionally a tincture, to which maple syrup, vegetable glycerine or honey has been added. These substances are added mainly to preserve the solution, but they also give the liquid a thicker and stickier consistency making it much more palatable to children. I prefer to use maple syrup and have done so successfully in my clinic for several years. Most children can be induced to take any herbal tincture by adding 25% or 50% maple syrup.

Syrups were traditionally made by reducing a decoction down to less than its original amount and then adding sugar or runny honey. If you slowly simmer your decoction down to half its original quantity, you will have what used to be referred to as a 3-power decoction. If you simmer your 3-power decoction down to half this amount again, you will have a 6-power decoction. By adding maple syrup to this, you get a 3 or 6-power syrup. Try to find organic maple syrup (instead of sugar).

## Dosage Guide

As for tincture.

**Onion and Garlic Syrup:** Use vegetable glycerine and lemon juice or maple syrup and lemon juice. Chop organic garlic and onions, or put them into the food processor or liquidiser. If you use fresh organic garlic and onions you can use the whole plant. Cover with vegetable glycerine and $1/2$ litre of honey, if it is of very good quality – i.e. the bees should not have been fed on sugar during the winter and the honey should not have been heat-treated. Some rainforest honeys are good for this, or maple syrup. Add one tablespoon of lemon juice. Alternatively you can liquidise the onions, garlic and syrup together, which is quicker but requires more syrup.

## ELDERFLOWER AND ELDERBERRY COMPOTE SYRUP

Just as fruit compotes are made throughout the summer in Europe, you can make herbal compotes, adding herbs as they come into flower or fruition. Use vegetable glycerine, runny honey or maple syrup with lemon if desired, instead of the brandy and sugar used in conventional recipes for fruit compotes.

Begin with elder flowers, which appear in June; their white, flat petticoats should be picked just as they burst out of their buds. Pull the white flowers off the green stalks and put them into a wide-necked container. You can add more every day or so, but each time cover the flowers with the vegetable glycerine or maple syrup. For a combined mix, a good ratio is roughly half a litre of vegetable glycerine to quarter of a litre of maple syrup to one tablespoon of fresh lemon juice. A cheaper version uses only vegetable glycerine with one tablespoon of freshly squeezed lemon juice added to every $1/2$ litre of glycerine.

Stand this mix outside to catch all available sunshine, but if the weather is relentlessly cold and grey then keep it in a warm, but not hot, place indoors.

As time goes by, the flowers will compact down and the upper part of the jar will contain only syrup. Add more flowers and fill the gap; however, never let the flowers rise above the syrup – this often proves difficult! Shake daily, preferably more than once, to avoid this, because if the flowers don't remain in the syrup, they will oxidize, turn brown and ferment. After at least two weeks, you can strain the syrup off from the flowers and then add more flowers to increase its strength.

In September and October the wine-red elderberries appear; collect these when fully ripe but not mouldy in any way and add these to the strained syrup, this time liquidising the whole lot in order to crush the berries. The resulting syrup is thick and full-bodied. Shake daily. You can likewise place it in any dwindling autumn sunshine, and strain and add more berries if you wish. The resulting brew, which is ready to consume by mid to late October, is so tasty that everyone who samples it will let you know immediately that they feel a little shivery – so make plenty!

## HERBAL CAPSULES

These are two types of empty gelatine capsules – those of vegetable origin or those of animal origin. To use, mix the powdered herbs together (if using a formula) and fill the capsules, fitting the two ends together. This is done by putting the powder in a saucer and scooping powder into both ends. Then push the two ends together, one will overlap the other. You can buy little machines to do this for you, or purchase them ready-made. Capsules are ideal for use in bowel remedies where the chemical constituents need to reach the colon. Otherwise tinctures, teas, decoctions or freeze-dried herbs are preferred because they will be fresher or reach the bloodstream more quickly. For people who cannot take large quantities of garlic, it can be freshly chopped and put into capsules; but use them immediately, otherwise the garlic will dissolve the gelatine. Capsules can also be useful for those who are unable to take hot cayenne on a teaspoon.

### Dosage Guide:

Adults: 2 capsules 2–4 times a day. Children 7–12: 1 capsule 2–4 times a day. Aged 3–7: 1 capsule twice a day. Under 3 years: Capsules are often not advised.

## OINTMENTS

These are used for their protective and emollient effect, liquefying when applied. Ointments are generally made from a mixture of herbs, oils (preferably virgin olive oil), essential oils and beeswax. The herbs absorb the oils, and the wax gives firmness to the ointment.

### How to Make Ointments

Pour olive oil onto the chosen powdered herbs. A good standard is 350g of olive oil with 300g of dried herbs. Place in a closed container (stainless steel, earthenware, unchipped enamel or glass) and either put into the oven and leave there at low heat (100°F) for an hour, or stand in the sun or some other warm spot for a week. Periodically, take a fork and stir the mixture. Leave for a further week to macerate (if using the oven method then heat up again before straining off). Do this by passing the mixture through a piece of muslin lining a large plastic or stainless steel colander; alternatively use a jelly bag and hang overnight. Finally, melt 50g of beeswax in a double boiler or very thick based saucepan using a very low temperature and add the herbal olive oil saturate. Have glass jars at the ready and put a little of the liquid into one to check that it is the correct consistency for use. Do not forget to label your ointments. See Chapter Eleven 'Other Items' for formulae.

### Dosage:

Apply 2–3 times daily or more frequently if necessary.

## Compresses

A compress is basically a herbal infusion or decoction applied directly to the skin using a piece of cloth, gauze or towel, always using natural fibres like cotton. Compresses can be made with any liquid at any temperature, but a hot herbal tea or decoction is commonly used. Other possible ways to make a compress are by using various vegetable oils, apple cider vinegar and essential oils.

To make a herbal tea compress, first make an infusion or decoction as normal. Then dip a piece of cloth in the solution, the size of the cloth being proportional to the area of the body you want to cover. Wring out excess liquid and apply this cloth to the affected area. You may wish to keep the fluid hot and keep dipping the cloth back into it when the cloth gets cool; this can be done every few minutes. Placing a heavy towel, cling film, or a hot water bottle over the compress will help it retain its heat longer. Replace when the heat has ceased.

A good way to increase circulation in any area of the body is to alternate the hot compress with a cold one. Place a wet, ice-cold cloth onto the area for a few minutes, and then follow with a similar application of a hot compress. You may decide at some point to leave the compress on for a long period of time. In this case, you will want to cover it with cling film and then extra towels, and definitely a hot water bottle. Leave on for up to two hours. Using these different temperatures encourages circulation in the affected area and will relieve congestion. While the hot compress pulls impurities from the body, the cold compress temporarily constricts the blood flow and circulation to the area. This can soothe discomfort caused by too much exposure to heat and will reduce unwanted swelling and pain. A mixture of the two will increase circulation three-fold.

## Poultices

A poultice differs from a compress in that, instead of the infusion or decoction being applied to the body, the herb or herb oil itself is applied. This can be done very simply by just 'bruising' a herb leaf and applying it to the skin; plantain leaves, mullein flowers and comfrey leaf poultices are good examples and are ideal for sprains. Another common method is to mix dried, cut or powdered herbs together and add water, apple cider vinegar or another appropriate liquid like olive oil, to form a paste, which is then applied to the skin. I have found that, by also adding some mucilaginous herb powder, such as slippery elm bark, to the mixture, a consistency that will adhere more effectively is obtained. With a non-oil based poultice, a little oil applied over the area to be treated will make the poultice feel more comfortable. When using a poultice on a 'hole' in the body, or on a deep wound, you will first need to clean the area with a minute essential oil and water solution – e.g. 1 drop of lavender and tea tree essential oil in 285mls water – before applying the poultice. Then you will need to add some anti-infection herbs to the poultice, such as turmeric rhizome, myrrh or thyme leaf. There is another rule for treating a wound: once the poultice has dried it may seem that some of it has disappeared or been absorbed into the body; don't clean the remaining poultice off – add a new poultice over the old one and keep 'feeding' the area. Once a poultice has dried onto a wound I consider it a part of the body, just like a scab – it will come off when it's time or it will grow into and become the flesh itself. There are, however, some types of poultice, especially drawing ones, which need to be changed frequently because they will have absorbed toxins that need to be removed from the body.

Poultices can be used to treat itching skin and other skin irritations and to draw out the poisons of stings and bites. They can also be used to heat an area (for example, a mustard plaster) and for glandular infections or congestion. A poultice can also be applied between two layers of gauze or light cotton if you don't want the actual herb to touch the skin for some reason. As a poultice dries, it becomes taut and draws out impurities. You can add drawing herbs or even refined clay, which increases this 'pulling' power. This is ideal for tumours and cancers; herbs like poke root may be used to assist in the treatment of breast cancer, while the addition of powdered charcoal will help purify the blood. A thin layer of olive oil can be applied to the skin prior to using non-oil based poultices in order to protect the skin from excessive drying.

Vegetable poultices have also been used widely over the years, using potatoes, onions, carrots, beets, garlic, cucumbers, aloe vera and a wide variety of greens. Cayenne, ginger, mustard and horseradish have all been popular for heating and stimulating poultices. Healing and soothing poultices made from comfrey leaf, slippery elm bark, marshmallow root, aloe leaves or gel, calendula flowers, lobelia herb and mullein flowers have been used extensively. Seed and grain poultices have also been used over the years with very soothing effects, along with fruit poultices using bananas, figs, apples, papayas and melons. Plantain leaf is a prime drawing herb used in poultices and is also a blood cleanser. Every kitchen contains an onion and this can be heated in the oven and placed over the affected area for pain relief.

## CASTOR OIL PACKS

Castor oil packs are useful for easing pain and inflammation. They can also relieve congestion and draw out toxins. Construct a muslin or flannel pack to size and soak it in warmed castor oil. The temperature on the body should be as hot as is bearable as the heat will force the castor oil into the area. After placing on the body hold in place and cover with clingfilm and a hot water bottle. The duration that the pack is left on will vary. Some packs are changed for new ones every hour or so in order to keep them hot. Some may be left on overnight, or just for 30 minutes in total. Otherwise a 30 minutes' pack done every 4 hours is another option.

## GARLIC PASTE FOR FEET

(An excellent aid for any respiratory disorders)
Peel 8 cloves of garlic and put in a liquidiser with equal parts of olive oil, water and slippery elm bark. Mix to a paste, then apply to the soles of the feet. Cover with fine muslin bandages and an old pair of baggy socks; you can even tie plastic bags over these. This paste should be checked every two hours to ensure that the garlic is not burning the soles of the feet.

## SUPPOSITORIES AND PESSARIES

Suppositories and pessaries are herbal poultices which are used internally. The base is generally made with a mucilaginous herb like slippery elm inner bark powder and a lubricant such as coconut oil or cocoa butter. Other powdered herbs are used for the particular problem and added to the base. These are inserted into body openings (vagina, rectum, nasal cavities, ears or mouth) in order to disperse their herbal constituents to internal areas. Suppositories and pessaries are made in the same way and are commonly used for rectal cleansing, vaginal infections, irritation, inflammation and general problems in the reproductive area.

When making a pessary, you will need finely powdered and sieved herbs in order to make the result as smooth as possible. The size of the pessary will depend upon the area that it will be inserted into.

Take a jar of coconut oil and place it in a bowl of hot water. In a short time the oil will melt. Mix the melted coconut oil with the finely powdered herbs until the mixture forms a pastry-like consistency. Form the herb mixture into the size and shape of pessary you desire.

Place the individual pessaries on a piece of waxed paper, stainless steel or a glass plate, and refrigerate them. Refrigeration will make them hard. When you want to use one, take it out of the refrigerator, hold it between your fingers for just a few seconds (the coconut oil will begin to melt) and then insert. Use some olive oil to lubricate the area of insertion first. When the pessary is inside the body, the body temperature, which is always variable, will cause the coconut oil to melt and the herbs will be dispersed.

**Vaginal Pessaries:** Use equal parts of the following in powder form; squaw vine herb, slippery elm inner bark, yellow dock root, comfrey root, chickweed herb, barberry root bark, mullein leaves and flowers, plus $1/2$ drop of geranium essential oil and lavender essential oil in a cocoa butter base.

**Candida Pessaries:** Use 9 parts slippery elm bark, 3 parts barberry root, 3 parts pau d'arco inner bark, 2 parts walnut husk, 1 part chamomile flowers, 1 part lavender flowers, and tea tree essential oil in a coconut oil base.

Start with a treatment of 7 pessaries, using one every night, or every third or fourth night. Insert into the vagina. If you wish, use a sanitary towel to protect night clothing, bed linen etc. but the more air allowed to circulate the affected area the better. The coconut butter melts at body temperature overnight (or longer, depending on the individual woman's basal temperature) leaving the herbs to be absorbed into the body. Any remaining herbs are easy to douche out every three or four days, or can be expelled by doing pelvic floor exercises in a bath containing a few drops of lavender essential oil and 5 tablespoons of cider vinegar. On dressing in the morning, use a natural sponge to prevent the herbs leaking out; you may even need the extra protection of a sanitary towel.

**Anal Suppositories:** Ideal for haemorrhoids. Use equal parts of walnut fruit, horse chestnut fruit, eucalyptus leaf, slippery elm bark, yarrow herb and a few drops of witch hazel essential oil in a base of cocoa butter.

## DOUCHES

Douches are herbal liquids gently inserted into the vagina (using a douche bag), usually in the form of a herbal infusion or decoction using vegetable, nut and seed oils, or aloe vera leaf gel.

An example of douche herbs would be a pre-made decoction of an equal amount of chamomile flower, pau d'arco bark, barberry root bark and lavender herb. This formula is capable of assisting in resisting a range of fungi and bacteria.

Douches can be used to wash out the residue of the pessaries and/or simply cleanse the area.

## ESSENTIAL OILS – THE COMPACT PHARMACY

Essential oils are extracted from flowers, grasses, fruits, leaves, roots and trees. There are, at present, over 300 different types of essential oils available which form an extremely efficient medical system. Many essential oils form the basis of modern pharmaceutical preparations.

Essential oils, wonderful benefits, must be respected. Applied directly and undiluted to the skin, they will burn, except in the case of lavender. Some people, having followed advice in books, have put neat essential oils (particularly tea tree oil) onto cuts, skin abrasions and skin problems. Tea tree burns are common because this essential oil has been advised for direct skin use. Some people are indeed all right, but a patch test is advisable.

If an essential oil has been applied directly in undiluted form and is burning, treat with aloe vera gel or olive oil, wheatgerm oil or any thick vegetable oil you have at hand. Do not use water as this will amplify the burning effect.

### Methods of Use and Dosage for Essential Oils

| | |
|---|---|
| Tissue and handkerchief: | Put 1 drop on and sniff when required. |
| Inhaled as a vapour: | Add 2–3 drops to a bowl of hot water and cover the head and bowl with a towel; keep your face 30cm above the surface of the water and inhale the vapour. |
| Massage oil: | Use approximately 4–6ml essential oil to 250ml base oil. |
| Baths: | Add a maximum of 8 drops. |
| Vegetable base oils: | Nut or seed oils are best: if in doubt use cold pressed virgin olive oil. |

## HERBAL OILS

Place your chosen and preferably fresh herb into a liquidiser, with a little olive oil or fractionated coconut oil – both are non-rancid, safe, stable base oils in which the herbs can be macerated. The cutting of the herbs will release the essential oils into the base oil. The ratio is approximately 100g of dried material to $^3/_4$ litre of oil but, if you use fresh material, use about 160g. Place this maceration in the sunshine and allow to steep for two weeks. Shake regularly. If you wish, you can strengthen it by straining the liquid, discarding the residual herbs and beginning the process again with a new batch of herbs.

For hot body oils and rubs, use 1 tbsp of each of the following herbs: English mustard seed, hot chilli powder, dried fresh ginger root powder and black pepper. Cover the ingredients with olive oil. Steep for 1 month and add essential oils of peppermint and camphor for extra heat.

Essential oils are being used increasingly today, and this demand has led, in some cases, to inferior quality. Toxins are sometimes not removed and occasionally the best bits of the essential oils are removed. Testing for oil quality is expensive but vital, ensuring that they are safe and reliable. Making your own in this way is easy and ensures high quality with no adulteration.

## SMUDGE STICKS

These provide a lovely way of 'fumigating' an area. The fragrance will change the atmosphere and help clean it. Native American Indians traditionally used wormwood and American sage. You can make your own version using a combination of English sage, thyme, eucalyptus, rosemary and wormwood.

Hold the herbs together in a tight bundle, then bind it even tighter using thick, pure cotton thread. Dry these thoroughly and quickly, otherwise they will become mouldy and unusable.

## POWDERS AND TALCS

These can be very useful for chickenpox, shingles, summer heat rashes, athlete's foot or any itching disease, especially where there are pustules that are weeping. You can even use it on weeping eczema.

Use 2tsp of arrowroot or cornflour (cornstarch) or fine maize flour. Mix with 1 dessertspoon of either a combination of finely-powdered black walnut inner hull, thyme leaf, barberry root bark and lavender herb; or any of these herbs singly.

**Vaginal dusting powder:** This is suitable for moist discharges and infections.
Use a combination of 7g fine white clay or bentonite clay, 12g arrowroot powder, 12g black walnut fruit powder, 12g barberry root bark powder or turmeric rhizome powder, 12g neem powder (if available) and 7g lavender powder. Either apply to the area as a powder or mix the powder with aloe gel and insert into the vagina. Aloe will cool the area in hot weather; however the powder will dry up and absorb discharge.

## BOOK LIST

*Aromatherapy An A-Z* by Patricia Davis (C. W. Daniel)

*Aromatherapy Handbook* by Danielle Ryman (C. W. Daniel)

*Making Tinctures* by James Green (Wildlife and Green Publications)

*School of Natural Healing* by Dr. J. Christopher (Christopher Publications)

'In a Nutshell' series

*Ginkgo, Echinacea, Hawthorn, Siberian Ginseng, St John's Wort, Garlic, Marigold, Saw Palmetto, Milk Thistle, Cranberry, Ginger and Aloe by* Jill Rosemary Davies (Element).

# FOUR

# FOOD AND NUTRITION

## THE HISTORY OF FOOD

Our body runs on the fuel it is provided with. When we were hunters and gatherers this fuel came in the form of wild collected foods, encompassing a diverse range of health giving chemistry, to include componants far beyond vitamins and minerals. For instance, archaeologists have found evening primrose seed on ancient European sites, leading us to believe that prehistoric men and women knew the value of the oil collected from these tiny seeds.

Archaeologists are also able to tell us of the diseases of ancient peoples. There is evidence to suggest that cancer, osteoporosis, rheumatism and arthritis were often exacerbated by their working and living conditions, but also partly because their dietary needs were not always met – just as with modern man. They did not, however, have high quantities of sugar literally eating away their vital calcium, magnesium, zinc and mineral supplies, with processed junk food creating a plethora of bowel diseases, cancer and other disorders. They had the stress of survival on a day-to-day basis, but the adrenaline they produced to deal with these situations was more readily burnt off. I rather feel that their instincts and needs were completely intact and, therefore, that their hormones, glands, brain and organs functioned with a more natural rhythm and balance. Modern-day man, by contrast, has become less instinc-tive and his balance less stable.

At whatever age, it can be difficult to make sure that nutritional needs are met. In the past, people had to travel and explore the great outdoors in order to find necessary medicine; but what do we do now? So much of what society considers food today should actually be avoided. It is strange to think that, in the average supermarket, at least 70% of the food for sale should not be consumed. Added to this is the fact that, in order to obtain what we require, we have to be prepared to spend a lot of time in the kitchen. (This was a way of life which our grandparents accepted without question.)

In the 1920s and 1930s, juicers, able to create a non-bulky and highly assimilable form of nutrition, became popular. The 1950s and 1960s saw the development of vitamin, mineral and other supplements made from animal parts, sea/land vegetables, minerals and other derivatives. More recently 'Superfood' drinks have been created using primary plants like algae and lichens – that is, using nature's potent forces.

Finally, at the beginning of the twenty-first century, people – not least, the leading supplement companies – are turning to combining supplements and herbs.

What should we choose? As a daily matter of course I would suggest good food with liberal amounts of culinary and wild herbs, with Superfood drinks to balance the effects of pollution and stress. For those chronic deficiencies picked up through tests and/or diagnosis, it is wise to choose supplements, Superfoods, juices, or a combination of them all.

Food builds us physically as well as nurturing us on a more subtle, unseen, vibrational level. Many great minds, not least those of botanists, archaeologists and herbalists, have recognised that, in the pre-farming era, health rested largely on the fact that humans consumed many different species of plants. This compares to the modern, genetically engineered and over-produced twenty or so species that are farmed today. It was this diverse array of plant chemistry that kept our systems honed and hardy and allowed our immune systems to act with force and spontaneity. It enabled our digestive systems to perform with vigour and digest almost anything. Since we stopped collecting and eating wild foods, which tend to be more bitter or sour (and altogether more rudimentary in their flavour), society has incurred a whole range of gut-based diseases which simply did not exist before. Many of our modern herbs were, originally, everyday foods, and it is the lack of everyday usage which has, in part, caused people to become physically weaker and more prone to an overall and ever-increasing degeneration of the body – not least through 'allergies'. Therefore, we should get back to using our known culinary herbs in earnest. In European homes, herbs such as thyme, marjoram, coriander, mint and garlic are or should be used at every opportunity, as should the inclusion of salads in the form of our garden 'weeds' – dandelions, chickweed, young oak leaves, fat hen and so on.

Being ill on an obviously physical level, like having a bloated stomach, arthritis or headaches, might lead you to believe that somewhere along the line your diet may have been responsible but, very often, it is easy to miss the more emotional and behavioural side effects of the wrong food input. Being poisoned, or else starved of the correct nutrition, can create anger, impatience, lack of interest and a whole array of negative emotions, which you may simply regard as being 'you'. Strip away the coffee, tea, alcohol, sugar, chocolate and, instead, supplement these with more healthy foods (which balance stomach flora and kills off any opportunistic parasites) and you may be surprised at who you meet! There are many herbs that greatly help this process of 'driven' addiction by altering the body's chemistry, balancing and over-riding unwanted cravings.

## THE OPTIONS

When I think about food for myself and my family, when I talk about foods with patients, I hope to represent the plant that flowers cheerfully, sways in the wind and has a good root system which grounds and stabilises it. Food is there to be enjoyed and you need to be creative and flexible in order to do so. The basis of this should be intuition and knowledge about what promotes good body chemistry and happy healthy beings.

Sometimes tremendous upheaval is needed in order to transform sickness into health. To many people it appears to be too hard to change long-established and often cherished patterns, tastes and beliefs. Changes in food can be bewildering and challenging and many people cannot, or will not, attempt such changes. Getting help to devise what is right for your own individual body type, body weight, health and culture will help this often difficult process. For some, the love and joy of nourishing their own bodies and respecting their own beings is simple; others find it more difficult. Some find it easiest to make changes when they are well. There are, however, some cases in which people become so seriously ill that a drastic change of diet may be their only option. In these situations, making this choice may prove to be a life-saver.

## BLOOD TYPES AND DIGESTIVE ENZYMES

Blood group tests are available which some professionals believe can give you an indication of foods which suit your genetic make-up; more simply you can just ask your doctor what blood group you are and then follow the general advice below.

Blood types can be broken down into Group O, Group A (which further differentiates into A1 and A2), Group B and Group AB.

### DIET FOR BLOOD GROUP O

Historically, the Blood Group O diet was apparently the first to evolve and is associated with hunter/gatherer societies. People who are Group O do well on diets that are high in proteins such as meat, poultry and fish. Dairy products, corn and most grains should be eliminated. Group O individuals are generally associated with higher levels of hydrochloric acid in the stomach, which helps to digest the higher amounts of proteins found with this type of diet. Fruits and vegetables should also be eaten in larger amounts to help balance the acid/alkaline content of the body.

### DIET FOR BLOOD GROUP A

Historically, Blood Group A individuals have adapted well to a vegetarian/agrarian form of diet, which evolved later and consists primarily of fruits, vegetables, nuts and grains. Generally, little or no meat should be allowed and then only as a condiment. Milk and cheese should also be eliminated, especially in type A2 individuals. Grains and beans contain higher amounts of naturally occurring agglutinins (lectins) which make their assimilation by the body more difficult. Larger amounts of fruits and vegetables are recommended for group A individuals, as they tend to secrete lower amounts of hydrochloric acid and thus absorb less. Raw fruits and vegetables are higher in natural enzymes, which promote digestion, absorption and assimilation.

### DIET FOR BLOOD GROUP B

Apparently, the Blood Group B diet evolved later than that of groups O or A and is associated with nomadic and herding societies. People who are group B do well with diets that are high in fermented dairy products. These individuals do better on ovo-lacto vegetarian diets. These diets are higher in products which contain milk, cheese and eggs. Natural agglutinins (lectins) in such foods as chicken, sunflower, sesame and buckwheat may cause problems for a group B person and should be used in moderation. Group B individuals are generally associated with lower levels of hydrochloric acid in the stomach and may need enzyme and hydrochloric acid assistance if higher amounts of proteins are ingested. Group B persons do well with a good balance of the different food groups allowed rather than a particular food type.

## DIET FOR BLOOD GROUP AB

Apparently, the Blood Group AB diet evolved last and is felt to be associated with modern diets. Because of the presence of both A and B antigens, group AB individuals are well adapted to vegetarian, grain and seafood diets, with small to moderate amounts of milk products. Natural agglutinins (lectins) in such foods as red meat, chicken, potatoes, tomatoes and many grains and beans may cause problems for a group AB person and should be used only in moderation. Group AB individuals are generally associated with lower levels of hydrochloric acid in the stomach and may need enzyme and hydrochloric acid supplementation if higher amounts of proteins are ingested. Group AB people do well with a good balance of the different food groups allowed rather than a particular food type or group.

(See the *Eat Right Diet* by Peter D'Adamo with Caroline Whitney (Rider) for further information on this subject.)

## ORGANIC FOODS

The word 'organic' has become semi-meaningless, due to the excess of acid rain etc. now prevailing. However natural a farmer or gardener tries to be, what drops from the sky does count! But the term 'organic' still indicates that something has been grown in chemical-free ground and is still worth pursuing.

A friend of mine, who used to work in a mortuary, told me years ago that bodies are taking a lot longer to decompose, due to the preservatives they ingested with food while alive. The very thought horrified me; the idea of the 'walking preserved' is a chilling one. The days of preserving foods and growing foods with the use of toxic substances are not, however, as recent as we might assume. In 1953 Professor Ehret talked about sulphur-dried foods, benzoid of soda, salicylic acid and sulphuric acid which were being used to preserve canned foods.

Consuming preservatives, pesticides, nitrates and other substances used by farmers is dangerous to every cell in the human body. The major concern is, of course, for children. The Soil Association has drawn attention to the fact that a one-year-old could easily receive a maximum lifetime's dose of eight pesticides from just twenty commonly eaten fruits, vegetables and grains. The Soil Association is trying to unite farmers, the Department of Agriculture and the Drug Administration Agency in an attempt to utilise beneficial organisms and crop rotation instead of some pesticides. Nerve gases are still used by farmers. They are commonly known as organo-phosphates. These chemicals enter the food chain via vegetables, grains and cattle feed, and are also transported by the wind. Many cases of motor neurone disease are now being reported amongst young children (and adults). Often these are farmers' children who I, in turn, see in my clinic. Let us not forget household pesticides and those used in our gardens; these at least could be dispensed with.

The major sources of pesticide residues in the Western diet are meat, poultry and dairy products. 'Pesticide' is a generic term that includes insecticides, herbicides (weedkillers) and fungicides, among other agents. One chemical commonly found in household, agricultural and commercial-use pesticides is 2,4-D, a key ingredient found in Agent Orange, the defoliant put to widespread use during the Vietnam war. Frequent use of herbicides, particularly those containing 2,4-D, has been associated with two to eight-fold increases in non-Hodgkin's lymphoma in studies conducted in several countries. Other agents, including triazine and organo-phosphate pesticides, have also been shown to increase cancer risks. Pesticide use has increased 33-fold since the 1940s and there has been a ten-fold increase in potency. Dr. Sheila Zahm of the U.S. National Cancer Institute has recommended that pregnant women avoid exposure to all pesticides, which is not easy if you live in an area surrounded by fields being sprayed throughout the year. The foetus is particularly susceptible to genetic damage, chromosomal aberrations and carcinogenicity. Infants are also at higher risk.

The food most likely to cause cancer from herbicide residue is beef. The frightening thing is that extremely few slaughtered animals are actually tested for toxic chemical residues. In America the figure is as low as one in every quarter million. Levels of DDT in non-vegetarian mothers' milk in America have been found to be as high as 99%, as opposed to levels of 8% in vegetarian mothers!

It is not surprising that staphylococci infections are much more rampant and that resistance in humans is now really low. Penicillin used to be able to deal with them, combating them successfully and leaving only 13% resistant; now the figure is more like 91% resistant, the reason being the breeding of antibiotic-resistant bacteria in factory farms due to the routine feeding of antibiotics to livestock. At present, one can expect 80% of all farmed livestock and poultry to receive drugs regularly. Milk is also affected by residues of sulphur drugs – tetracycline and other antibiotics have been found. One hopes that the government will step in.

Doctors and health workers are aghast at the hijacking of antibiotics by the animal feed industry. They have been left with fewer resources with which to fight disease as our bodies acclimatise to antibiotics via the food chain, making their use less and less effective. Through the addition of hormones to increase speed of growth and size of animals, our fertility and balance is being put into chaos, producing disease and distortions.

All plant life has a vibration and a gift beyond visible food sustenance – both aspects are important. It has been shown that foods grown in loving, positive atmospheres produce more nourishment in nutritional and vibrational terms.

## BUYING ORGANIC

The Soil Association can put you in touch with local fruit and vegetable growers from whom you can buy directly; or contact the headquarters of Friends of the

Earth. Alternatively, you could ask your local health food store for information. A typical winter selection of vegetables in a family box consists of organic onions, potatoes, mushrooms, Brussels sprouts, two types of cabbage, cauliflower, leeks and carrots. In the spring, summer and autumn there are beans, peas and other seasonal variations. If asked, they will often provide fresh organic fruits and other specialist items. The boxes are made up not sooner than a day or two before delivery. Organic fruits, vegetables, nuts, seeds and grains have a very much longer shelf life than their pesticide-laden counterparts, so even if you need to buy in quantity at some distance you can be sure that they will retain their vitality longer. Store them in a cool environment away from sunlight.

Organic farmers represented 1% of British agriculture in 1995, but, in the same year they received only 0.01% of the £1.5 million assistance for farming in Britain; so when I pay a little more for organic foods I know I am helping to compensate for this lack of government assistance to growers. I am also keen to support those in other countries, including Spanish organic growers who produce the lemons and avocados which British farmers are unable to produce.

If you cannot afford the little extra that organic foods cost, then add garlic to your normal supplies; with its sulphur compounds and antioxidant chemistry, this will detoxify some of the harmful effects. There are also fruit and vegetable wash concentrates which help remove chemicals, waxes, dust, atmospheric pollutants and exhaust fumes. For those who are able to do so, growing your own is cheap and fun using an allotment or your garden.

## HERBS AND SPICES

Herbs and spices are the hormonal, glandular, immuno-protective and procreative parts of plants. They aid our digestion and add flavour. To me they also represent fun, colour and health. They are masters at dancing with our taste buds. They are nature's aid to the relaxation of stomach muscles. They also encourage better production of balanced and sufficient gastric juices. They contain elements which help counter-balance toxic foods. Some contain anti-fungal, antibacterial and anti-viral ingredients, giving some help to harmonise food combinations that might otherwise 'fight it out' and cause indigestion and wind; still others help the liver with its job of constantly negating and purifying.

You can grow fresh herbs and spices and use dried or freshly imported ones. Those who shy away from garlic because of its smell should add freshly grated ginger to it and, providing you wash regularly, keep generally healthy and don't get constipated, the garlic odour will be minimised.

The spice and herb section of any kitchen is one of the major medicine cupboards for any household. This section should be used for everyday eating and staying healthy. The whole kitchen should be full of live, healing and tasty foods, but herbs and spices have a special gift. Remember that by adding these to all meals and rotating their use, you are bringing in a diversity of healing chemistry; thus reducing the likelihood of disease in general.

**Aniseed** *(Pimpinella anisum)* is a sweet spice. It is excellent for breaking up mucus in the body and for the relief of griping in the bowels, also colic and flatulence. It is also very calming; soothing to the nervous system and alleviating sleeplessness.

**Caraway** *(Carum carvi)* is an excellent aid to digestion and relieves indigestion.

**Cardamom** *(Elettaria cardamomum)* is the king of spices; it warms the body and soothes indigestion and wind.

**Cayenne** *(Capsicum minimum)* is a medicinal and nutritional herb. It is the purest and best stimulant. It is an excellent food for the circulatory system as it feeds the necessary elements into the cell structure of arteries, veins and capillaries so that they regain elasticity. It also regulates blood pressure. Used most beneficially raw, it rebuilds the tissue in the stomach and heals stomach and intestinal ulcers (the opposite is true of cooked chillies). It also produces natural warmth and, in stimulating the peristaltic motion of the intestines, aids in assimilation and elimination. Cayenne peppers have white seeds which are the hottest part; they are good for colds and flu.

**Cinnamon** *(Cinnamomum zeylanicum)* is available as bark, shoots and sticks. The bark is mainly sweet, but also slightly hot and bitter; the shoots taste very different and are not so sweet. Both are warming and tonic. Cinnamon and whole barley grain soup is good for all kidney problems, balancing water volume, general tone and function, and helping to cleanse the system. Cinnamon and cloves complement each other in cooking, warming and speeding digestion. Nausea, flatulence and diarrhoea can be helped with these.

**Cloves** *(Eugenia caryophyllata)* are a stimulant and are effective for warming the body, increasing circulation, improving digestion, alleviating nausea and vomiting and clearing phlegm. They are also capable of inhibiting viruses and fungi and parasitic eggs. Use sparingly as the flavour is strong.

**Coriander** *(Coriandrum sativum)* is the queen of spices. As a seed it is a good thickening agent. It is stimulative, digestive and considered universally useful and healing.

**Cumin** *(Cuminum cyminum)* is 'cooler' than some spices but it still warms and aids digestion. It is one of the best spices for the relief of flatulence. It is also a stimulant and anti-spasmodic, useful to the heart and uterus.

**Fennel** *(Foeniculum vulgare)* assists digestion and increases metabolic processes in general; it alleviates wind, bloating and spasms and speeds up digestion. It dissolves and disperses mucus and fats. The lungs benefit from this when taken as a tea.

**Fenugreek** *(Trigonella foenumgraecum)* is a useful 'healing' spice; it is very nourishing and considered to be a tonic. It balances blood sugar. It is a very useful thickening agent in foods – 3 cups of tea a day will help people gain weight. It will also calm an acidic or ulcerated stomach and increase milk flow for mothers with poor production. It also strongly supports the pancreas.

**Garlic** *(Allium sativum)* is the paragon of blood cleansers and, with its abundance of sulphur (80 different sulphur compounds), it is capable of killing viruses, bacteria and fungus. It can calm and feed the nervous system and help correct faulty digestion. The fresh juice is effective for cramps, spasms and seizures. Combine it with ginger, French tarragon or marjoram to prevent wind. Combined with onions it is very beneficial for colds and flu, but simmer rather than boil it or it will lose much of its goodness. Those with high cholesterol will find that it is lowered with garlic. It is a major antioxidant, proven to help reduce the incidence of cancer and many other diseases. Garlic juice, diluted 1 part in 125,000, inhibits the growth of most types of bacteria. In fact, the odour alone does this. Garlic is nature's own broad-spectrum antibiotic, but works without killing off friendly bacteria as drug antibiotics do. In addition, garlic is positive for your heart, as it lowers blood pressure and reduces clots and platelet aggregation. Garlic not only encourages white blood cell formation but also produces a bacterial agent that halts tumour growth. Garlic protects the body from toxic chemicals, harmful food additives and rancid oils. It is also helpful in the treatment of AIDS where lymphocyte clumping encourages the spread of HIV from cell to cell. Cooked and raw garlic should be a part of everyday life, eating between one and three cloves daily. (However 1% of the population cannot tolerate it).

**Ginger** *(Zingiber officinale)* is one of the most versatile herbal stimulants. It is of great benefit to the intestines, circulation and stomach. Use as a tea when you are feeling sick or headachy. It enhances the effect of all other herbs and spices. Make your own ginger honey (organic, cold-pressed) and use instead of marmalade. **Avoid use if you have high blood pressure, or in cases of extreme inflammation or dry skin or liver inflammation.**

**Lemon** *(Citrus limonia)*. Not only delightful in flavour, the lemon is one of nature's best kitchen healers. Gypsy lore says it is among the five foods which should always be in the kitchen. Using the whole organic ones, the fresh skins can also be used. Lemon juice can be added to so much – including teas. Rich in vitamin C, a natural antioxidant, it encourages the immune system. Suck on an organic lemon if you have swollen glands.

**Marjoram** *(Origanum marjorana)* is a stimulant, antispasmodic, antiseptic and carminative, a combination of opposites which brings balance. It relaxes the lungs and digestion and expels mucus wherever it may be situated. It is helpful in many bowel disorders, easing, soothing and healing. It can be used for cramps, nausea and sickness and adds a slightly lemony flavour to all dishes.

**Mustard** *(Brassica alba, nigra and other species)* is a stimulant, alterative and rubefacient which is excellent for the digestive system. The best mustards are those made from whole grains and mixed with apple cider vinegar rather than white wine or malt vinegar. Add it frequently to salad dressings and when cooking rice and other grains. Use the seeds whole on steamed cabbage, carrot and parsnip to add crunch and spicy heat!

**Nutmeg and Mace** *(Myristica fragrans)*. Mace is the outer covering of the nutmeg. Nutmeg and lettuce soup is very good for depression and nervous disorders. Mace is an antiseptic and is delicious in sweet dishes. Sprinkle nutmeg and mace on cooked fruit, use with cinnamon in sweet dishes or grate onto potatoes, cabbage, onions and leeks. The effect is generally warming and soothing. Together they are supposed to be an aphrodisiac but be aware that in large quantities they can be hallucinatory. Nutmeg encourages menstruation and can be abortive in large quantities – therefore avoid during pregnancy.

**Parsley** *(Petroselium crispum or species)*. There are many varieties of parsley, all of which are incredibly tasty and health-giving. Parsley has a very high vitamin and mineral content and is very rich in chlorophyll. I used it a lot when making my babies their first foods. Millet and parsley was a much used combination for protein, iron, calcium, vitamin C, chlorophyll and many other nutrients. Try it in soups, stews or salads, not just as a garnish, to which status it is usually relegated. Parsley is a blood cleanser – its high iron content helps the blood. It also acts as a diuretic and digestive through increasing bile flow, so one could call it a digestive and a detoxifier. Do not make into strong teas if you are pregnant or suffer from heavy periods, as the oestrogen within it could be unsuitable.

**Pepper** *(Piper nigrum)*. Black pepper is anti-catarrhal, anti-mucus, anti-fungal, anti-bacterial and is also a natural preservative. It should be freshly ground and added after the food has been cooked; cooking changes its chemistry making it more aggressive to the stomach. White pepper produces acids and is almost a mature fruit when the skin is removed – use it only as a seed to flavour, and do not eat large quantities. Green pepper, like black pepper, is an immature fruit. Those with liver problems should only eat small amounts of it.

**Rosemary** *(Rosmarinus officinalis)* is astringent, bitter, highly stimulating and yet calming, which makes it useful for indigestion, colic, nausea, gas, nervousness and fever. It is also high in calcium and is a natural antiseptic.

**Sage** *(Salvia officinalis)* is an antispasmodic, antiseptic and astringent, and is helpful for slowing fluid secretions. Consequently, it is helpful in cases of excessive perspiration, night sweats, milk flow and vaginal discharge. It has a slightly bitter taste, so limit its usage and certainly never consider it as a single herbal tea. It needs careful dosage but is invaluable if used correctly.

**Thyme** *(Thymus vulgaris)* is useful in cases of lack of appetite, chronic gastritis and diarrhoea. It is highly antiseptic and can activate and strengthen the immune system, and it warms and tones as it works. (However, excessive amounts can cause depression if made into daily teas.)

**Turmeric** *(Curcuma longa)* is one of the most useful and versatile spices. Not only is it an excellent cleanser of the liver due to its bitter taste but it is also highly antiseptic and, as a blood purifier, is useful for eczema, pimples and a variety of other skin complaints. It is helpful for all circulatory problems and menstrual regularity; it also keeps all kinds of undesirable bacteria and infection at bay. It is also an antioxidant.

Note: As you have probably realised, foods and spices in their different states – fresh, whole and powdered – all have different flavours. Whole, unprocessed spices last the longest. If you are buying powdered ones, buy only small quantities at a time; alternatively buy whole ones and grind your own in a coffee grinder. Perhaps the main quality of most culinary herbs and spices is that their essential oils all help with digestion, relaxing stomach muscles, speeding digestion and killing off unwanted amounts of fungi, bacteria and even parasites in some cases. They are generally tonic, feeding and health-giving. Don't forget others such as bay leaf, basil and chives.

## DIGESTION

This is the most important subject of this chapter and perhaps the book, for without proper digestion much ill health and many diseases can be created. The digestive system comprises the mouth, spleen, pancreas, stomach, liver, gall-bladder, intestines and the colon. There is much work to be done by each of these; for instance the mouth secretes digestive enzymes and the entire digestive tract is populated by symbiotic bacteria whose job it is to break down the partially processed food, and assists its decomposition by fermentation.

A few helpful tips on eating are:

Don't eat if you are angry or frightened; eating should essentially be a feeding, nurturing and sensuous experience. If you are tired but hungry, choose easily-digestible foods that need little chewing, like soup, broth, soft fruits or vegetable/fruit juices. A relaxed state of mind means relaxed stomach muscles and an easy production of balanced gastric juices resulting in proper assimilation and easy, natural elimination. A before-dinner joke is as important as an after-dinner one; laughter is the best relaxant I know. That, or simply take some deep breaths. Mothers with babies and young children often have enforced strange and disturbed eating routines, especially when nursing; therefore they need extra support and help at this time.

See 'The Digestive System' in Chapter Nine.

## FLAVOURS

'**Bitter**' flavours, which are first tasted in the mouth, help the immune system that lies within the gut, aiding production of white blood cells, generally empowering immune responses and helping to fight many diseases of the immune system from candida to AIDS. Bitter flavours help to burn up excess fats in the body, quickly providing the energy to do this. For the very underweight, few bitter foods should be consumed unless they are being used for a specific reason like ridding the body of worms.

We owe it to ourselves to eat bitters and sours. The taste helps to de-stress and calm the nervous system, balancing and grounding, preventing over-extensive output of nervous energy.

Bitters include: gentian, artichoke, olives and olive oil, dandelion leaves, chicory and nasturtium leaves. As a digestive aid they are often put with aromatics to help cool, calm and soothe the digestive tract like cinnamon sticks, fennel seed and ginger root. The European Swedish bitters and liqueurs can be consumed to aid pre- and after- dinner digestion.

Bitters often come in the form of wild greens in spring, but they are still available in the summer.

'**Sour**' heals and nurtures the liver and gall-bladder by deep cleansing and cooling them down, making the digestive process largely passive, which in turn has a positive emotional effect. A cleansed and cooled liver and gall-bladder readily releases the positive emotions of joy and happiness. These are two important emotions for the well-being of the immune system in general. Include limes, lemons, sorrel, sauerkraut, pineapple and apple cider vinegar. *Pineapples are sour/sweet and the bromelain in them is a prime digestive, scavenging for and helping to finish off half-digested foods.* The taste helps to de-stress and calm the nervous system, balancing and grounding, preventing over-extensive output of nervous energy.

You can pickle your own foods easily, using apple cider vinegar. This type of vinegar helps regulate the balanced output of stomach acid, correcting 'over' and 'under' active conditions. The sour flavour can really be exciting and chillies, which couldn't ordinarily be eaten raw, can be when softened by the pickling process.

'**Salty**' heals and nurtures the kidneys, adrenals, bladder and thyroid. It is in all sea vegetables like kelp, nori, wakame and so on. Parsley and celery are considered salty and make an excellent 'dried and sprinkled-on' substitute. Do not use too much salt as the kidneys will suffer. The dangers of high salt intake are so well publicised that it is almost more important to say, these days, that a little good quality salt should be consumed – some people need more than others.

'**Spicy**': This really sums up two flavours, hot and pungent. It supports and nourishes the lungs and colon, opening both and allowing them to operate with the ease they should. This category includes hot peppers, mustards and horseradish. They generally aid circulation, encouraging the delivery of oxygen and nutrients and the expulsion of waste products and toxins.

'**Neutral**': This taste includes, among others, rice, potatoes, sago, arrowroot, banana, yam, turnip, parsnip and millet. It nurtures and grounds the body, feeding and toning. It is one of the most unifying of all flavours, providing harmony and balance.

'**Sweet**': The sweet flavour heals and nurtures the stomach, spleen and pancreas, thus improving digestion, if used in a balanced way. Some positive sweeteners are real maple syrup, brown rice syrup, barley syrup, cold pressed organic honey, date syrup, whole liquorice, stevia herb, peppermint leaf and certain culinary herbs.

Sugar inhibits the ability of white blood cells to destroy bacteria. Just two teaspoons is enough to diminish our immune system response dramatically; teaspoon for teaspoon, and also consumes calcium, stripping the body of one of its most necessary minerals. If sugar is to be used, then real cane sugar is rich in essential minerals and vitamins and provides a better alternative than most. Blackstrap molasses are sweet and loaded with iron and calcium which also makes them a good substitute for sugar. Try using a little liquorice on occasion. Stevia, which is 300 to 500 times sweeter than sugar, does not feed yeasts, fungi and other unwanted gastro-intestinal micro-organisms and it helps improve digestion by stimulating the pancreas. Made as a tea and kept in the refrigerator, a small amount could be added to herbal teas. Both this and liquorice are very useful for hypoglycaemic people who need a sugar boost.

We all start life with a sweet tooth – breast milk is sweet and, as such, it nourishes and replenishes and is right for this vulnerable entry into life. With the constant availability of sugar reaching huge proportions over the last 30-35 years, 'sweet diseases' have increased and, along with them, parallel mental afflictions. It is not just our pancreas, teeth and waistlines that are affected, our whole emotional state also suffers. Artificial sweeteners are a further perversion of the problem – not only poisoning but also increasing appetite in many cases! It is always advisable to read labels in order to see how the food you buy has been sweetened. Never use artificial sweeteners – proven to be carcinogenic, in the 1970s they were banned in Japan by the government. Look at health store foods and see how many products have been sweetened by the inclusion of fruit concentrates. Even though this is far better than adding white sugar, it still represents work for the liver and other organs and systems.

**Putrid** fermented foods, like miso, sauerkraut and tofu support the immune system immensely and sustain the body. There is more on this later in this chapter.

## OILS (AND ANTIOXIDANTS)

The only oil that does not become rancid is olive oil. It is the only oil which benefits the heart, liver, gall-bladder (and cholesterol levels). It can also be heated and cooked with at low temperatures without diminishing its character and life force. Used raw, it is excellent with salads. It is 80% mono-unsaturated and, as such, does not present the health hazards of saturated or polyunsaturated fats. For occasional variance, there are other oils that can be safely used such as walnut oil, safflower oil, grapeseed oil, sunflower oil, hempseed oil and linseed oil.

Oils are attacked by oxygen almost within moments of harvesting and become rancid; more rancid, in fact, the older they become. This effect of oxygen excess causes a knock-on effect in our bodies producing free radicals, and it is these free radicals that attack, kill or damage our cellular structure. Many, many plants help stop this destruction due to containing chemical components that act as anti-oxidants. The liver is particularly susceptible to free radical damage because this is where fats accumulate and are processed. Avoid all foods containing fats and oils.

When you stir-fry with olive oil, keep the heat low and be sure to add water at any sign of drying out or over-heating. Remember, fried foods are basically too rich and indigestible to our systems and cause fermentation and stagnation. There is some recent data linking free radical damage to Creutzfeldt-Jakob disease. Scientists are also linking diseases like Alzheimer's and Parkinson's to free radical damage.

## WHOLE-GRAINS

These have always existed in their wild state but have now been genetically altered to suit mono-crop, mass farming. This has largely contributed to many of the allergy problems we see today, with wheat as the main culprit.

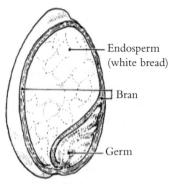

The whole grain

There are eight whole-grains readily available: rye, oats, millet, rice, quinoa, corn, wheat and barley. They are healthiest eaten in their whole state to retain maximum food value and roughage. Using a slow cooker is an ideal way to preserve their life force and nourishment, due to its low temperature but lengthy heating. Alternatively, soak them in a saucepan overnight. Pre-soaking will enable grains to be cooked at a low temperature for a shorter period of time. However, for those who do not have the time, try using a rice cooker which will cook the grains for you and then keep them warm for three hours if necessary. Whole-grains can be eaten with at least one main meal a day for balance. Whole-grains are rich in fibre and when fibre ferments in the large intestine, a chemical called butyrate is produced which blocks the action of genes produced by cancer cells.

If you wish to eat raw grains, then growing organic wheat grass and sprouting barley, rye and corn is wonderful. (Read *Light Eating for Survival by* Marcia Madhuri for details on how to do this).

## REFINED CARBOHYDRATES

These are grains that have had their outer husks (roughage) removed, leaving just their inner section. This tends to create body imbalances because the grains are themselves unbalanced. Refined carbohydrates have also very often been pre-cooked. Mucus is a natural coating of mucous membranes and soft tissue, but consumption of refined carbohydrates creates too much of it. This excess mucus clogs and tires the whole body and exacerbates digestive problems in turn, catarrh, asthma, and much more. Its sticky consistency invites infection. Sourdough rye and mixed-grain breads, Ryvita, rye bread, rice cakes or Manna (sprouted seed bread) are healthy alternatives to the average loaf!

## MEAT

Meat isn't what it used to be. Herbivores and poultry are now injected with antibiotics, fed on hormones and synthetic proteins, and were, until recently, even fed dead animals as a 'recycling' policy, making them toxic to our bodies and especially to our livers. Beef contains high quantities of creatine, a member of the caffeine and theine family, which are heart and kidney stimulants. Pork is very high in fat (67.4% on average) and very low in protein (only 9.4%). All meat putrefies in the intestine and strips calcium from the body. If you wish to eat meat, then strive to find organic suppliers and avoid eating huge quantities, putting slivers rather than big chunks on your plate, more in keeping with our sedentary lives. Always cook this meat with herbs like oregano and thyme to reduce parasites and microbes in general.

A 95g portion of red meat typically contains 100mg of cholesterol, even after it has been skinned. The excessive fats found in meat raise cholesterol and uric acid levels in the tissues and interfere with the proper metabolism of carbohydrates. They encourage diabetes and dull the brain by causing clogging of capillaries, reducing the amount of available oxygen. Some cultures balance their meat consumption by mixing lean meat with grains, seeds and vegetables. Meat, being a heavy protein, requires maximum digestive abilities and, if the body is too sick or undernourished to do this, then toxicity and further sickness will result.

Genetically engineered meat could make headway. These genetic creations are believed to be the future of meat, with extra meat and less fat being the goal; but some unpleasant side-effects have been observed. I find it wholly frightening. It is not natural selection and runs contrary to bio-diversity.

If you want to move from meat-eating to vegetarianism or veganism, take it very slowly over a period of a year or more to give your body time to adjust. It is also important to make sure you know where to gain adequate vegetable protein which is vital for growing bodies. Organic meat is certainly an option, but ensure that the machinery used in the slaughter houses has been thoroughly washed and sterilised to prevent the risk of cross infection, which according to meat inspectors is prevalent.

## MEAT PROTEIN VERSUS VEGETABLE PROTEIN

Levels of protein consumption currently far exceed official recommendations. Excessive animal, dairy and egg protein can lead to many problems from high cholesterol levels to excessive uric acid formation, cancers, calcium loss and many more ailments.

We need amino acids for growth, repair and the production of hormones and enzymes. Yet an excess of amino acids (the basic component of all proteins) forces the elimination of very important trace elements like zinc, calcium, magnesium, iron and chromium, all of which are vital for emotional and physical well-being. The shedding of calcium, for instance, wears away the nervous system and depletes bone mass.

If you are going to eat meat and fish, then consume only $^3/_4$ kg (750g) of flesh foods per week (approximately 100gms per day). For less active or non-growing bodies, this could be reduced by about half. All meat dishes, particularly those containing red meats, increase the likelihood of uric acid forming in the body, causing arthritis, rheumatism and bowel diseases. Poor digestion of even fresh foods can cause tremendous stagnation and create harmful bacteria and toxins. However, having said that, a balanced intake of protein in some form is essential. A totally vegetarian diet, without due care and attention being paid to alternative protein intake, is just as dangerous as an excess of animal protein. Lack of protein will produce visible symptoms like allergic sensitivity, bronchial and nasal congestion (lots of clear mucus), tiredness and cold extremities among others. These symptoms could continue for as long as one to two years after you change to a better diet.

## PROTEIN NEEDS AND PERCENTAGES

The World Health Organisation suggests 4.5% of daily calories should be provided by protein. The USA Food and Nutrition Board suggests 6%.

### VEGETABLE PROTEIN

Chlorella and bluegreen algae are extremely rich in proteins (higher than meat), but here are some others: spinach, broccoli, mushrooms, lettuce and pumpkin.

In order to obtain the twenty-two amino acids essential for complete protein and for adequate body function use a combination of any grain and seed/legume.

The approximate amount of protein needed for adults is 50g daily. Children require about 75g daily.

*Some Ideas for Grain & Seed/Legume Combinations:*

| | | |
|---|---|---|
| $^2/_3$ Rice | plus | $^1/_3$ Broad Beans |
| $^2/_3$ Millet | plus | $^1/_3$ Sprouted Alfalfa |
| $^2/_3$ Corn on the Cob | plus | $^1/_3$ Lentil Stew |
| $^2/_3$ Barley | plus | $^1/_3$ Runner Beans |
| $^2/_3$ Rice | plus | $^1/_3$ Sesame Seeds |

## DAIRY PRODUCTS

Foods under this heading generally cause more concern and apprehension than any other. I see more sick people who have overindulged on dairy products than any other single food grouping. Milk and cheese are particularly damaging to children and they can contribute to sinus problems, heart problems, allergies, colds, constipation, chronic fatigue, headaches, obesity and dental deterioration. Many of us do not have suffi-cient natural lactase to break down the digestible lactose present in dairy products into digestive sugars, which are assimilable.

Dairy products often contain high levels of bacteria that can remain in these foods even after cooking and even pass into unprotected food stored nearby. They do, of course, contain all the pesticides and herbicides the cattle have grazed on, unless they are organic.

**Yoghurt**, although made from milk and therefore potentially just as harmful, does have the benefit of containing live cultures. Make it from organic goat's milk if you decide to eat yoghurt.

**Butter** is almost free from mucus-forming substances and can be consumed, but use small amounts as it contains roughly 83% fat and 1% protein! But don't forget that it is basically rancid and has lots of free radicals. Avoid margarine completely.

**Cheese** is in a concentrated form and is often salted. Migraine headaches are frequently caused by cheese consumption due to the presence of the protein tyra-mine. Cheese causes excessive mucus production which clogs up the intestines and other areas, such as the lungs. This mucus forms a coating on the inner lining of the stomach which hardens, making an impermeable layer thus preventing the absorption of nutrients. It can cause similar damage in the bowel, producing chronic constipation.

**Milk** and cheese have a history of causing allergies, such as hives and skin rashes. This is because they over-stimulate certain stomach cells producing a hydrochloric acid deficiency resulting in proteins entering the bloodstream. In fact, milk neutralises the hydrochloric acid necessary for food digestion, causing excessive mucus build-ups which inhibit absorption of vital nutrients from all foods. In addition to this, fifty per cent of the protein in cows' milk is indigestible anyway. The late Dr. Spock, the well-known child psychologist and nutritional expert, latterly advocated the withdrawal of milk from children's diet. In the book *A Diet for a New America* by Tom Robinson of the billionaire ice-cream family, milk and other dairy products are cited as creating osteoporosis. Cows tend to graze on fields sprayed with pesticides. One pesticide that has been banned in Israel is lindane, an organochloride insecticide related to DDT. Fourteen other countries have banned lindane, with its use being restricted in still more. In Britain, however, lindane continues to contaminate our milk and put our women at risk of breast cancer – the biggest killer of women between the ages of 35 and 54 in Britain. Search out organic milk perhaps.

**Calcium (and Magnesium)**. Sources are regularly found in common foods and herbs. The recommended daily allowance of calcium is 800–1200 mg, with sufficient sunshine or other sources of vitamin D to aid proper absorption of the calcium. The recommended daily allowance for magnesium is 350–450 mg.

Calcium rich herbs and foods include valerian root, pau d'arco inner bark, kelp, wakame and hijike seaweed, nettle leaf, raw almonds (soak overnight and remove the outer skin before eating), dried figs, walnuts, raspberry leaf tea, boneset tea, fresh parsley, carrot juice and sunflower seeds. Magnesium rich foods include all of the above and Irish moss, oatstraw and turmeric.

All four recipes below are rich in calcium and magnesium.

### Coconut Milk
1 cup grated coconut meat, 2 cups water, honey to taste if wished; liquidise and sieve.

### Almond Milk
$^1/_2$ cup almonds (remove skins and pre-soak in the refrigerator), 4 cups water; liquidise and sieve.

### Cashew Milk
1 cup cashews, $3^1/_2$ cups water; liquidise and sieve.

## EGGS

Eggs, like milk and cheese, are often alternatives to eating meat for vegetarians. Like milk and cheese, they are very mucus-forming and cooked eggs deposit inorganic sulphur in the bowel. Therefore, if you wish to eat eggs, confine yourself to two free-range eggs a week. Eggs contain protein but so do vegetables, grains, beans, nuts and seeds in their correct combinations, while the B vitamins often missed in non-meat eating can be obtained from vegetables, herbs and yeasts.

Eggs are potential causes of diseases like arthritis, gallstones and kidney stones, so, if you suffer from any of these, or have a tendency towards them, avoid eggs altogether. It is not advisable for women with gynaecological problems such as menstrual difficulties or abnormalities of the womb and/or ovaries to eat eggs, as their consumption enhances this type of problem.

Eggs and flour are frequently the traditional binding elements in foods. Rice, corn, potato and lentil flours can replace wheat. Other excellent binders include arrowroot or cornflower. If a slightly spicy thickener is required, use ground coriander.

## FISH

Fish now consume waste products that we liberally dump into the oceans year after year: drugs, radioactive materials, chemical waste and heavy metal accumulations (particularly lead, cadmium and mercury). Most of the fish in our rivers and lakes are equally poisoned in contaminated water. The notion of fish being a more digestible protein than meat (with almost no fat content) is becoming more irrelevant by the day. Trout and salmon, now 'grown' in fish farms (fin to fin), live in water contaminated with antibiotics, anti-fungals and other chemicals used to combat the diseases caused by unnatural overpopulation.

Chemical pollutants in the sea provide a nightmare scenario, but nitrate discharges into the sea are high and sewage discharge causes oxygen depletion, resulting in aggressive algae growth which suffocates fish. Instead of using fish oils to decrease plaque build-ups in the vascular system, use linseed oil or hemp oil which are richer in essential fatty acids like Omega 3 and 6.

## DRINKING

What we drink is as important as what we eat. Drinking forms a large part of all our lives.

**Coffee and Tea** both contain caffeine, a strong stimulant. Tea also contains theine, which is an additional stimulant, and tannin, which lines the stomach with an impermeable wall making it difficult for assimilation and digestion to take place. Both drinks also contain theobromine − a harmful chemical which particularly exacerbates female gynaecological disorders. Tea and coffee affect our adrenal glands and long-term consumption can often lead to 'worn out' adrenals. The kidneys, too, are adversely affected. Coffee, in particular, will make the heart 'race' and palpitations and tachycardia are common. Yet these effects tend to go on constantly, so that most people do not notice the gradual degeneration of their bodies. Often, they are unable to remember what life was like before, or imagine what it could be again.

(When coming off tea, coffee and alcohol refer to 'Fasting and detoxifying' in Chapter Six.)

**Decaffeinated Tea and Coffee** can provide a vital interim step for those wishing to come off the real thing. Spring water decaffeination is the safest process and the labelling will show if this has been used.

**Herbal Teas**: These are lovely made from fresh or dried (and preferably loose) herbs. Try them with the most natural sweeteners, such as pure honey or lemon juice – or drink them just as they are. Herbal tea-bags are very useful but confine their usage to the office or for quick convenience on odd occasions. Tea made from fresh, loose herbs is fresher – no tea-bag or dried herbal tea will come close to it for quality.

To dry your own herbs for teas, pick them as young as possible and preferably first thing in the morning. Dry in the air and away from direct heat or sunlight, covering with a brown paper bag to help preserve all their healing components. Store away from light.

**Alcohol**: All alcohol adversely affects the body, especially overloading the liver, but the purest alcohols are the best, such as 80% top-quality vodka or brandy or even good champagne which is double fermented and organic. Anybody with liver problems, gall-bladder problems, stomach, pancreas or spleen problems should not drink alcohol at all.

**Water**: Water cleanses and revitalises the whole body. This is the best liquid to give you your daily needs. Its consumption tends to be overlooked and its delicate taste underestimated. Often, it is just a question of having a bottle there when you need it – in the office or beside the bed. The habit grows on you. Well over half your body is made up of water and you need it to constantly cleanse and regenerate all your cells and organs. Drinking a glass of water first thing in the morning helps clean out the body, especially helping to remove acids or foods left in the digestive tract overnight. If your airways are blocked or mucusy in the morning, add to your water some fresh lemon juice. It is best to drink half an hour before a meal and half an hour after. This means that your digestive juices will not become diluted. Becoming excessively thirsty is a sign that you should seek professional help.

It's difficult to tell exactly what is filtered out by the local Water Board or by home water filters. Regularly found in tap water in the past was a chemical called nonylphenol which mimics oestrogen and causes disruption in the endocrine, nervous and immune systems of both people and animals. There has been a 30% increase in prostate cancers over the last 20–30 years and many more male genital deformities are occurring. This has been coupled with a huge drop in male fertility.

Buying bottles of water can be useful for easy access to good quality water. Compared to the rest of Europe, Britain buys the least amount of bottled water – we are still committed to our tap water it seems (according to 1998 statistics). Some people opt to use some kind of home water filter. This system generally relies upon regular changing of filters and cleaning of equipment to ensure that the bacteria levels themselves do not become a hazard. Not all filters are capable of removing all the undesirable chemicals. Water distillers are yet another choice. They remove approximately 99% of impurities such as arsenic, barium, cadmium, nitrates, chlorine and chloroform. They work by placing water inside the unit and heating; as the temperature rises, light gases start to discharge through the ventilating system. When the water temperature reaches boiling point (100°C), bacteria and viruses are killed and the boiling water produces steam. As the steam rises into a stainless steel cooling coil, chemicals, salts and other water contaminants are left behind. As the vapour is cooled it re-condenses as water. This water passes through an activated carbon filter in the spout and the purified water is then collected in the storage container. Meanwhile, the contaminants are left behind in the stainless steel interior and can easily be cleaned away. They appear as a greeny, yellowy-grey sludge!

## Home-made Barley Water

Barley water rejuvenates the kidneys. To make, use half a cup of whole barley to five cups of water, add quarter of a cinnamon stick, some grated ginger, simmer for 20 minutes, then, after cooling, strain, add fresh lemon juice for extra flavour and drink once a day.

## VEGETABLES

Vegetables should be organic and a proportion should be eaten raw. When cooking, use a steamer, as the vegetables retain their colour, shape, texture and flavour, not to mention all the vitamins and minerals.

### SEEDS AND SPROUTING

Whole, stir-fried, soaked and sprouted seeds are a wonderful source of nutrition. Choose pumpkin (rich in copper, zinc and phosphorous), alfalfa (rich in all vitamins, minerals and trace elements, and fibre), sunflower – there are many to choose from. If you combine sesame, sunflower and pumpkin, you can arrive at a total protein supplement. Sprouting is easy to do. If you have

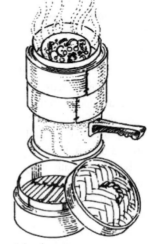

*A bamboo steamer*

never tried it before, start with alfalfa seeds because they sprout very quickly. Directions come with any sprouter box you buy from a wholefood or health food store.

### GRASSES

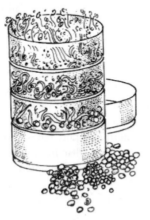

*A salad sprouter*

Try growing organic wheat, rye, alfalfa, corn, millet or barley in a tray with a little soil exposed to the sunlight. Once it has reached a height of one inch, cut it off and add to salads. It is incredibly rich in minerals, vitamins and enzymes. It is also tasty, cheap and versatile. For in-depth advice on this, read *Light Eating for Survival* by Marcia Madhuri. Wheat grass is often dried commercially and can be found in good quality organic nutritional drinks.

## Seaweed and Green Foods

Seaweeds are rich in minerals and trace elements, especially when harvested from the least-polluted waters. These seaweeds are vital to a vegan diet and important to most others. (It is in seaweed and algae that sunlight is most easily accessible to us. The plant structures are simple and the sun's energy is readily released with minimal digestion). Seaweeds are rich in iodine, calcium and sodium – which are vital for the proper functioning of the thyroid – and in kelp, nori, dulse and wakame. Spirulina algae, which is not quite a seaweed but is very similar, is rich in protein, chromium, manganese, niacin, riboflavin, thiamine, vitamin A and zinc, is also vital. Both can be sprinkled on to food for a salty flavour and much-needed nourishment. Many green foods have a high chlorophyll content which is highly therapeutic. In fact, the chlorophyll content of any edible, non-sprayed weed will provide more nourishment than the average non-organic shop-bought vegetable. For instance, just 4 or 5 dandelion greens contain approximately 14,000iu of vitamin A compared to only 33iu in the same amount of supermarket Iceberg lettuce. You need only a few dandelion leaves to gain a good daily intake of vitamin A compared to the pounds of Iceberg lettuce you would need to achieve the same result!

## FRUIT

According to some archeologists, ethno-biologists and zoologists, we were originally designed to be fructivorous, i.e. fruit-only feeders. Our eye-placement and dexterous hands reflect this. Early man also lived in rainforests where fruit was readily available throughout the year. According to Dr. David Forman of the Imperial Cancer Research Fund's Epidemiology unit at Oxford, fruit can substantially reduce the risk of stomach cancer. He says that a 30%–50% lower risk of cancer can be achieved by eating one piece of fruit a day, and one third of the annual deaths from cancer could be prevented this way. Many fruits contain large amounts of digestive enzymes – papaya and pineapple in particular (these are used by the supplements industry to enhance digestion). Proper digestion is essential for good health, so, on several levels, returning to increased fruit consumption is a healthy move. When fibre ferments in the large intestine, a chemical called butyrate is produced which blocks the action of genes produced by cancer cells.

Fruit is not only tasty, but is also full of fibre, minerals, vitamins and enzymes. If you feel cold in the winter, add paprika, powdered ginger, cinnamon and other warming spices. Generally we eat more fruit in summer than winter, a natural choice if we are not to feel too cold and watery; but fruit is vital at any time. They are best in season but can also be dried or bottled for use out-of-season. Keep an unpeeled onion in your fruit bowl and its sulphur content will keep the fruit fresher, preventing bacteria spreading as quickly between the fruits, and thus delaying decay.

## JUICES (VEGETABLE AND FRUIT)

Perhaps our greatest authority on the subject of juicing is N. W. Walker, author of *Fresh Vegetable and Fruit Juices*. He died relatively recently aged about 120 years, having helped many people. He said: *'By juicing the vegetables and fruits one is keeping the vitamin, mineral and fluid content while discarding the fibre. This means that the goodness of the alkaline vegetables or fruit can be assimilated by the body in about 15 minutes instead of hours.'*

Who would chew through ten raw carrots, five sticks of raw celery and two raw beetroot at one sitting anyway? You couldn't. The juicing process also sets free a lot of the food value which can remain permanently locked up in those whole raw vegetables whose molecular structure is too complex. For instance, the vitamin A (beta carotene) in carrots is not surrendered except in light steaming or juicing of the vegetable.

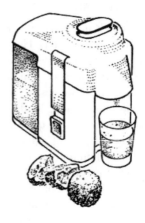

Juices are one of the best ways I know of bringing sick and depleted bodies back to health, and for the

*A fruit and vegetable juicer*

healthy to enjoy ever-increasing vitality. They are also important for growing children, especially for calcium intake. Live, organic fruit and vegetable juices supply us with organic vitamins, minerals and antioxidants which are very easily assimilated by our bodies. It is preferable to have your own juicer and to use organic ripe fruits and vegetables – preferably locally grown and in season. However, other fruits are also highly recommended.

The greatest part of the vitamin and mineral content of a fruit or vegetable lies just beneath its outer layer. It is vital, therefore, to juice the skin as well if it is organic. Also include the white pith, which is rich in immuno-stimulative chemistry. It is very important to chew the juices. This sounds funny but they are more than water, they are food, and should therefore be well mixed with saliva and chewed for quite a while before swallowing to allow the greatest assimilation.

Cooking kills many enzymes, alters nutritional food values and changes the food from alkaline to acid. However, fibre, as everyone knows, is vitally important to one's diet for peristaltic movement and cleaning of the intestines, so sufficient whole raw food must be eaten as well.

## ORGANIC SUPERFOOD

Nutritional Superfoods are made solely from dried organic plant substances which have a high nutritional value, rich in vitamins, minerals, amino acids, trace elements, antioxidants and more, which are assimilated in roughly fifteen minutes. They nourish at a highly potent level and relatively small amounts go a long way! They are targeted to give an all-round range of necessary nutrition and to provide 'bedrock' care at the deepest level, giving the body true nourishment upon which the varying chemistries found in medicinal plants can be added. They are ideal for young growing bodies, the elderly, the pregnant or simply just as a good beginning to the day for everyone. However, they are vital where primary feeding is essential, especially in all forms of wasting diseases, including cancer and M.E.

Superfood comes in a powdered plant from which can be easily stirred into or liquidized with fruit juices and freshly squeezed lemon juice.

Superfood is good for convalescence of any kind, as it supports the body and involves minimal digestion. It is also excellent for the young – toddlers, children and teenagers, giving them the building blocks for healthy, vibrant growth. For teenagers worried about weight, yet needing nutrition, this is the ideal food. For students, often away from home, taking Superfood makes a good daily addition to canteen food. Anybody can use it as a quick meal substitute.

For men and women prone to low blood sugar levels, perhaps associated to candida, this is a good food which is capable of supplying a calorie-free 'in-between' meal. It is ideal for supporting women pre-menstrually, helping to balance the liver, hormones, sugar levels and mood swings, non-active yeast flakes.

Key ingredients in quality Superfoods include: spirulina, blue-green algae, chlorella, barley grass, alfalfa grass, wheat grass, purple dulse seaweed, non-active yeast flakes.

**Spirulina Blue-Green Algae:** Indeed the most concentrated, nutritious food on the planet. It is the highest natural source of complete protein known (75%).

**Chlorella:** Second only to spirulina in food value, it is an extremely concentrated source of nutrition and complements spirulina well. Alfalfa grass and wheat grass are wonderful healing grasses that are rich in vitamins, minerals, enzymes, phytochemicals and chlorophyll.

**Purple Dulse Seaweed:** It is an extremely rich source of assimilable minerals. It contains most of the minerals and trace minerals known.

HINTS AND TIPS FOR QUICK USE

For Superfood to be used for breakfast, make up the night before, leave in liquidiser overnight in refrigerator and re-mix in the morning just before drinking, or leave in the glass and simply stir.

**Wintry Cold Weather:** Add in a knob of fresh root ginger.

**Hot Summer Weather:** Chill the fruit juice first, so you have a cool drink, or alternatively add ice cubes to the drink.

**Low-Calorie Version:** Don't use fruit juice, instead add just the juice of 2 fresh lemons and spring water.

## IMMUNITY THROUGH FERMENTED FOOD

Beneficial bacteria are vital for our health; they inhabit the intestines, teeth, hair, appendix and other places. They help digest food and create vital vitamins. Also, importantly, they inhibit the growth of disease-promoting pathogens and sustain the correct amount of beneficial ones. One's diet provides the balance of beneficial intestinal bacteria, which support the continued growth of 'friendly' bacteria. Therefore fibre, as found in raw fruits and vegetables, is vitally important, along with sauerkraut, pickles (with apple cider vinegar), olives, yoghurt, soya sauce, tamari and sourdough bread, all of which create beneficial micro-organisms. It has also been scientifically proven that these foods are natural antibiotics and anti-carcinogens and are wholly capable of breaking down and recycling toxins, much as the liver does.

Intestinal micro-flora (i.e. that of the colon, lower small intestine and stomach) are generally heavily populated; a swarming and diverse environment containing many hundreds of differing species of beneficial bacteria. It is their unique ability to quickly change with varying external environments and varying internal metabolic conditions that keeps us alive!

These rather intelligent micro-flora can help extract nutrition from everything we eat, while at the same time also stimulating other aspects of our immune systems. They also inhibit the growth of pathogenic organisms by competing successfully for available nutrients in the intestines. If healthy they will also form a beneficial covering over all the intestinal inner linings. Having enough beneficial micro-flora helps digestion, primarily by cutting down on the amount of ammonia produced, which can cause wind, cramping, spasms, etc. Excessive production of hormones and steroids within the body can be balanced by having sufficient levels of beneficial micro-flora. Intestinal micro-flora also have the ability to keep the inner lining of every cell active, energised and able to reproduce.

**Fermented Foods:** Eating fermented foods and having daily access to beneficial micro-organisms is vital. For example, try non-active yeast flakes, e.g. Engervita, which are ideal for those with yeast intolerance.

**Rejuvelac (Home-made intestinal flora):** Bowel flora is vital to enable the body to digest and assimilate foods. Rejuvelac contains B complex vitamins including B12, also vitamins K and E, lactic acid and water-soluble minerals. Good rejuvelac has a somewhat lemony and sour odour and flavour. For variety add your favourite herbs or seasonings. Find a warm place to ferment, between 60–80°F (15–28°C). Use one cup of grain to two cups of water. Wheat is more commonly used but you can also try millet, rye, oats, brown rice, barley or buckwheat. Always rinse the seeds first and use the best quality organically-grown seeds. Soak the seeds for twenty-four hours, and keep covered. The rejuvelac is the water left after this process. Drain and refrigerate the rejuvelac. Drink one or two cups daily, adding lemon for flavour. It can also be added to any cooking. Add the same amount of water and repeat the process, using the same grains. They can be re-used about five times.

**Home-made Sauerkraut:** (N.B. Generally, bought varieties contain malt vinegar or preservatives) You will need a stone crock with fitted lid, a glass sweet jar with plastic lid, or any large commercial glass jar – all are ideal for sauerkraut making. Use organic cabbage and add green seaweeds like nori or wakame, herbs and seeds e.g. cumin, caraway, thyme, marjoram, juniper, ginger, turmeric and coriander. Pour boiling water into the container to sterilise it, then empty out. Finely cut the cabbage. Add herbs and spices. Add some tamari to give a salty flavour and to ensure a good fermentation process. Put into a jar and cover the mix with whole cabbage leaves to within 2–3 inches from the top. Finally put the lid on and weigh this down with a brick (or similar weight) to make sure no air enters.

Keep at a temperature between 70° and 80°F (20–29°C) for three to four weeks. Open the sauerkraut every two to three days and remove any 'scum', which may have been produced. When opening the lid use a pre-boiled spoon and ensure you have clean hands. Use pH strips from the chemist to test. When the pH level has reached 3 to 7 and remained there for a week, it will be ready. When it is ready, you can if you wish, add apple cider vinegar to it. This will ensure an almost indefinite shelf life. Keep it refrigerated. This is a successful recipe which I have used on numerous occasions.

**Sourdough Bread:** Sourdough bread contains at least a hundred beneficial micro-organisms. The resulting bread contains almost no gluten. Sourdough breads use a 'starter' made from flour and potato. Sourdough starters are easy to make – although you have to leave the mixture for a long time before it is ready to use.

**Soya Fermentations:** Miso (a fermented paste made from soya, barley and other grains) provides a tasty, salty and very energising food source. It can make a good and quick gravy, form the 'body' behind soups, stews and dahls, and be spread on bread or rice cakes.

**Engervita:** Engervita is a sprinkle-on 'non-active' yeast product which can be used instead of grated cheese and being 'non-active' can be eaten by those with candida. It lends a nutty flavour to any dish. Its beneficial bacteria are Saccharomyces cerevasiae. It is also packed with B vitamins, protein, amino acids, enzymes, minerals and trace elements.

## FOOD ALLERGIES

Allergy testing can be useful in order to highlight specific foods causing food allergies, but don't forget to look at the primary causes which can often be sluggish digestive abilities and make changes via balancing digestive enzymes which are not function-ing correctly. Cleansing programmes and herbs to support and stimulate enzyme pro-duction and general health of digestion related organs, cleanses of major organs and other natural regimes will help. Allergy testing on its own can be limiting and will eventually exhaust the patient because it achieves its results through avoidance. A body which has become weak and poisoned can only cope with a few foods but this does not mean that 'that is it' for the rest of one's life. A balance has to be struck in which a very broad range of foods becomes tolerated as strength of digestion is built up, giving greater diversity and, with it, good health. (Refer to sections on digestion throughout the book.)

## FOOD COMBINING

One of the most noteworthy exponents of food combining has to be Dr. Hay who, over 60 years ago, devised a 'nature-cure' food approach, based on separating out certain food combinations. He ate many vegetables, fruits, nuts, unrefined grains and, to a small degree, meat and milk. He said that surplus acids are neutralised by the alkaline salts i.e. sodium, potassium, calcium and magnesium (all found in fruits and vegetables) and he suggested that acid wastes pile up in the body tissue, creating many problems, when our alkaline reserves are grossly depleted. He suggested eating one totally alkaline meal a day. For some people, a closer look at food combinations can be very useful and, in some cases, vital. Perhaps one of the simplest ways to aid successful digestion is to separate foods completely, perhaps by eating fruits at breakfast, vegetables at lunch and either protein or carbohydrates at dinner.

## COOKED AND RAW FOODS

Cooking foods can be looked at on two levels.

Cooking destroys many vitamins, enzymes, minerals, nucleic acids and chlorophyll. After a cooked meal, white blood cells increase in the stomach, thereby decreasing the body's immunity and leaving it more open to infection. In addition, cooked food is more likely to ferment or decompose in the intestines, resulting in toxicity. The stomach works at a temperature of 105°F (40°C) and food that is cooler or hotter than this can slow down the stomach's ability to function.

On another level, cooking adds certain energies into food, which creates a feeling of nourishment and warmth. Cooking is vital for foods which would ordinarily be indigestible or even toxic if left raw (including meat and some grains and beans). It is also useful for people with decreased stomach energy, resulting in a lower metabolic rate and a reduced ability to digest their food. Anyone with a compromised spleen should take care that raw foods do not further weaken their spleen and pancreas. However, many people will thrive on raw food, which often makes the work of the pancreas easier. Eating only cooked food is unhealthy. Therefore it is suggested that a 70% to 80% raw food diet is a good programme to follow in the summer, or in hotter climates, while a 30% to 40% raw food programme is appropriate in the winter. Our bodies do not like feeling damp, cold and chilled and hot food can balance this.

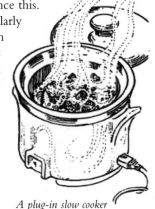

Cooked food kills white blood cell activity, particularly in the stomach. Yet excessive raw foods will weaken some people by depleting spleen and pancreas function. Steaming is less aggressive than baking, and slow cooking in a slow cooker, in which the temperature does not rise above 130°F (42°C), will ensure hot and wholesome food which is still very much alive. Sprouted barley seed and cooked barley create very different feelings inside us and it is worth experi-menting with each to see how you feel – grounded, tranquil, 'high', stodgy, elated or earthed. Climate, geography and season will also influence your choice of food preparation.

*A plug-in slow cooker*

Many foods become sweeter and more nurturing when low-heated – e.g. onion and turnip. I use a cook pot that keeps an even low temperature for four to six hours, but you can also use low-bake or low-steam methods. You simply need to plan ahead a little. Low-heated food has the comfort value of cooked food while retaining its nutritional value.

## KITCHEN BASICS

### Cooking Base
Use 4 cups virgin olive oil, $^1/_2$ cup apple cider vinegar, 12 cloves chopped fresh garlic and 2tbsp finely grated ginger and blend. Use in all savoury recipes.

### Potassium Broth
Fill a large pot with 25% potato peelings, 25% carrot and beet peelings, 25% chopped onions and garlic, 25% celery and greens. Add hot peppers to taste or cooler herbs like thyme and marjoram. Add enough spring water to cover the vegetables and simmer on a very low temperature for 1 hour. Strain and drink the broth. Use organic vegetables.

## BOOK LIST

*Conscious Eating* by Gabriel Cousins
*Diet for a New America* by Tom Robinson
*Fresh Vegetable and Fruit Juices* by N.W Walker (Norwalk)
*Healing with Wholefoods* by Paul Pritchard (North Atlantic Books)
*Eat Right Diet* by Peter D'Adamo with Caroline Whitney (Rider)
*Light Eating for Survival* by Marcia Mudhuri (21st Century Publications)
*Nutritional Herbology* by Mark Pederson (Wendell W Whitman Company)
*Prescription for Natural Healing* by James and Phyllis Balch (Avery)
*Rejuvenation through Elimination* by Dr. John Christopher (Christopher Publications)
*School of Natural Healing* by Dr. John Christopher (Christopher Publications)
*Staying Healthy with Nutriton* by Earnest Haus
*The Nutrition Desk Reference* by Robert Garrison and Elizabeth Somer (Keats)

## RESOURCES

Bio-Dynamic Ovens **Caradoc Ltd.**, Woodman Lane, Clent, Stourbridge, West Midlands, DY9 9PX. Tel: 01562 886 858

Juicers and Water Distillers, **Wholistic Research Company**, Bright Haven, Robins Lane, Lolworth, Cambridge, CB3 8HH. Tel: 01954 781 074

Suppliers of Organic Superfood – **Herbs Hands Healing**, The Cabins, Station Warehouse, Station Road, Pulham Market, Norfolk, IP21 4XF. Tel: 01379 608 007 Tel & Fax: 01379 608 201

Food Therapy video by Dr. Shamin Daya and workshop details on nutrition available from:

**Food Therapy Co.** 57 Harley Street, London W1N 3DD. Tel: 07000 388 388

**Hipp Organic** – Organic Baby Food, Hipp Nutrition UK Ltd., 165 Main Street, New Greenham Park, Newbury, Berks., RG19 6HN

**The Soil Association**, Bristol House, 40-56 Victoria Street, Bristol, BS1 6BY. Tel: 0171 490 1555

**Friends of the Earth**, 26-28 Underwood Street, London N1 7JQ. Tel: 0171 490 1555

# FIVE

# NATURAL HEALING METHODS

These various methods will support and/or radically promote the healing process.

## BODY WORK

### SKIN BRUSHING

Skin brushing is a most effective technique for cleansing the lymphatic system through physically stimulating it. It also stimulates the bloodstream and is excellent for poor circulation. It gives you a refreshed, uplifted feeling on completion and makes you feel alive and energised. It takes no longer than five minutes, so don't

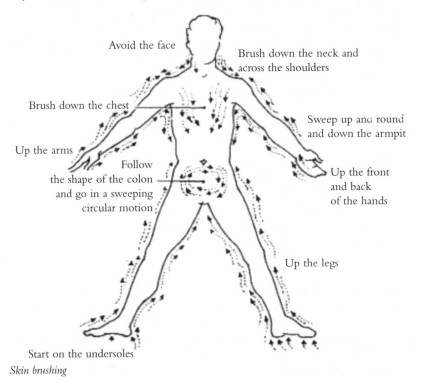

Avoid the face

Brush down the neck and across the shoulders

Brush down the chest

Sweep up and round and down the armpit

Up the arms

Follow the shape of the colon and go in a sweeping circular motion

Up the front and back of the hands

Up the legs

Start on the undersoles

*Skin brushing*

skimp and try to do it in less – it can be done while running the bath water. Use a skin brush made from natural vegetable bristles (nylon or animal bristle will be too rough and will damage the skin), with a long but detachable handle, so that you can reach your back if you are ordinarily unable to do so. Always keep it dry and strictly for this job, washing it in warm soapy water every so often.

Do not touch the face. Make bold movements, passing only once over each part of the body in a sweeping motion: start by brushing the soles of the feet and work up each leg, over the bottom, avoiding the genitals, and up to the middle of the back. Then start at the fingertips and brush up the arms, armpits, across the shoulders, down the chest and the top of the back. Brush down towards the colon. On reaching the area below the navel, you can use brush movements starting on the right hand side, going up, across and down, following the shape of the colon. Women should brush their breasts (it helps guard against lumps) but avoid the nipples, covering them with the fingertips. Basically, you work towards the heart and then bring all toxins towards the colon.

The face should never be skin-brushed in this way, as this treatment is too harsh for it. Wet exfoliation, especially in grimy towns and cities, is a good alternative. This should be done as part of your daily washing routine. Use a lotion containing oatmeal and abrasive particles like sand, aduki beans, silica, or pumice. One treatment a day is quite enough for the face, preferably at the end of the day to remove grime, grease and other residues.

## MASSAGE

Think for a minute, what is massage? It is being in contact with our body. When we experience physical pain our natural reaction is to touch the painful part of our body. This forms the basis of massage. It is one of the oldest methods of healing – massage was used as long ago as 3000BC in the Far East where the positive benefits of applying oils and rubbing the body to prevent or relieve pain and illness were widely appreciated. In ancient civilisations scented oils were almost always used – heralding the birth of aromatherapy massage.

Massage is commonly used as a tool to relax and release tension from the body and can be very effective when both the body and mind are taken into consideration. It can be used to relieve many common ailments, including sinusitis, headaches, insomnia and hyperactivity. The physical act of massage helps the body to eliminate waste materials and to process and use food in the best way for the body itself. It also stimulates the muscular and nervous system and improves blood circulation. In addition, massage can have profoundly positive effects in those with depressive or anxious personalities as it can promote a feeling of calmness and serenity. With this new-found calmness, people are often able to begin dealing with those underlying problems that initiated the anxiety or depression. Massage can be used in many other positive ways, including calming fretful babies and the rehabilitation of those with long-term incapacity problems (including those who are bedridden) – for example, lymph massage is often used in post-operative recovery from breast cancer.

Massage can be practised in many ways. Just stroking your own or other people's bodies is a type of massage; this contact is incredibly important in order to gain some understanding and love for the human form. There are, however, four main categories of massage that are widely recognised:

Effleurage – stroking
Friction – pressure
Percussion – drumming
Petrissage – kneading

Most masseurs use a variety of the above styles, depending on each individual case. Generally, they also use other personalised styles combined with other natural healing methods. This is often reflected in their choice of essential oils and carrier oils.

## Reflexology and Foot Massage

Reflexology is a technique of diagnosis and treatment. It is believed to have partly originated in China approximately 5000 years ago. Dr. William Fitzgerald introduced reflexology into Western society. He applied ten zones (channels) to the human body and these zones were considered to be the energy paths along which a person's 'vital energy' flowed. The zones end at the hands and the feet. Therefore, when pain is experienced at one point in the body, it can be alleviated by applying pressure to the corresponding energy zone in the hands or feet. Today, in the main, practitioners tend to concentrate on the feet. There are many uses for reflexology including pain relief. You can simply massage your own feet, which will go a long way towards relaxing, centering and grounding you. You can use any oil that you like the smell of, massaging your feet dry or simply rubbing them in the bath.

## Chiropractic

The word chiropractic has its origins in two Greek words, 'kheir' meaning 'hand' and 'praktikos' meaning 'practical'. Chiropractic is used for pain relief through manipulation and corrects many problems in the joints and muscles, especially the spine. Spinal disorder can cause widespread problems throughout the body, e.g. the hips, legs and arms, and can also be the root cause of sciatica, a slipped disc or other back problems. It can also be responsible for conditions that on the surface have no relation to the spine, including catarrh, asthma and constipation. Chiropractors use their hands in a skilful manner in order to perform different manipulative techniques. The process will extend the joints to their fullest and then, with a short push, extend them further; this in turn relaxes the muscles around the joint and gives optimum movement and freedom to the area which was previously restricted in some way. This may sound painful but it should not be.

## SLANT BOARD TREATMENT

A slant board treatment can help the spine, circulation, reproductive system and more. It is really pleasant to use – place a strong piece of wood (long enough to accommodate your height), on the floor, with one end raised by six inches or a little higher. You will be aiming at a height of two feet eventually. You can go straight to two feet if you are fit and able. If not, then listen to your own body and capabilities. Lie with your head towards the floor, feet on the raised end of the board. This will take the weight off your feet, relieve congestion in the hips, bowel, stomach and lower back and also bring blood to the head. Begin with 2 or 3 minutes building up to 20 minutes – again take this at your own pace.

*Do not use the slant board if you are pregnant, or have high blood pressure, stomach ulcers or heavy menstruation. There are also other times when it isn't advisable, so ask your practitioner.*

You can buy slant boards or 'tip-ups' from the Wholistic Research Company (see the end of this chapter for the address). Alternatively, you can buy boots that hook over a bar, from which you hang upside down like a bat. You can also practise shoulder stands and head stands, which will have a similar effect.

## BREATHING

Correct breathing can really transform your whole life and is the basis of all meditation, sports, singing and other techniques. Insufficient, strangled, shallow breathing, gained through a life outweighed with illness, stress or fear, will make your quality of life and emotional outlook much worse. You can learn breathing by joining a yoga class or by practising easy counting techniques.

## BELLY BREATHING

Do this by lying down in a warm place or by sitting comfortably in an upright chair, or stand at ease with your shoulders relaxed.

- Gently become aware of your breath.
- Gently breathe into your belly or tummy by pushing it out like a balloon and breathing in through your nose. Count one.
- Breathe out by 'deflating' your tummy and exhaling through your mouth. Relax the jaw and let go. Do this for a count of two.
- Continue doing this for 2 minutes initially, slowly building up to 20 minutes. You can also build up your breathing time to a count of 6 when breathing in, and a count of 12 when breathing out.
- Sometimes you may feel a little tired or even dizzy after breathing so deeply, so take your time and breathe normally for a few minutes before attempting to move around again.

## EXERCISE AND MOVEMENT

### BAREFOOT WALKING

Walking barefoot on grass, sand, leaves, or pebbles has a grounding effect on the body. It helps to discharge static electricity from the body, calming the nervous system. Those who have tried this when they have been feeling particularly nervy, excitable or tired have found that they feel calmed, rejuvenated, grounded or, indeed, lightened: it has a very balancing effect.

**Dancing** seems to come more naturally to women who, from young girls, like to move with grace and rhythm. However, I'm not sexist and believe dancing is a lovely meditation and joy for all.

**Power Walking** (that is, walking very fast for sustained periods) is not as jerky for the body as jogging but is more balanced than running and easily sustained. Alongside yoga it is one of the powerful ways of exercising and moving the lymph system.

**Any Exercise** is vital. Whether your preference is for football, swimming, tennis, whatever, it doesn't matter – just do it!

## HYDROTHERAPY

Water treatment, or hydrotherapy, is a very useful and natural way of improving circulation around the body. It complements exercise and massage but can also act as a substitute for people who are not able to exercise or cannot obtain massage. Very cold or very hot water and the steam thereof forces the blood to circulate more effectively and this brings nutrients and oxygen into and out of organs, easing congestion and stagnation.

### HOT AND COLD SHOWERS

Try a cold shower after a hot shower or bath, adjusting the water slowly in order to acclimatise yourself. Direct the jet onto the area you wish to treat, this will encourage circulation and thus facilitate healing. If you do not have a shower unit, a cheap shower hose that fits over the taps will be adequate. A jug also works if nothing else is available, but the jet from a shower is far better. After the initial shock and gasp caused by the cold water, you will get accustomed to it; then continue for at least a couple of minutes.

Swim whenever you can, in unpolluted sea where possible. When using swimming pools be careful of the chlorination as the gas given off by chlorine is very toxic and will greatly affect those with allergies and a low immune system. Otherwise, wash the chlorine off afterwards with thorough showering, using lavender or other essential oils to aid the process. Do a smell test afterwards. If you can still smell chlorine on the skin or hair then return to the shower!

## SAUNAS

These encourage perspiration, effectively opening the pores of the skin, driving water, toxins and unwanted debris from the body via profuse sweating. Saunas should not be used by the weak or frail, the very young, elderly or pregnant, or by anyone who has certain heart conditions, or high or low blood pressure. Frequent showering is vital during sauna sessions; concentrate the water stream over the top of the head as the skull heats up tremendously and this can cause nausea or sickness.

## SITZ BATHS

These encourage circulation and oxygen to the womb and other associated areas and are very useful for fertility, endometriosis, PID (pelvic inflammatory disease) hip problems, sciatica, congestion and so on.

They can be hot or cold baths in which the water line reaches the hips, womb and ovaries, but stays below the kidneys (so as not to chill them if the water is cold). The navel acts a good guide level. Once you are in the water, swing both legs over the side of the bath. Alternatively, lower yourself into the water bottom first, keeping your legs over the side of the bath. Whether you have the water hot or cold will depend on the particular problem you are aiming to treat. Sitz baths focus on encouraging circulation, increasing oxygen flow and relieving any congestion or stagnation there might be in the lower abdominal area.

With cold sitz baths, where it may be difficult to stay in the water for any length of time, shout or scream, as this will relieve the shock and numbing effect of the cold water. Wear a jumper and socks if the bathroom itself is cold. Begin by staying in the water for one minute and progress to 5 minutes as you get used to it. Very importantly, ensure that you warm up very quickly after a cold sitz bath. Placing a hot water bottle over the area, going for a run or sitting near a fire can all achieve this.

## FOOT AND HAND BATHS

Water may be used as a medium to carry herbs to all areas of the body by soaking the hands and feet in it. The water is placed in bowls of varying temperatures – if the person feels hot, as is often the case with skin diseases, then cold water is used. Hot water would be appropriate with other conditions like flu. Herb decoctions or teas, essential oils, mustard, Epsom salts or cider vinegar can be added to them. Soak your hands or feet in the solution for at least 20 minutes in order to absorb the plant extracts via the skin for topical or internal healing. You can use two bowls at once, each containing different herbs or varying water temperatures. One may be hot and the other cold – you can alternate between them. The famous French herbalist Maurice Messague used these for healing very successfully and reading his book *Of People and Plants* will enlighten you in a whole system of healing for every known disorder.

## COLD SHEET TREATMENT

This is a natural healing technique used to merge the effects of sauna with hot and cold. It is especially effective for use with very chronic diseases, ideally when an acute stage arises. **However, it should only be attempted with professional advice and help** (see below).

The cold sheet treatment accelerates the movement of white blood cells by up to 64 times. This is exactly what happens when a natural fever reaches 103°F or 104°F. The good thing about the cold sheet treatment is that the body heals itself, setting its own temperature. Some people do not have a temperature gain at all at the cold sheet stage. This indicates that the body has produced what it requires.

## BOOK LIST

*Of People and Plants* (his life story and descriptions of the use of foot and hand herb baths) by Maurice Messague (Newleaf)

## RESOURCES

**For Skin Brushes and Slant Boards** Wholistic Research Company, Bright Haven, Robin's Lane, Lolworth, Cambridge, CB3 8HH. Tel: 01954 781 074

The British Chiropractic Association, Equity House, 29 Whitley Street, Reading, RG2 0E9. Tel: 01734 757 557

British Association for Applied Chiropractic, The Old Post Office, Stratton Audley, Near Bicester, Oxon, OX6 9BA. Tel: 01689 277 111

McThimoney Chiropractic Association, 21 High Street, Eynsham, Oxon, OX8 1HE. Tel: 01865 880 974 (Please send SAE for information)

For further details about **The Cold Sheet Treatment** (and a list of practitioners who are trained to help with this treatment) contact: The Selfheal School, The Cabins, Station Warehouse, Station Road, Pulham Market, Norfolk, IP21 4XF. Tel & Fax: 01379 608 201

# SIX

# CLEANSING AND DETOXIFICATION

## USING CLEANSING AND DETOXIFYING PROGRAMMES

You would not own a car and assume that simply by giving it oil, water and petrol it would keep functioning efficiently. You would realise that, at some time, it would need a complete oil change and a service. Interestingly, however, many people do not take similar steps to ensure that their bodies get the correct fuel and care. Yet they expect them to run efficiently. Detoxifying is like home-servicing an engine, a self-help programme to keep your body functioning well. Yet emerging is a new breed of people prepared to give them a try and finding the results worthwhile.

Decreased immunity due to an increase in toxicity is evidently the key health issue of our time and will continue to be so for the foreseeable future. However, detoxifying and cleansing programmes can help redress this problem. Cleansing the body of toxins, by excreting, transforming or neutralising them, frees the body. Every organ and system can sigh with relief as burdens are lifted, excess toxic baggage is towed away and the effort of digestion is reduced to a minimum while nourishment is still provided.

What exactly are these toxins? They can be excessive mucus, abundant free radicals, fungal and other microbial infestations, parasites and worms, in fact anything that blocks tissues and suffocates cells, causing stagnation and the diseases which often arise out of an immunally or digestively compromised body. Free radical damage is a common factor in chronic disease. Free radicals are irritants which cause tissue to inflame, blocking normal, free-flowing function at every level. Whatever the toxicity, and whatever the cause of it, the effects can manifest themselves in many ways. Cancer, diabetes, diverticulitis, obesity, fatigue, immune weakness, sexual disorders, swollen joints, headaches, candida and depression are just a few examples.

Good health relies entirely upon a correctly functioning gastro-intestinal tract, which assimilates nutrients from food and swiftly removes toxic substances. Because this area creates harmony and balance, it stands to reason that foods, or lack of them, can be the major mechanisms through which the body is healed or remains sick. Exercise, hydrotherapy and herbs have a supportive role in healing and should be used alongside healing food programmes and other supportive therapies, e.g. acupuncture, radionics and kinesiology.

63

## EXERCISE

Exercise will always speed up the detoxification process because it helps to remove toxins by increasing circulation.

## MASSAGE AND SKIN BRUSHING

This helps move the body by stimulating the skin and is a very valuable aid to health.

## HYDROTHERAPY

Simple hydrotherapy should include hot and cold showers, sitz baths and saunas. It encourages circulation, promoting the movement of toxins and the delivery of nourishment to all cells, organs and systems.

**General examples of herbs that may be chosen include:**

**Blood cleansers** – burdock root, red clover flowers, plantain leaves and lemons.

**Diuretics (Water movers)** – corn silk, dandelion root and leaves and celery seed.

**Laxatives (Colon movers)** – barberry root bark, cascara sagrada bark and turkey rhubarb root.

**Liver supportives and cleansers** – milk thistle seeds, buplerum herb and dandelion root and leaves.

**Immune enhancers** – echinacea root, thuja herb, garlic cloves and chamomile flowers, olive leaves, oregano leaves.

**Supportive and tonic herbs for the whole body** – Siberian ginseng root, Astragulus root, pau d'arco bark and schizandra berries.

## FOODS AND CLEANSES TO SUIT THE INDIVIDUAL

Before undertaking cleansing and detoxification programmes there are several things which need to be taken into consideration in order to determine what kind of cleanse is most suitable for you. However, in all cases, the body will require building and toning and then maintaining. Every programme should include the use of water, juices, Superfood, herbs and specific foods.

Very often, only a selective grouping of foods should be eaten during this type of programme. They should be specifically chosen to clean and detoxify the system which needs initial attention. It is important to remember that it is not the variety of food types which is important but, in this case, the quantity of the food type you are consuming. Often vegetables are chosen for these programmes because they clean out the bloodstream, lymph system, kidneys and colon, whilst putting as little strain as possible on the digestive system and pancreas.

Ayurveda and other cultural healing systems look at body types and then advise on the duration of, and methods used for, a detoxification or fasting programme, that is appropriate to the individual. For instance, thin, hypermetabolic constitutions burn up material quickly and the metabolism slows down. As this decreases the likelihood of excessive detoxification, this type of person should be given a shorter programme. People who have a slower metabolism and greater body weight can cleanse and fast more frequently and with increased intensity. People who are of medium height with red tones to the skin and hair and who maintain good levels of body warmth will find fasting and detoxifying programmes an easy and productive process. If you wish to clarify your body type, consult an Ayurvedic practitioner. However, you can also simply start a cleanse and then stop if you are too overwhelmed physically and emotionally and return to it at a later date.

*N.B. Excessive fasting can slow down the metabolism and break down muscle, possibly leading to subsequent undesired weight gain.*

## THE DIFFERENCES BETWEEN FASTING AND DETOXIFICATION

### WHICH IS BEST FOR YOU?

Fasting involves total abstinence from food, with only water being drunk. This is a very good way of healing the body because only pure fluids, which do not require much processing, are entering the system, thereby giving the body a complete rest. However, fasting should only be considered if you have a lot of experience of cleansing programmes.

Detoxification through cleansing involves more than water and can, in many ways, be more effective. It is certainly a more appropriate choice for the majority of people.

Those who are pregnant or breast feeding should only choose a modified, lighter and shorter cleansing programme using juices, raw foods and herbs which are acceptable and complementary to pregnancy, along with gentle hydrotherapy. All should be professionally supervised and should not, in any circumstances, include enemas or colonics. People who should also avoid fasting programmes include those with a sluggish metabolism and congested organs, those already weak and depleted (as fasting can lower the body's resistance even further), those who are malnourished, those with low blood sugar levels, diabetics, and those contemplating strenuous tasks for their bodies in the near future.

## EXCESSIVE DETOXIFICATION

Excessive use of laxatives, colonics, enemas, fasting and cleansing programmes can cause nutritional losses resulting in protein, vitamin, mineral, fat, fibre and trace element deficiency. Remember you are aiming to achieve equilibrium in your body, not trauma.

For many relatively healthy people it is simply pleasant and rejuvenating to perform a cleanse at the onset of each season. Choose cleanses to fit the weather and your mood. The consumption of lots of juiced root vegetables, raw hot chillies and ginger, accompanied by plenty of potassium broth and warming herbal teas should be used in autumn and winter while, for the spring and summer, watery vegetables and fruits like melon and cucumber, along with an abundance of green salads, would be ideal.

For those wishing to cleanse only twice a year, the first cleanse should take place in spring. This is traditionally the best time of year to cleanse. It helps to replenish your energy and to shrug off the excesses of winter. Spring itself gives us the fresh ingredients for the cleansing, e.g. spring greens (the sour variety), dandelion leaves, young nettles and new hawthorn shoots. Such plants can be used to thin the blood before the onset of summer heat. There are striking similarities between spring and autumn, for example the damp nights and the golden days that give us green grass of such piercing vernal freshness. During the transitional season of autumn, you will again be able to find young dandelion leaves shooting up everywhere, and the nettles that have been cut down all summer will also begin to produce green tender growth. Therefore autumn is a good time of year to cleanse the liver in preparation for the work it will have to do throughout the winter months, when the body and immune system are called upon to endure the cold and the possible increase of infections.

## HEALING CRISIS

This is so called because it can feel like a physical and emotional crisis and almost always accompanies these cleansing methods. However, if you do not experience a healing crisis, it does not mean that the cleanse has failed. Your body is simply eliminating toxins in a different way. The whole process is a natural one whereby the body is healing itself by expelling excess toxins. However, you may initially feel as though your illness is becoming worse because of the unpleasant symptoms you are experiencing; in some cases it may remind you of the worst periods of any chronic illness or acute disorder you have experienced.

Many things can happen during a healing crisis, from headaches to aching limbs or rashes. Whatever form the reaction takes, it is a sign that toxins and stagnant materials which were previously poisoning the body are leaving it. The liver and colon are important areas to clean out and can release huge amounts of toxins accumulated over many years. The bowel can easily congest under the new regime being introduced, unless careful advice and herbal help is given, so gentle laxatives are usually needed to accompany cleansing. Constipation at this stage works directly against what you are trying to achieve and making sure the bowel is moving freely will speed up the general detoxification process. The crisis stage may last 3-4 days but should never exceed seven days. This is an important guideline to follow, as ongoing symptoms would indicate that something else is amiss.

A healing crisis can be slowed down if it is too dreadful by eating cooked food and reducing the number of days taken for the cleanse. Do not feel that you have failed because of this but accept that your particular body needs to adjust more slowly and that you need to allow it to detoxify in smaller, less strenuous stages.

Initially, in the wrong hands and with certain diseases, a healing crisis could become a real crisis, resulting in excessive loss of weight from an already underweight and sick body. There is much to consider, physically, genetically and emotionally before embarking on a cleanse, just as there is when choosing the right food programme. It is vital to look not only at your body type and constitution but also at what your body is doing at the time. Under professional skilled supervision, body weight can be allowed to drop in certain situations but, in these circumstances, daily massage with feeding oils and other natural healing therapies should be used as back-up in order to maintain and support the body.

A one-day cleanse can provide a gentle start, allowing you slowly to progress to 3 days, 5 days or longer at later dates, as you become more experienced and your body has fewer toxins to expel. Drinking water and lemon juice will flush toxins through more quickly and, within a few days, the worst will usually be over. For the fit and able, extra exercise will help alleviate headaches and body aches by increasing circulation, thus moving and expelling the toxins more rapidly. For those who are sick and weak and find exercise almost impossible or very debilitating, cold showers are a perfect substitute. Alternatively try a little yoga – deep breathing helps the lymph system work more efficiently. The fit and able must do all of these.

## SPEED OF ELIMINATION

It is important to keep in mind that 'fast elimination is not necessarily the best elimination'. Excessive toxins forced through an organ can result in overload and crisis.

A critical rule to observe is: *cleanse a little, build a little.*

The body's systems all have their own capacity, their own delicacy. A car engine doesn't run on jet fuel. Healing is the careful creative use of purifying elements. In a classic system, W. H. Cook described four groups:

*Slow organs (e.g. liver) require slow remedies.*
*Rapid action organs (e.g. kidneys) require active remedies.*
*Sudden conditions require prompt and strong herbal remedies.*
*Slowly appearing conditions require slow, steady herbs.*

(From *The Textbook of Modern Herbology* by Terry Willard)

## INTUITIVE FASTING AND CLEANSING

This follows no specific rules. You comply with your body when it says, 'I'm not hungry, I don't want to eat, even though it's meal time.' An intuitive fast can be for a single meal or for a day, and it's up to you to find some way of making it comfortable for others around you. Do not make the mistake of letting them cook you a meal and then turning it down! As meals are important social occasions, only you can decide when this is convenient. Never eat when you are excessively tired, angry or upset or when you are feeling overworked or depressed. Always eat when you are feeling relaxed and balanced. Some fruit or vegetable juice or light soup can be taken when you are feeling not quite able to digest but are still in need of food.

## ONE AND THREE-DAY CLEANSES

A one-day cleanse can be a gentle introduction to general cleansing. One day is not usually sufficient to induce the effects of excessive toxin release; if you do feel uncomfortable in any way on the night of the cleanse, there is no need to worry as you will feel fine after eating a meal the next day. Eating naturally prevents detoxification.

A short detoxification gives the body time to rest, shut down and do some repair work. It is usually perfectly safe for anyone to try. Choose a time when you have to do little or no work either on the day of the cleanse itself or the next. Weekends are usually ideal. Choose the same day or days each month. The mind has a chance to rest and relax as well as the body, and the detoxification makes eating afterwards all the more pleasurable!

Firstly, drink a glass of pure, organic prune juice or fresh plum juice and then purified water with a little cayenne, apple cider vinegar or lemon juice in it and add a teaspoon or more of olive oil in order to cleanse the toxins from the liver. It can all taste surprisingly pleasant. You can also drink blood-cleansing teas. Include herbs like nettle leaves, cleavers herb, burdock root and red clover flowers. Drink lots of spring or distilled water to encourage the process. (Diabetics will not be able to undertake these cleanses.)

The next day, make your first foods fruit, then vegetables, building up to grains and the heavier proteins towards the end of the day. If you felt good on this one day, you may want to go on for a further two days, making it a three day cleanse.

## A ONE-DAY LIVER CLEANSE

A liver cleanse is specifically aimed at cleansing this organ and is something that can be done at any time of the year. It simply involves swapping your normal breakfast for a liver drink for one morning (or for three consecutive mornings as above). This cleanse can give one a really spring-like lift, whatever the time of year. Everything associated with spring can be reproduced with this cleanse (after the possible healing crisis) i.e. renewed energy levels, a greater feeling of joy, the desire to sing like spring birds, and even the emergence of new creative ideas as sloth and slowness ebb away. If you are feeling sluggish or out of sorts, this method of cleansing is paramount. People with liver and gall-bladder dysfunction will definitely benefit from it. According to iridologists, those people who have brown or yellowish eye colours will particularly find relief with this gentle flushing process. It can also help those people with a history of either prescribed or recreational drug-taking. Cleansing your liver should lead to an improved sense of well-being. It is especially effective in breaking down cholesterol in the bloodstream by preventing fatty deposits from forming along the walls of the arteries. Herbal cleansing once or twice a year will significantly help those people with an above normal cholesterol level.

Start by cutting out all coffee, tea and alcohol for three days. This will prepare you for cleansing and already the body will begin releasing toxins, so do drink plenty of water to help flush them through.

Four foods are essential to the treatment: olive oil, garlic, lemon juice and ginger.

**Virgin Olive oil** helps to oxygenate your body internally; in its unrefined, uncooked state it is a prime antioxidant. Virgin olive oil is a monounsaturated fat, which means that it does not clog your arteries with fatty deposits. It also increases the body's levels of High Density Lipo-proteins (HDL) or 'good cholesterol'; this allows the blood to absorb more cholesterol so that it may be eliminated by the liver. Therefore it is important to choose the best quality oil, that is organic, virgin (first pressing) olive oil.

**Garlic** is rich in sulphur and will help the liver perform and clear out better, as well as aid in keeping cholesterol and other levels in check.

**Lemon juice** is a wonderful blood cleanser and helps clear out excess acids.

**Ginger** will help ease any nausea associated with the cleanse and help to warm the whole body. However, leave it out if your liver feels hot or inflamed.

To carry out a gentle flush of the liver, you will need to make up a drink to be consumed each morning on an empty stomach.

For one person you will need: 8fl oz/200ml organic apple juice, 2 or 3 freshly squeezed lemons, 8fl oz/200ml spring, distilled or filtered water, 1 clove of fresh garlic, 1 tablespoon of extra-virgin olive oil, $^1/_4$ inch/1cm fresh ginger root.

Lemon juice is a citrus acid that becomes alkaline in the stomach, thereby aiding the cleansing of the digestive tract; it will also emulsify the olive oil. Should you be unable to consume any citrus at the time, use a teaspoon of turmeric instead. The garlic is best crushed before it is put into the liquidiser. Liquidise all the cleanse ingredients until they form a well-blended, smooth liquid. Transfer this into a glass and drink it slowly; you can drink some organic apple juice afterwards if desired. Fifteen minutes after this, drink a hot cup of peppermint tea (using fresh leaves from the garden if they are available) or dandelion coffee with cinnamon sticks, cardamom, grated ginger, a little liquorice or any other flavouring that you have readily available.

If you feel a little headachy, this is because you are flushing your system. It will help if you drink plenty of fluids, especially water, and take some exercise. If you are unable to exercise, try hot and cold showers or massage.

## ONE-DAY KIDNEY FLUSH

Pick a day when you can relax and keep warm. Start the morning with the juice of one lemon or lime, one litre of spring water and a pinch of cayenne. Drink it all and, fifteen minutes later, drink a cup of kidney tea containing dandelion leaves, parsley leaves, uva ursi leaves and corn silks. Also take kidney tincture if you have some to include all or some of the following herbs: dandelion root, marshmallow herb, rehmannia root, astragalus herb, chickweed herb, lobelia herb, burdock root, corn silks, Siberian ginseng root, gingko leaf, parsley leaf and uva ursi leaf. These herbs help to release overly stored water in all the cells of the body, as well as cleansing and healing all round.

At lunch time, drink diluted fresh raw vegetable juices if you have any, or simply eat a large raw salad of sprouted seeds, dandelion leaves, lettuce, grated beetroot and grated carrot. Use olive oil, apple cider vinegar and lemon juice, with a little cayenne and black pepper, for salad dressings. Have a cup of barley water (see recipe in Chapter Four) with your salad. Continue the day with more raw juices and raw foods (but in winter avoid raw food and especially fruit if you feel the cold). In total, you should drink three cups of barley water, three cups of kidney tea and approximately 15ml of kidney formula. Also drink plain water at times, aiming to drink three to four litres of liquid in total.

## ADVANCED CLEANSING PROGRAMMES OF FIVE DAYS OR MORE

Before you begin advanced cleansing programmes you must be proficient in the shorter and less intensive cleanses. The five-day programmes achieve cleansing at a very deep level and will make huge differences to your well-being. Get plenty of help, support and advice prior to, during, and after the cleanse. Make sure all the ingredients for the cleansing programme have been obtained and prepared before you begin.

## A THREE-STAGE HERBAL COLON CLEANSE

**Do not attempt when pregnant or breast-feeding.**

Read through the section on the colon ('Body Systems' in Chapter Nine) for vital further information.

Cleansing the colon is a good initial step, because efficient waste disposal is essential in order to prevent the accumulation of debris and disease. Many modern bowels are accustomed to fast food, which is highly processed, and a variety of problems can arise from this, ranging from bowel complaints to less obvious problems in other parts of the body. Antibiotics, vaccinations and depleted digestive juices will also make the colon less competent and more prone to imbalance, premature ageing and a lack of efficiency.

You can buy many different herbal colon cleansing programmes from health food shops. They all basically serve the same function. However, be careful to choose ones that have not been bulked out with a lot of psyllium husks. The programme below is one that I choose to use with my patients and have found to be most successful over many years.

Between the herbalists Dr. John Christopher and Dr. Richard Schulze, three formulas have been designed for thorough colon cleansing, which lasts between 2 and 3 weeks or months, depending on the speed at which you take the programme. If this entire programme is not appropriate for any reason such as work commitments or children, it can be modified and used on a 2-day basis just like the short liver and kidney cleanses, using the capsules and powders to suit individual needs. Below is described the programme, which should be directed and supervised throughout by a practitioner, with initial checks for suitability before commencement of the cleanse.

## The Three Stage Programme

**Formula A:** This is very strong formula, made for the modern bowel, which can be used on a weekly or daily basis on its own but is also a vital part of a three-pronged approach to the cleanse. I've known patients on massive doses of very strong bowel drugs who were experiencing painful side effects like wind, while still having very irregular movements. They have found this formula excellent; it is strong but gentle, containing powders of : 2 parts cascara sagrada bark, 1 part each of garlic cloves, barberry root bark, aloe leaf gel, cayenne pods, senna pods, ginger rhizome and $1/2$ part of chamomile flowers. Mix these together and place into capsules (see Chapter Three for details).

People who may need to use this are those who are constipated due to an inherited lazy colon or through fibre and water deprivation or those who use morphine and other opiate drugs for pain relief. However, there can be many, many other reasons for constipation. The number of people with lifelong genetic and behavioural tendencies toward this condition is rising by the day, as 'junk' food consumption increases. The herbs help to retrain and regulate bowel function, promoting natural peristalsis; they also facilitate water absorption in the bowel and encourage liver, gall-bladder, stomach and pancreatic function. These herbs also clear out some of the old pockets of stagnant and potentially viral, parasitic, fungal and bacteria-harbouring faecal matter. Should the bowel be inflamed, bleeding and with pockets, this formula can still be used but with the addition of individually chosen herbs like meadowsweet herb, marshmallow root and slippery elm inner bark. At first the formula may not quite suit the individual, but minor changes can be made until it does, e.g. using stool protectors and softeners.

**Formula B:** Once constipation has given way to regular bowel movements, the bowel is ready to be cleansed in a different way. This formula is based on Master Herbalist Dr. Christopher's formula and is designed more for daily maintenance. Dr. Christopher originally had a dysfunctional and chronically constipated bowel. He wanted to design and use a herbal formula, containing no laxatives, which would maintain, strengthen and gradually improve his bowel after he had cleansed and removed most, if not all, of the old faecal matter with strong herbs and healing clays. Combine it separately with psyllium husks, linseeds and plenty of water on a daily basis.

The herbs he used, which now have over 50 years' use, included:

2 parts cascara sagrada bark – this herb, used in correct quantity, is a gentle peristaltic tonic.
$1^1/2$ parts barberry root bark – a liver and bowel herb.
1 part cayenne pods – help circulation and peristalsis.
1 part fennel seed – alleviates wind and toxicity.
1 part garlic bulb – protects against fungus, virus and other microbials.
1 part ginger rhizome – warming and circulating.
1 part liquorice rhizome – digestive and tonic.
1 part lobelia herb – antispasmodic, relaxing.

1 part red raspberry leaves – stops bleeding, 'feeds' the bowel, provides mucilage which protects.

1 part turkey rhubarb root – gentle, tonic and laxative.

1 part turmeric root – assists the immune system and liver.

1 part wild yam root – a prime digestive (alleviates wind) and liver herb.

$^1/_2$ part chamomile flowers – soothing, anti-microbial and re-establishes bowel flora.

Mix these together and place into capsules (see Chapter Three).

Many people use this formula on a daily basis, aside from using it on a bowel cleanse, and it is quite safe to do so.

**Formula C:** The third herbal formula (by Richard Schulze) is designed to draw and detoxify within the bowel. It was based on Russian and Native American Indian herbal use of clays and herb powders and is used alongside the above two formulas but on a more limited basis.

The formula is made with the following powdered herbs: 6 parts each bentonite clay, apple fruit pectin and linseed, 4 parts slippery elm inner bark, and 2 parts each sycamore charcoal, marshmallow root and fennel seed.

This formula draws out poisons, toxins, heavy metals (like lead and mercury) and even removes radioactive materials such as Strontium-90. The formula removes over 2000 known chemical and pharmaceutical drug residues. Another of its incredible abilities is that of softening hardened faecal matter so that it comes away from the colon wall easily and painlessly. At the same time it soothes and heals the stomach, intestines and colon itself.

Bentonite clay is able to absorb forty times its own weight and gently eases out old faecal matter, stale bile and other unwanted residues. The clay is derived from volcanic ash and contains montmorillonite which is a molecule 1/500 the size of those that make up water (hydrogen and oxygen), making it a far superior cleanser to water. These tiny molecules are capable of getting into the incredibly small nooks that water simply can't enter, which is vital for a thorough cleanse. Most toxic material is positively charged, while bentonite clay carries a negative charge. Therefore, toxins are immediately neutralised.

The pectin in apples removes radioactive substances from the body and generally detoxifies. Flax seed and slippery elm inner bark lubricate, nourish and cleanse. Marshmallow root similarly soothes and its calcium and magnesium content feeds the nervous system. Slippery elm and marshmallow share an ability to regenerate tissue. This is useful in a bowel condition where certain areas have worn very thin or where old deoxygenated flesh is being exposed for the first time in years after being cleaned. Fennel seed is rich in phenols, which act in an antibiotic capacity. Charcoal cleans the bloodstream supplying the bowel. Psyllium husks provide gentle, healing fibre.

This formula can be taken a $^1/_2$ tsp at a time (once or twice daily), mixed in juice, not just as part of a particular cleanse but by way of gently and consistently cleansing.

*Please Note: Because bentonite clay is so strong, any drugs prescribed by a doctor and upon which you rely, for instance for the thyroid or blood pressure may become less effective. You may be able to temporarily increase your dose, but you must consult your doctor first. Otherwise you need to 'negate' the shortfall and should not rely on any hormone contraception during this time. Account must also be taken of any drugs being taken, as these will have a bearing on the outcome of the cleanse. How other organs and systems are functioning is also important. Some sort of healing crisis is to be expected and, for this, a support network of friends or relatives can be of great help.*

## WEEK 1

Begin with Formula A just after supper. Should your bowel not be in need of these strong herbs (which is unusual), then take Formula B instead. Do either for one week. You will, however, need the stronger Formula A later on in order to help push through the Formula C herbal powders. You must decide upon the amount of nightly capsules by trial and error, no one can really advise upon this. However, after the first night of taking the formula, you should notice an increase in your peristaltic bowel action and in the amount of faecal matter that you eliminate, the consistency of which should be softer. If you do not notice any difference in your bowel be-haviour or the difference wasn't dramatic enough, the dosage should be increased to two capsules the following night. You can continue to increase your dosage every evening by one capsule until you notice a dramatic difference in the way your bowel works. It has taken most of us years to create a sluggish bowel, so be patient and allow time to get the dosage right.

By the end of the first week you should know what your optimal dosage is. Contact your herbal practitioner should you experience any pain. You should, in fact, keep in regular contact anyway for individual advice and encouragement.

## WEEK 2

At the beginning of the second week start using Formula C, which is to be taken five times each day, one hour after a light breakfast of fruit/vegetable juices or Superfood (see Chapter Four). Mix one rounded teaspoon of the powders with enough liquid (e.g. 150mls) including fresh lemon juice and spring water, to make it a drinkable con-sistency. Do the same at mid-morning, lunch time, mid-afternoon, tea and supper so that you are consuming a total of five rounded teaspoons each day. Once you have started on the Formula C herbs/powders, take Formula A nightly at the required dose to successfully ease them through. If you have already been taking these, increase the dosage you discovered during the first week by one additional capsule (or more) in order to make sure the clay and other herbs are moved effectively through the bowel. If you are taking these for the first time, you will need to experiment with the dose – begin with 2 capsules, increasing or decreasing the amount as necessary.

Should the amount of 5 teaspoons a day of formula C produce uncomfortable sen-sations (excessive bloating for instance, due to the expansive nature of the clay) then tailor the amount to suit. A quarter teaspoon, 1 teaspoon, 2 or 3 teaspoons would still produce an effect. Formulae A and B would need adjustment and the cleanse would take longer, which does not present a problem. If a quarter to 1 teaspoon is all that were possible, then only minimum amounts of formula B would be necessary.

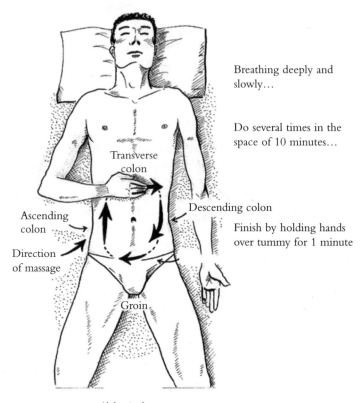

Breathing deeply and slowly…

Do several times in the space of 10 minutes…

Descending colon

Finish by holding hands over tummy for 1 minute

Transverse colon

Ascending colon

Direction of massage

Groin

*Abdominal massage*

You must also:

Drink plenty of pure water, herb teas, fruit and vegetable juices during the colon cleanse – a minimum of two and a half litres and up to four litres of liquid each day.

This bowel cleanse **must** be accompanied by a good diet, bereft of coffee, sugar etc. and containing some raw foods but, if you want to eat more 'normally', then include whole-grains and steamed vegetables. Organic linseed is a nice addition to a fruit breakfast, or it can be taken on its own. Occasionally use psyllium husks instead (the fluffy, soft tops of the large plantain found growing in Asia). Both plants soothe, heal and attract water into the bowel. Mucus-forming foods must be avoided as they can cause excessive stickiness in the colon, slowing down the passage of the faeces and pasting old faecal matter to the walls of the colon. It is important to remember that excessive mucus clogs the whole body, not just the colon, so avoid animal products, eggs and cheese.

## WEEK 3

Now switch back to the more toning Formula B colon capsules. These will help regularise the colon again after the onslaught of the cleanse which really forces peristalsis. For those normally constipated, it may be necessary to stay on these capsules for some time; it is better to use them than to slip back into old ways.

*Note:* This bowel cleanse can be repeated every so often, on professional guidance, depending on the severity of the original condition. It's difficult to imagine the unseen processes taking place in your body. The only feedback you will have on your cleanse is your healing crisis, the look of your bowel movements and how you feel afterwards – often the brain clears and you feel more emotionally positive. However, for those with long-term problems, several cleanses will very likely be needed. Each cleanse will leave you feeling more energised and generally stronger, more balanced physically and mentally and less prone to allergies.

During the colon cleanse, a professionally administered colonic or enema will be of great use. A colonic is a gravitationally-fed enema which is pumped into the bowel, using many gallons of water, to 'sweep' the bowel clean. Water and herbs chosen for the individual are gently coaxed round the entire large intestine. It rarely hurts, except perhaps if an air pocket develops, and then some extra wild yam herb in the water will expel the gas within moments. People's needs vary according to their bowel problems so the number of colonics required will vary; a good therapist will use lots of herbs in the water. An individual with many old pockets will obviously need more sessions than someone who has a lesser problem. Colonics are particularly useful for people with old pockets full of putrefied and decaying faecal matter of many years' standing. Those with candida or parasitic infestations will also find colonics useful and a good colonic therapist will be able to tell you how infested you are.

## ONE OR FOUR-BAG 'HIGH' ENEMA

Enemas are useful for cleansing the bowel during and after the three-stage colon cleanse and for the majority of people unable to obtain a colonic. You can do a one or four-bag high enema: The four-bag enema treats the entire length of the colon, from the anus to the ascending colon and ileocaecal valve, whereas a one-bag enema may well only fully reach the descending colon. The enema ensures that all traces of clay and toxins are removed from the body.

1. Using your specifically chosen herbal tinctures, mix 50ml with 300ml of cider vinegar and 650ml warm spring water.
2. Ideally make up 4 litres of mixture and keep 3 litres in flasks to keep warm while you use the first litre.
3. This first litre goes into the enema bag (it is advisable to use $^1/_2$ litre of cold-ish water initially for a few seconds, this contracts the bowel and makes it easier to 'hold' the subsequent warm herb litres). The bag is hung on a bathroom door hook or some convenient place high up so that, using gravitational force, it can feed into the bowel.
4. The bathroom should be warm with towels placed on the floor. Lie down on your back and using Vaseline jelly or ointment, grease the end of the tube and insert into the pre-lubricated anus. Then turn slowly onto your left side and get

comfortable as the litre slowly goes in. Stay on your left side and gently massage your stomach, easing all the fluid in. Relax and breathe, so as to keep the fluid in as long as possible. Finally let it go into the toilet.

5. Now repeat with another litre bag of fluid, but this time stay on your back, encouraging the fluid to go into the transverse colon; you will still need to start on your left side in order to get the fluid in. Massage, breathe and finally let go.
6. Continue with the third litre, but this time, having started on your left side, move onto your back and then onto your right side; massage, breathe and finally let go.
7. When using the last bag, repeat all these movements in the same order, then stand up and massage the area over the ileocaecal valve (the spot on the right hand side of your bowel where worms and faecal matter often collect). There is sometimes quite a strong and forceful reaction to massage of this area, so do stay in close proximity to the toilet! Finally, let it go; you have finished. Well done.

## DOS (AND DON'TS) OF ENEMAS

- Do use during and after sickness.
- Do use during and after cleanses.
- Do use drops of lobelia herb on the tongue to relax you before and during the enema, and add a little to each enema bag.
- Afterwards thoroughly chew foods and juices to re-establish good digestion.
- Remember to take some type of acidophilus to re-establish intestinal flora.
- Don't get addicted to the washed-out sensation or feeling thinner. You do lose several pounds of weight for a few hours but this is due only to reduced water levels in the bowel, which will soon rebalance.

### INTESTINAL FLORA AND PARASITES

Intestinal flora is vitally important in colon function as it aids many essential processes (see page 90 for more information). Sufficient amounts are needed of this beneficial flora which require fibrous foods to multiply. Antibiotics kill intestinal flora and it takes between 6 and 12 weeks to re-instate it to normal levels. Take daily probiotics to help cope with the release of unfriendly flora and to rebuild friendly intestinal flora. Many companies sell them either by mail order or in health shops. Also drink chamomile flower tea or tincture; eat plenty of garlic and oreganum as they have natural probiotic action and kill off various antibiotic-resistant strains of bacteria. Soil organisms are also now being sold to help repopulate the gut and these will also kill parasites, which is a bonus as parasites very frequently hide in dirty bowels. There are many herbs to assist parasite removal. This is just one formula – 2 parts wormwood leaves and 1 part walnut hull, with cloves to remove the eggs. The cloves for parasitic eggs was originally researched by Hulda Clark.

Parasitic diseases and the general systemic nature of parasitic invasion of the body are more prevalent than many people believe. They range from microscopic organisms, to threadworms, to the well-known tapeworm. One in six people is believed to be host to some kind or another of them and far from being a problem of 'other countries', it is prevalent in the West. They can be the end result of a weakened, sickly body, unable to fight their introduction, or conversely they can be introduced in to a relatively healthy body and cause a slow or rapid decline which shows baffling symptoms yet causes sometimes disastrous results.

These parasites do not kill directly, but they can cause a range of uncomfortable and debilitating symptoms according to the type of parasite. Some lodge and 'coat' the inside of the small intestine, resulting in a prevention of absorption of nutrients from food. Others directly attack components of the immune system and can lower resistance drastically and even dangerously. Amoebiasis and giardiasis (amoebas and giardia) are two conditions now fully recognised as causing long-term illness. A book to help understand this complex and far reaching subject is, *Parasites: An Epidemic in Disguise,* written and compiled by Stanley Weinberger (published by Healing Within Products, USA).

Specific herbs are very powerful and best used with other specific programmes, such as bowel cleanses and liver cleanses and immune support, specifically. Apart from the afore-mentioned wormwood and black walnut, there are other very powerful herbs: artemesia annua (vera), well known for malaria prevention and treatment as well as being a profound anti-parasitic. Olive leaf (olea europaea) is another wonderful and competent parasitic.

## THE LIVER

### A FIVE-DAY CLEANSING AND DETOXIFICATION PROGRAMME

This involves 3$^1$/$_2$ days of a purifying food programme (using raw foods) with 1$^1$/$_2$ days of juice fast in the middle. It should only be undertaken after the successful completion of the one-day version.

Drink at least 4 litres of liquid per day during the cleanse (if you weigh over 10 stones increase this quantity by approximately $^1$/$_2$ litre per extra stone). As you drink, keep a note of how much liquid you're consuming so that you consume enough before bedtime.

### Day 1

Breakfast: On rising, drink at least $^1$/$_2$ litre, preferably 1 litre, of spring water. This is a great way to start your day. The water rinses your digestive tract and flushes out any leftover food or acids.

Within 1 hour prepare a liver and gall-bladder flush: mix in a liquidiser 200mls citrus juice singly or as a combination (1 lemon, 1 lime and enough orange, grapefruit or tangerine to make 200mls) or apple juice. Then add 2 freshly squeezed lemons and add another 200ml of spring water (so it totals 400ml). Add one or more cloves of garlic, one or more tablespoons of organic cold-pressed virgin olive oil and one piece of fresh ginger root. This sounds rather strange but, in fact, tastes like an exotic salad dressing and sits easily in the stomach. However, if you need to split up the juice, the water, the herbs, and the olive oil and garlic, then do so, but consume each within a few moments of each other.

You can add 5ml of liver formula to this drink or dose it separately. This formula or one similar would be appropriate: 3 parts each of milk thistle seeds, buplerum herb, wild yam tuber, 2 parts each of artichoke globe, barberry root bark, dong quai root, gentian root, rosemary herb, dandelion root, turmeric rhizome, 1 part each of agrimony herb, burdock root, ginger rhizome, lobelia herb and ½ part mugwort herb.

Fifteen minutes after this drink, consume two cups of tea made from a variety of general cleansing and specific liver herbs, e.g. plantain leaves, liquorice rhizome, carob pod, cinnamon sticks, star aniseed, damania leaf, mullein flowers and fennel seed.

If you are hungry before lunch time you may have fruit, diluted fruit juices, or fruit 'smoothies' (i.e. banana, apples, grapes, cinnamon, cardamom and vanilla essence, rose water or lemon juice blended together in the liquidiser). Stop all fruit or fruit juices at least 1 hour before lunch: it is best, while on this programme, not to mix fruit and vegetables together.

**Lunch:** make a salad incorporating a dressing of olive oil, raw apple cider vinegar, lemon juice and any herbs and raw spices of your choice. Organic mushrooms, olives, dandelion leaves in season, parsley, chicory and watercress are very beneficial and tasty. Drink potassium broth (see under 'Kitchen Basics' in Chapter Four).

**Afternoon snacks:** raw vegetables, diluted vegetable juices, sprouts, potassium broth, herb teas. All vegetable food must be stopped by 4.00pm.

**Dinner (5.00pm or later):** diluted fruit juices, whole fruits, fruit salads and herb teas.

## Day 2

As Day One.

## Day 3

Today is your first day to fast. Repeat day 1 procedure up to and including lunch, then begin fasting taking no solid food after 1.00pm. After 1.00pm continue with diluted vegetable juices, potassium broth and herb teas.

## Day 4 (Fasting day)

This is the only complete day of fasting. Start with your water, morning drink and herbal tea. Take diluted fruit juices and herb tea until noon, diluted vegetable juices, potassium broth and herb tea mid-day and afternoon, then diluted fruit juices and herb tea again in the evening.

## Day 5

Today is the day to break your fast. Continue the fast until 1.00pm and then you can have some fresh fruit. Chew it very slowly and mix each mouthful with plenty of saliva. Remember, breaking your fast is a very important part of this programme. Chew your food well and eat until satisfied, not full. You can always eat more later on if you are still hungry. After 4.00pm you may have a vegetable salad, and fruit again in the evening.

## Day 6

Start the same way as Day 1 and then ease your way back into a good diet over a few days. This schedule can be done on a week-on, week-off basis until you feel that any deep-seated imbalances have really changed.

### Things to do every day
- Skin brushing, bathing or showering with lavender essential oil.
- Hot and cold water showers.
- 30 minutes minimum of vigorous cardio-vascular exercise to get your blood moving, preferably in fresh air.
- 20 minutes of belly breathing exercises twice daily, preferably once in the morning and again in the afternoon.
- Take a detoxification tincture containing red clover flowers, plantain leaves, wild yam tuber, sarsaparilla root, uva ursi leaf, ginger rhizome, liquorice rhizome and myrrh resin. 1tsp. three times daily
- It is vitally important that you seek advice on bowel cleansing during this programme.

## THE KIDNEYS

### A FIVE-DAY CLEANSING AND DETOXIFICATION PROGRAMME

A kidney cleanse can be done at any time of year, but if a liver cleanse is also contemplated, do the kidney cleanse first. Very cold, damp weather is not an ideal condition in which to clear the kidneys, but as long as you keep warm and well wrapped up, it can be done during any season. Emotionally, you may feel weepy, vulnerable and watery. Those who have felt like this have also felt that past issues were somehow accessed and flushed away.

You must consume at least four and a half litres of liquid a day, plus 3 cups of barley water (see recipe in Chapter Four).

Keep vegetables and fruit separate on this programme.

**On waking,** drink at least half a litre of distilled water. This flushes the digestive tract.

**Prepare a morning drink in a bottle:** For the kidney and bladder flush use the juice of 2 lemons or 1 lemon and 1 lime, 1 litre of spring water, a pinch of cayenne pepper. You can, if you wish, add 5ml of kidney herb tincture to the morning drink or take it separately. Herbs to choose would be similar to (or the same as) this formula: 2 parts each of dandelion root, marshmallow root, rehmannia root and 1 part each of chickweed herb, lobelia herb, gingko leaf, astragalus herb, burdock root,

Siberian ginseng root, parsley leaf and uva ursi leaf. A little maple syrup may be added to taste. Fifteen minutes after this drink, consume 2 cups of a tea made from dandelion leaves, parsley leaves, uva ursi leaves and corn silks. This really gets the kidneys awake and livened up.

If you are hungry, drink fresh fruit juices, fruit and herb teas until noon. Leave for one hour, then begin on vegetables or vegetable juices, using olive oil dressing with apple cider vinegar, spices and herbs. Also have some potassium broth (see under 'Kitchen Basics', Chapter Four). It aids the body in ridding itself of toxins. Eat only vegetables, salads, vegetable juice and herb teas until four o'clock. Leave one hour before switching back onto fruit.

**Supper:** Fresh fruit, fruit juices, herb teas.

This programme can be followed each day but it is desirable to incorporate a day or two fasting in the middle. For instance, on a 5-day programme, stop all solid food after lunch on the second day and stay with liquids only, including the potassium broth, until supper time on the third or fourth day, then take a little fruit and ease back into eating vegetables and fruit as before.

Every day, take 30 minutes of energetic exercise in the open air to get the cardio-vascular system stimulated, and cultivate positive thoughts. This is a time to nurture yourself and find out how to make the most of the food programme – don't plan to do this programme in a busy week.

On this programme, the kidneys are stimulated and supported and, although it might seem that they are working overtime, they are relieved of coping with a heavy, exhausting diet with too much inorganic material and too little liquid. The adrenals also benefit. Distilled water, being 'empty', can carry out of the body a much greater load of inorganic material which might otherwise collect in the kidneys forming stones and irritation. Traditionally, the kidneys are associated with the emotion of fear and they are also the seat of energy in the body. Purging this negative emotion is very important and has a radical effect on the general outlook on life.

## WEIGHT LOSS AND WEIGHT GAIN WITH CLEANSES

This is an essential issue for many people. There is no doubt that underweight and overweight conditions are, like any disease, partly due to inherited genetic patterns. Thyroid function, amino acid performance, metabolism in general, liver function and the well-being of the stomach and pancreas will all have great bearing on how well or badly we store or loose our fat supplies.

We would all love to be just the right weight but few of us are. Those of us who are overweight know only too well that it is unhealthy and slows us down; those who are underweight would love to be more formed, muscular, 'filled-out' or simply to be warmer and have more energy. Obviously a whole body tuning will help to compensate, using cleanses and organic foods. Taking plenty of water helps remove excess toxins, which are always stored in faulty tissue. Eat less, but eat well.

Desired weight loss is aided by spirulina, kelp, evening primrose oil, chickweed herb, dandelion root and leaves and burdock root, whereas desired weight gain is aided by fenugreek seed tea or decoction, marshmallow root and slippery elm inner bark.

Weight can plunge during cleanses in those with chronic diseases when switching to new food programmes. This can be unavoidable but olive oil massages will help 'feed' the body. Slippery elm inner bark, fenugreek seed tea or decoction and miso gruels will help to feed and nourish and keep undesirable weight loss at bay. Superfoods like algae, wheat and barley grasses will ensure proper nutrition while (or if) weight loss is occurring. Eventually the weight will creep back on and metabolism will be optimal as all organs and systems find a greater harmony and well-being.

Young women heading towards anorexia, or indeed those already anorexic, may be unnecessarily force-fed stodgy food in an attempt to fatten them up when, in fact, good nutritious juices, broths and Superfoods would keep them feeling light and slim until more solid food is introduced, whilst herbs can help immensely.

## TOXIC FAT-STORES

Weight loss can also be achieved by bearing in mind your possible need for particular herbs for hormone balancing, constipation and treating a sluggish liver. Whichever way you look at it, fat holds on to toxins even if you are not overweight. Our fatty tissues attract toxic substances from petrol, chlorobenzine, tap water, herbicides and car exhaust residues. We also take in toxins from paints, petrol and lacquers. These can cause fatigue, headaches, tiredness, reproductive problems, immune deficiency problems, dizziness, eye discharge and many other conditions.

## 21ST CENTURY REASONS TO CLEANSE

Toxic bio-accumulation isn't just a steady build-up in the fat-stores of the bodies of overweight people. Most people have fatty tissue, especially women. All these toxins can be potential cancer promoters. There are at least 50,000 environmentally harmful chemicals in use causing daily problems and most of these are unlikely ever to be investigated. There are approximately 50,000 pesticides alone used around homes, schools and work places. Levels of car exhaust fumes are steadily increasing: approximately 30,000 new cars are put on the road worldwide every 24 hours. This knowledge should give us a strong incentive to take regular care of our bodies by cleansing and detoxifying just to keep pace with all the poisons that flood our systems, no matter how careful we try to be.

# HINTS AND TIPS WHEN ELIMINATING CERTAIN FOODS

| | |
|---|---|
| Food | **Coffee** |
| Effects | Coffee is a strong masker of flagging energies and these will now |
| Emotionally | be felt, sometimes making it hard to concentrate. You may feel sad, depressed or angry as the liver starts to detoxify. You can also feel dizzy, anxious or nervous. Irritability, insomnia and depression can also be a result. |

| | |
|---|---|
| Effects Physically | The bowel will become more lazy due to a lack of morning peristaltic stimulation, via the coffee. Headaches (throbbing, pressure), sickness, nausea (vomiting) and other such 'liverish' side-effects may be felt. |
| Tips and Procedures to help the detoxification process | Reduce the daily number of cups and gradually decrease the strength of the coffee used. Decaffeinated coffee can be an intermediate crutch, but only briefly. For energy 'lows', through lack of coffee's stimulating effects, take rosemary herb tea and prickly ash berries and bark tincture until the crisis is over. A few drops of lobelia herb tincture will help balance and calm nerves, decreasing the overall need. Ensure the bowels are moving daily and that the liver is supported via liver drinks once or twice a week. Drink plenty of water and herb teas – dandelion root, chamomile flowers and burdock root – in order to flush the body out. St John's wort flowers can help some people with depression (and valerian rhizome will aid sleep if needed). Dance or exercise in some way will speed the release of toxins from the body. Saunas will help. |
| Food Effects Emotionally | **Tea** Tea is a stimulant like coffee but it doesn't kick the adrenal glands quite so hard, so, in some ways it's a little gentler on the body and, of course, the emotions. |
| Effects Physically | Lack of tea will slow down bowel function to a degree and low energy will be a problem. Because tea contains a lot of tannin you will gradually benefit from improved digestion and iron absorption. |
| Tips and Procedures to help the detoxification process | The body won't feel as toxic as when coming off coffee. Please follow suggestions for coffee as many of them will apply. Try green tea for a greater flavonoid and antioxidant-rich alternative to help flagging energy. Finally, switch to other herbal teas. Those that will be stimulative are rosemary herb, lavender flowers, peppermint leaves, prickly ash berries – alternate daily. |
| Food | **Alcohol** (People with a recognised problem will need to attend AA or take the 12 Steps Programme) |
| Effects Emotionally | Vulnerable, craving, depressed, sad, angry and low. Anxiety, paranoia and irritability. Fuzzy-headed and generally emotional and/or aggressive. |
| Effects physically | Shaky, low blood sugar due to a lack of sugar alcohol. The liver will be reflecting gastro-intestinal difficulties, headaches, nausea (vomiting). Fevers, chills, cramps. Hallucinations and seizures at worst. |

| | |
|---|---|
| Tips and Procedures to help the detoxification process | Read information on coffee – most of this will apply. Use St. John's wort herb to help with depression if it is appropriate. Milk thistle seeds will help to protect the liver cells and encourage their re-growth. Support nutrition. Drink Superfood because heavy drinkers are used to 'empty' calories and nutritional deficiency is probably present. |

| | |
|---|---|
| Food | **Wheat** |
| Effects Emotionally | Irritability and muddle-headedness as the various allergies manifest from the wheat intolerance. |
| Effects Physically | A relative feeling of relief as the symptoms slowly subside. |
| Tips and procedures to help the detoxification process | Try sourdough and rye bread, rice, quinoa, sweet corn etc. instead of pasta. Read information on coffee for extra tips. Use herbs to help better digestive powers, e.g. gentian root and liquorice root. |

| | |
|---|---|
| Food | **Sugar** |
| Effects Emotionally | When sugar is eaten, an instant high will ensue. However, afterwards the level of sugar in the blood drops, leaving you feeling vulnerable, weepy, angry and chaotic, depending on the individual. Hyperactivity and poor concentration. |
| Effects Physically | Low energy. You might also suffer blackouts if weakness in the pancreas and spleen is critical. |
| Tips and procedures to help the detoxification process | Read information on coffee – use applicable suggestions. Always keep blood sugar as balanced as possible; use liquorice tincture or tea, or chew a liquorice stick and sip stevia herb tea which is 300–500 x sweeter than sugar. Chew on bitter foods to re-direct taste and to 'strengthen' e.g. dandelion leaves, dandelion coffee, olives and chicory coffee. Support nutritionally to provide plenty of zinc, vitamins B and C, chromium, calcium, magnesium, and amino acid L-Glutamine. |

## BOOK LIST

*Textbook of Modern Herbology* by Terry Willard (Wild Rose College of Natural Healing)

*The Cure for all Cancers* by Hulda Regehr Clark, PhD, ND (New Century Press)

*Parasites: An Epidemic in Disguise* by Stanley Weinberger (pub. Healing Within Products, USA)

## RESOURCES

**Probiotics Acidophilus:** Bio-care, Lakeside, 180 Lifford Lane, Kings Norton, Birmingham, B30 3NT. Tel: 0121 433 3879

**Nature's Biotics Soil Organisms:** Springfield Pharmacy, Mr. J N Patel, 124 Sheen Road, Richmond, Surrey TW9 1UR. Tel: 0181 940 2304

**Enema bags, Acidophilus:** Archturus Healthcare Ltd, Strathenry House, Leslie, Fife, Scotland 1LY6 3HY. Tel.: 01592 620865. Fax: 01592 626965.

**Herbal Suppliers and Superfood:** Herbs Hands Healing, The Cabins, Station Workhouse, Station Road, Norfolk, IP21 4XF, England. Tel: 01379 608 082 Tel & Fax: 01379 608 201

# SEVEN

# IMMUNITY

## THE IMMUNE STORY

I have heard many stories from history and traditional peoples about the use of plants, fire, air and water to help the body physically defend itself – and also the reverse. Let's listen to a few.

Frenchwomen who packed lavender essential oil for the perfume trade in the seventeenth century didn't catch typhoid and it soon became evident that lavender, just by handling it, could prevent this. The French are still known to use a great deal of lavender eau de cologne. Only twenty years ago, it was often used in place of a bath, with the name stemming from the French 'to wash'.

When a small band of thieves was captured in France staggering under the weight of gold, silver and jewels they had plundered from the graves of the rich (many of whom were unlucky victims of a plague which often killed off entire villages at a time), they were given a choice – they could escape the punishment of death if they told how they had avoided the plague while being continually in such close proximity to the very infectious dead. They disclosed all! The secret was simple: they collected a variety of wild thyme, marjoram, rosemary and lavender, depending on their availability. They crushed the leaves and rubbed them over the entire body, releasing the pungent green, oily, sap. A daily, or twice daily, treatment had kept them free of the plague. What we now realise scientifically is that 'knowing' it would work, would also have increased their 'happy hormone' output, thereby increasing the body's own abilities to defend itself.

Our family home is a cottage in Norfolk, which was originally medieval; it had most of its south-facing windows blocked off during a very virulent plague. Knowing that the plague came from London to the south, the owners believed that a southerly breeze would surely blow the disease in through openings as you slept.

Europeans deliberately gave blankets infected with smallpox to entire American Indian tribes with dire consequences. This is still common practice in modern warfare. Much of the world still lives in fear that someone will eventually use smallpox as a lethal weapon.

Dirty water carries disease, especially wherever public water order breaks down – in war, earthquake, political upheaval or famine. This still accounts for a large proportion of disease and death worldwide. Today the two major water-borne diseases are typhoid and dysentery. The World Health Organisation estimates that 2.1 million people are killed by these two diseases alone each year; most of these fatalities being children.

We often think we're steps ahead, only to find we're steps behind. A classic example of this was the law passed in the 1980s which insisted that all chopping boards in catering kitchens must be made of plastic. Years later it was discovered that plastic chopping boards harboured unchallenged germs in tiny cutting grooves, whereas the natural essential oils, resins and gums within all wooden ones were natural and on-going germ destroyers, constantly being released when chopped upon! It appears that wood is a living organism, rooted or unrooted.

Human beings, like other large species, evolve slowly. Microbes do not. They adapt and mutate incredibly quickly and, even if the world's wealthier countries eventually find some way to control them, they will still go on killing the inhabitants of poorer regions until those people finally become immune. The 1.7 billion people who were infected with tuberculosis bacillus in 1993, but who nevertheless didn't develop the disease, can illustrate this. Every year, 100 million people contract malaria. Two children die of it every minute, due to the collapse of a number of programmes set up to eradicate it. The standard drugs being used are simply not as effective as they once were.

Many 'old' or poor world diseases have returned to and are spreading in the developed world – dengue fever, diphtheria, salmonellosis, pneumococcus and listeriosis have all become more and more resistant to antibiotics. In fact, the National Institute of Health in the USA has called it an epidemic of microbial resistance. Infectious diseases are still the world's biggest cause of death, killing at least 17 million people each year. According to the World Health Organisation up to half the 5.72 billion people on earth are at risk of endemic disease.

Tuberculosis has made a big comeback, killing 3.1 million people a year with an ever-more lethal strain of the disease that some say is potentially more dangerous than AIDS. The number of cases of hepatitis B has risen dramatically. Acute and chronic respiratory infections have risen to 4.4 million new cases a year. These alarming increases may be due to a combination of pollution and the overuse of antibiotics – sending out a clear message that we need to learn how to take care of ourselves.

An American professor called Pavel Ewald has published a book called *Evolution of Infectious Diseases* in which he strongly suggests that diseases long ascribed to genetic or environmental factors are actually caused by infectious diseases. He lists many: Alzheimer's, most forms of cancer, polycystic ovary disease, multiple sclerosis, Hashimoto's Thyroditis, cerebral palsy, Lupus erythematosus, rheumatoid arthritis, many bowel diseases and many heart and circulatory diseases. Of the latter, he talks of the links between chlamydia, pneumoniae and heart disease where this live bacteria was found in arterial plaque fresh from operating tables. The same bacterium was found in a similarly high ratio of Alzheimer's sufferers. He suggests that as time goes by there will be more and more examples of chronic diseases with an infectious etiology – Helicobater pylori bacterium (the cause of stomach ulcers and disorders) being just one example.

## THE LAYOUT OF THE IMMUNE SYSTEM

Immunity is not just a matter of balance, of germs versus our particular micro-flora and whether they can cope with invasion on a physical level. Looking at it like this initially, however, can help us to understand the modern view of the immune system.

The immune system is the name given to particular cells and microbes in the blood, lymph, and other organs which defend the body against disease, harmful foreign microbes and antigens that come into contact with them in the body; or indeed on the skin. The skin is our first line of defence – the armour of the body.

The immune system itself is a wonderful, subtle and powerful system in which bone marrow, spleen, liver, thymus, tonsils, appendix, stomach and adrenal glands have important roles to play. The system is intelligent and sensitive: for instance, chemicals issue from damaged cells in a form which allows them to pass through blood capillary walls and 'eat' microbes by a process called 'phagocytosis'. Their numbers increase according to the condition, as they are able to determine the severity of the situation. Certain cells can produce a chemical called interferon, which is useful because it limits the replication of a virus. Other cells secrete histamine, which causes blood vessels to dilate and which, in turn, helps the healing process. Others still increase their numbers during allergic responses alleviating the condition by neutralising histamine.

Different cells destroy foreign bodies. They are known as antigens and enter the tissues to become macrophages (or 'big eaters') which can multiply as needed in affected organs. These 'big eaters' are capable of isolating affected areas while they deal with antigens.

Cells have to be 'educated' and activated. Once they have been, their job is to find and destroy all invasive organisms, such as viruses and bacteria, that enter and endanger the body. They form what is commonly called the white bloodstream – the lymphatic system. This is a fine network which runs through the entire body, flowing in only one direction – towards the heart.

T-cells are produced for fighting abnormal cell structures, for example cancer cells, cells invaded by virus or transplanted tissue (as in heart transplants). They also fight pollen, fungi, bacteria and some large molecule drugs like penicillin. It is the T-cells that are counted in chronic disease situations like AIDS, where people who have less than two hundred of them are considered 'auto immune deficient'. In so-called 'auto-immune' diseases, the T-cells may act against themselves by mistake. B-cells are activated by microbes and toxins. When they come into contact with a specific antigen they secrete antibodies called immunoglobulins. Both B- and T-cells are capable of carrying out two jobs: one is to recognise antigens and remember previous encounters, while the other is to produce antibodies in response to this.

## CURRENT IMMUNE PROBLEMS

One of the current world – but mainly Western – immunity problems stems from the overuse of antibiotics in animal feeds. These enter the human food chain and weaken our immune systems by killing valuable flora. Doctors now recognise the dangers of this. The number of patients who contract food poisoning via contaminated meats and dairy products is constantly increasing. They cannot be treated with the available antibiotics because humans have built up resistance via their food intake. Cases of food poisoning are rising by thousands each year. In fact, the Department of Health today regards salmonella as an epidemic, as it is now resistant to commonly used antibiotics. Pork, sausages, chicken, take-away restaurant food and meat pastes are all in the higher risk category. Intensive farming methods using antibiotics, steroids and hormones are damaging both human and animal immune systems. It remains to be seen if recent 'clean up' laws in abatoirs help to abate this trend (1999). A report from The World Clearing House for Information on Scientific Investigation of Disease Control said that the number of new strains of bacteria which are highly resistant to antibiotics is rising rapidly. The fifty doctors working on this report fear that resistant germs threaten to increase the likelihood of routine deaths from infection to a level comparable to what was experienced when tuberculosis and pneumonia were virtually at epidemic levels.

## VACCINATION

I frequently get asked about vaccination and I generally suggest that it is a good idea to read a lot about the entire immune system, to research the 'ins and outs' of individual vaccines and their short and long-term side-effects before making a decision. After that, I would suggest a look at alternatives. These must include living an immunally strong lifestyle and developing an ability to react well under potentially stressful and emotional conditions. In other words, you will be embarking on a lifestyle of responsibility. However, I have seen enough problems associated with vaccination to make me personally very wary and thus generally avoid their use within my immediate family. I have had many children in my clinic suffering from lung complaints, digestive problems, bowel infestations, brain diseases, fungal and parasitic infestations, brain and speech breakdowns and more. These conditions have been traced back particularly to the Measles, Mumps and Rubella (MMR) vaccin-ation. It would seem that such a huge immunal assault on the very young often proves too much, and the body adversely reacts in a variety of ways.

Vaccination works because of the immune system's ability to recognise and respond, but it can 'tie-up' the body's B- and T-cell memory capacity to such an extent that the body's immune function ceases to be free to deal with any new challenges. Natural coding, whereby immunity is achieved through overcoming normal infections one by one in childhood, is more subtle: between 3% and 7% of memory capacity is tied up through natural coding instead of the 70% when a vaccine is used. (This was revealed in data collected by the Humanitarian Society in 1983.) Never allowing our immune system to 'self-educate', to recognise and remember for itself, is dangerous. This may happen if antibiotics or vaccinations have been overused. Triple vaccines have been banned in some countries because of the increased danger of over-stimulating a child's immune system. In Britain, however, it is still considered safe and acceptable. Although one brand of triple vaccine was removed recently because of apparent links with meningitis, Britain still continues to use this type of triple vaccine.

Instantaneous allergic reactions to vaccinations can be caused by excessive immune responses. This happens through the combining of antibodies with antigens to form allergies, which in turn stimulate cells to produce histamine. Excessive histamine can cause breathing difficulties and, indeed, bronchial spasm, which to a baby can be highly dangerous. Yet these immediate and worrying problems are minimal in comparison to the longer-term effect of vaccination and its overall strength.

If you decide to immunise your baby with the live polio vaccine, make sure you wash your hands carefully in essential oils after all nappy changes for three months after he or she has received the vaccine. Also, keep your baby out of contact with the following people because they are at high risk of contracting vaccine-induced polio: those receiving radiotherapy, cytostatic drugs, systemic gluco-corticoids like cortisone, potent corticosteroids for the skin, and those taking Adreocorticotrophic hormone (ACTH), or other immuno-suppressive drugs; those with congenital immuno deficiencies and those with a history of paralytic disease.

If you or any other adults wish to be vaccinated, make sure you have the killed vaccine, which has a higher safety record than the live vaccine. Live vaccines are definitely considered riskier for adults. Also take them separately (and spread the timing out) even if you have to pay to do so. Multiple vaccines are cheaper, but they overburden the immune system incredibly.

## AUTOMATIC DEFENCES

We have many automatic and natural defence systems for dealing with viruses, bacteria, fungi and 'foreign bodies'. It is generally believed that viruses are different from bacteria in that bacteria operate outside cell walls while viruses choose a host cell in order to replicate themselves. Some can mutate – e.g. HIV dodges the memory system in order to survive. With all viruses there can be the added problem of secondary bacterial infection. Although modern drugs can deal with fungal or bacterial infections, they used to be unable to invade viruses and to penetrate cell walls inhabited by viruses. However, some are now able to overcome certain viruses' sophisticated defence systems. This development could lead to the production of entire 'families' of antiviral drugs in the future, which could have a similar outcome to the story of our modern antibiotics – see below. Should an antibiotic be given to a person with a virus, and should it enter the cell wall, aggressive side-effects can take place; these may include severe nausea, dizziness, imbalance and emotional swings.

## ANTIBIOTICS

Once reserved for life-threatening situations, antibiotics have now become abused substances, generally via the dairy and meat food chain. Repeated courses of anti-biotics can disturb the immune system so much that they can become ineffective and G.P.s are now much more aware of this and avoid them where possible. Repeated use of antibiotics in children, toddlers and babies can lead to severe conditions, which may include cases of unresolved tonsillitis (often resulting in surgery to remove the tonsils), chronic respiratory problems, skin disorders, middle ear infections, allergies and hyperactivity. These are problems which, originating in childhood, may be reflected in a difficult and sickly transition into puberty, with deeper problems like M.E., cancer and other virulent immune disorders occurring in adulthood.

We now know, in terms of specific side-effects, that prolonged use of Neomycin can cause liver malfunction, Tetracycline can stain children's teeth yellow, Chloromycetin can interfere with the production of red blood cells and Chloramphenicol can cause potentially fatal underproduction of bone marrow. It is now generally understood that repeated use (i.e. three to four courses of broad spectrum antibiotics in the course of several weeks or months) can so deplete a patient's immune system that chronic illness can set in very fast. This opinion is often reiterated by many enlightened doctors, nurses and members of the public. Indeed the NHS has produced a laminated pamphlet for public distribution, warning them that they should not overuse antibiotics. It is now generally understood that once the 'good' bacteria in the gut are gone – destroyed by antibiotics – yeasts and moulds can quickly overpopulate the body, leaving it in a weakened state. What is less well-known is that, at this point, the body is vulnerable to a variety of other conditions ranging from digestive disorders, liver and gall-bladder problems, spleen and pancreas dysfunction, to hormonal imbalance, thyroid insufficiencies and bowel disorders.

We have created antibiotic-dependent cells in our bodies; we have coded our memory cells so that they are constantly looking for antibiotics. In other words, our cells have become 'drug-addicted'. Thus, antibiotics that once worked now have little or no effect. In some parts of Africa and the Philippines penicillin won't work at all. In other countries, where once one medium dose of penicillin would have worked to clear gonorrhoea and staphylococcal infections, it now takes two huge doses of penicillin together with another antibiotic to deal with these conditions. MRSA stands for Methicillin Resistant Staphylococcus Aureus, a form of staphylococcus aureus (SA). SA are the most common type of bacteria which can infect humans. About a third of the population are colonised 'harmlessly', but it liberally passes to the vulnerable, especially in hospitals and care centres.

Probiotics are organic substances for life as opposed to antibiotics (which kill germs, very often indiscriminately). Ecobiotics treat intestinal flora but, very often, ecobiotics are also called probiotics – a term first used by a woman called Monica Bryant in 1986. Vets have administered probiotic bacterial supplements for a long time to treat animals. It is only comparatively recently that these substances have been put to use with humans. What we now realise is that a balanced colony of beneficial bacteria will prevent intestinal toxicity and give good general protection from infection. The highest numbers of beneficial bacteria in the body are situated in the small and large intestine, perhaps as many as 1,000 billion micro-organisms. This volume of flora can easily weigh around four to five pounds! All bacteria have different actions, some living permanently in intestinal walls, others moving through the system, working as needed. This protective bacterial colony deals with invasive parasites, yeasts and so on. Its other jobs include helping to break down bile in order to inhibit pathogenic organisms, assisting complete digestion and helping to reduce toxic residues that encourage putrefactive bacteria. They assist in the making of B vitamins and important enzymes for digestion – particularly lactose.

Where do probiotics come from? Some come from milk products, but others from lactic-fermented vegetables and other sources. Ask your supplier for one that is suitable for you and appropriate for the problem at hand. Soil organisms are also being used very successfully to balance our own flora, reinstating 'the peck of dirt' that used to be considered vital for our well-being according to the old European saying.

## HOW WE THINK AND FEEL IS THE IMMUNE SYSTEM

The key to an effective immune system is the general well-being of our mind, body and spirit. Being sick is not due simply to one problem, it is a collection of many factors. Some diseases are regarded as being modern, such as depression due to stress, pollution and so on. We become frightened by them and perhaps even feel guilty about them. These negative feelings are also factors in disease. Cancer is often talked about as a modern problem too, but archaeologists and scientists have told us that the skeletons of ancient peoples and animals have repeatedly shown signs of cancer, proving that this is an inherently old problem affecting all living creatures.

In lectures to student doctors on the immune system in top American hospitals, great emphasis is usually laid on 'state of mind' as being the key to the health of the immune system. Medical experts have discovered through extensive research that the main, fundamental drive to the immune system is the hypothalamus, and that what dictates its performance is the way we think – that is, whether we are happy or sad, positive or negative. It is also important to look at the health and well-being of the adrenal glands, which support the hypothalamus. A stressed, overworked, unhappy life can lead to disease, whereas a positive attitude, happiness and relaxation are vital in overcoming disease. In this modern era of gene testing it is important to realise that we can all possess mutant genes with a potentiality towards cancer. Not only can we be responsible, in part, for whether or not they get switched on, we can also have the power to switch them off.

For those who are enlightened about positivity and who know about negativity and pain, the subject becomes something of a meditation itself. Maintaining genuinely good and positive feelings in any situation creates vibrations, and these vibrations create different auras and body chemistry. Kirlean photography and chromatography can reveal these normally invisible things. Body chemistry creates smells and fragrances which attract or repel and will affect you, other people, animals, insects, plants, stones – anything that has a vibration of its own. It is possible to hurt yourself with your own bad, angry or depressed feelings because, by bringing this kind of emotional pain into your own heart, you cause a kind of internal poisoning. If your childhood has been spent alongside parents or close relations who were often sad, angry, in pain or depressed, this can affect your adult system. Your present immunity pattern may have something to do with early negative vibrations. However, recognition that a parent or close friend was indeed emotionally disturbed can have a liberating effect. You can accept that this was the way it was in the past, and then move on.

We are beginning to explore such taboo subjects as sex, hopefully creating a society that is less sexually ignorant and more sexually loving, mature and aware. Children treated with love and respect, who are accustomed to being listened to and responded to with freedom of knowledge about their bodies, their sexuality, life and death, are more likely to grow up feeling relaxed in relationships, and with the ability to recognise 'unhealthy vibrations' in other people more quickly, rather than becoming victims who are unable to move on. People who have known and been surrounded by positive experiences as children will have that valuable asset, self-esteem. They will feel a balanced confidence and, being more whole, will be able to cry, laugh, grieve, feel, play, be silent, be noisy and experience all the rainbow of emotions without becoming overly stuck in any one corner.

There are various ways of learning the art of maintaining genuinely good feelings most of the time and this brings your lifestyle into the spotlight. Do you enjoy your job, your lover, your children, your neighbours? If not, then change one or other of them, or change yourself. But, whichever initial approach you take, you'll need to spend time on yourself. Some form of meditation will have to become a part of you and your life. Without this, emotional or physical pain will be an unwanted companion. Understand that bad feelings hurt you, bad feelings against someone vibrate most strongly back at you, so it is vital to transform this state. Counselling and voicing your problems can be very helpful, but to remain stuck in this mode for years merely becomes another excuse to avoid yourself. Meditation has the knack of allowing you to gain an understanding of yourself.

Physical pain is nagging, but is made worse by wishing to jump out of it. Exploring and settling with it can bring about a huge transformation. Of course terror, fear and/ or anger usually hinder this transformation but, with time, guidance and practice, it can become a reality.

## BREATH, TRANQUILITY, LAUGHTER, SOUNDS AND IMMUNITY

Like a contented baby who breathes with sublime bliss from its belly, we too can learn to breathe deeply again. Breath is the basis of any silent or moving meditation, just as it is the basis of dancing, singing or laughing. Breathing from the belly is something we do in deep sleep. Most of us, during our waking hours, return to the more shallow breathing area of the rib cage. This method utilises only one third of our lung capacity. Oxygen is so strongly connected to good health that it is helpful if we can learn to discipline ourselves to return to the more contented and balanced breathing, using the diaphragm and our entire lung capacity. Fear and anger are emotions that create controlled, frozen or spurted breathing patterns, high up in the chest. Outrage generally comes from the area of the gut, the belly. Laughter also comes from the belly and is always a strong, spontaneous medicine. At about the age of three, a child's breathing moves more into the chest rather than from the belly. This is a good time to remind children about belly breathing, using it on occasions to calm grief, anger, fear and other strong emotions. Adults, set in patterns developed and acquired during the course of life, often need more consistent practice. Breathing is a meditation on its own and many old cultures still practise this. It is also the basis of all life: real, full life.

Perhaps the most attractive thing we are all capable of doing is laughing – whether at jokes, clowning about, watching funny movies or slapstick humour. I make it my business to have these around me because I have always been attracted to laughter-making entertainment and find it vital for my own well-being with the work I do. Very often, after a day spent treating the pain and distress of others, laughter provides almost instantaneous medicine. I'm a great fan of comedy and have got a growing collection of humorous videos, so that I can get a 'quick laughter fix' to balance all the other more serious things in life.

In the USA, where many new positive theories come from, music is being used directly for pain relief, relaxation, psychiatric problems and blood pressure reduction. Here in Britain and on the N.H.S. a hospital in Oxford is at present offering treatment using music for stroke patients, together with massage at meal times to help digestion, and at night time to aid sleep.

## USING HERBS FOR OUR IMMUNITY

Please refer to the section on 'Immunity through Fermented Food' in Chapter Four. This will give you further insight and a more comprehensive understanding of this subject.

Herbs that help the immune system can be used on a vibrational or a physical level, utilising the chemistry of plants. Each plant has individual traits and diverse uses as a means for empowering the immune system. Some help to create interferon and T- and B-cells, some assist the utilisation of oxygen which keeps cells alive and healthy, still others act as antioxidants, preventing free radical damage.

Sometimes it becomes difficult to know where the categorisation of immune herbs begins and ends. However, the choices are progressive and we will start with supporting the body both physically and emotionally.

**Adaptogen herbs:** These belong to a category of herbs which can help you to adapt more quickly to whatever is new in your surroundings, be it emotional, physical or environmental. They can help to strengthen and change hereditary weaknesses. When the common cold virus came to Greenland from America many Eskimos died. The virus was so alien to them that their cells couldn't cope. Their adaptability was overwhelmed for there were no cell immuno memories. The next generation fared better, something common to all disease throughout history. This is an extreme example of a situation in which adaptogen herbs would be used.

In order to be classed as an adaptogen there are three qualifications the herb must possess:

It must increase the body's immune functioning abilities using a wide range of actions, rather than just one specific action. It must restore and maintain balance in all body systems at no expense or aggravation to them. It should not produce side-effects.

In general terms, adaptogens are described by the herbalist Christopher Hobbs as working by: supporting adrenal function, thus counteracting the debilitating effects of stress; increasing the concentration of enzymes that help produce energy in the body's cells; helping cells to eliminate waste by-products of the metabolic process;

providing an anabolic effect that helps build muscle and tissue, helping the body use oxygen more efficiently and enhancing the regulation of biorhythms.

Some famous adaptogens are Siberian ginseng root, schizandra berries, reishi mushroom and pfaffia bark.

The Russians have probably done the most research into adaptogens. They have concluded that there are also secondary adaptogens – herbs that are not quite as strong, but which are nevertheless very useful. These secondary adaptogens help to balance and normalise the immune system, nervous system and hormone system. Those most recently studied include gotu kola, wild oats, astragalus and burdock.

Adaptogenic herbs can be used daily as food, in herbal teas, as tinctures or in capsules. They are ideally suited to being combined with other plants as they mix well and remain balanced and supportive.

**Siberian Ginseng** *Eleuthero (Eleutherococcus senticosus)*: This beautiful plant is a herb of our time and, if used on a more widespread basis, could help balance major deleterious immune trends through its ability to fortify against environmental pollutants and radiation. It helps to regulate blood-sugar levels and influences and nourishes the pituitary and adrenal system. It protects the liver and helps eliminate drug residue from the body. On a daily basis, Siberian ginseng increases our ability to resist infection; it has also been shown to suppress cancer cells by enhancing phagocytosis and the production of leukocytes. It is a good long-term tonic which should be used by those suffering from many conditions ranging from M.E. to cancer and all the various auto-immune diseases including multiple sclerosis. I use a mixture of this and milk thistle seeds to treat and support those turning around from drug and alcohol addiction. Additionally, it increases endurance, by improving the cells' ability to use phosphorus-containing molecules and by disposing of lactic acid and other unwanted and often-harboured by-products of metabolism. It is wonderful for stress and one teaspoon of tincture before breakfast can really help the quality of one's day and of one's night sleep. You can take up to three doses daily. It is a good idea to stop for two days in every ten and then repeat the cycle for up to nine months (or longer under supervision). Siberian ginseng also affects the cortico-adrenals and will therefore have a slight hormonal effect – which could be oestrogenic, but is more likely to be simply an endocrine tonic and balancer.

Although it is called a ginseng it is in no way related to true ginsengs, either by its action or its botanical structure. It got its name purely because it gives vitality. In order to avoid confusion it may be wiser to refer to it by one of its other common names, Eleuthero.

**Echinacea** *(Echinacea angustifolia)*: This is a well-known herb which is cultivated in Britain, America and Europe. The only place it still grows in its natural habitat is North America. Pronounced eke-nay-shuh, to sound most like its original Native American Indian name, it is capable of rallying the top defences of the immune army. Native American tribes have been aware of the benefits of this herb for many centuries. While white Americans grudgingly accepted its medicinal value towards the end of the 18th century, it has only comparatively recently reached Europe. It was used as a major immuno stimulator by the indigenous peoples who loved this pretty purple/pink-rayed flower with its attractive centre. They sucked on the root, with its tingling, almost metallic taste, all day when they were sick.

The tingling is caused by a chemical called isobutylamine. Many herbal scientists have said that the tingling is incidental to its healing properties but full-time practitioners have proved time and again that it is actually vitally important. Echinacea angustifolia is the preferred species. The tingling and numbing of the tongue should be the deciding factor when buying the tincture. Alternatively, you could make your own.

As with all herbs, the quality of the tincture is of the utmost importance; some echinacea tinctures on the market are weak and ineffectual. Some people have told me that echinacea has made no difference to the way they felt; however, further investigation has revealed that they had bought poor quality tincture. Tinctures are relatively easy to make if you have a quality benchmark to be guided by; otherwise you can buy them from reliable suppliers. You can also consume teas and decoctions or simply chew on the crude root.

*Please excuse the 'older' names which follow, I am aware that some may have changed:*

Sioux, Cheyenne, Comanche, Pawnee and other tribes all over America traditionally used echinacea to help in many ways, from stimulating energy or soothing toothache to treating deadly rattlesnake bites. Echinacea can be put directly onto bites, stings and cuts, and enters the bloodstream that way. If the white blood count is very low and general immunity is severely depleted, echinacea cannot work fully unless vitality-building herbs and foods (and other immunity stimulants) are used alongside it to build up the bone marrow reserve. It should categorically never be used with auto-immune diseases as this will only exacerbate the out-of-balance immune response, provoking it to 'eat itself' and thus lower immune levels even more.

It was a hard battle to get echinacea accepted by the medical profession. They viewed it as a type of 'quack' medicine. Yet by 1914 it was scientifically proven to activate phagocytes (immune cells that disarm invading microbes and help recycle bacteria and other wastes in the body). Recognised in Germany during the 1930s, it has been welcomed back in a new wave of interest there and is now being used more than ever. Germany is the largest producer and importer of echinacea in Europe, using the superior fresh tincture from wild organic plants in America. More recently they have been growing their own and making fresh tincture from this. They also produce hundreds of medicinal products with echinacea as one of their ingredients. Up-to-date, scientific data shows that echinacea broadly acts by doubling or tripling the number of T-cells in the body (although some tests have shown that it can increase available T-cells by 10 times and some research has shown an increase of up to 15,000). It also activates areas of the immune system which are only motivated in serious conditions (macrophage production); it also vastly increases the amounts of interferon, interleukin, immunoglobulin and other important natural chemicals present in the blood. Echinacea actually boosts the number of immune fighter cells and then stimulates these into action by mimicking the function of the cell wall which gives a signal to the body that an immune response is needed; a group of chemicals called polysaccharides is responsible for this. Short-term benefits include the treatment of colds. It also speeds up recovery from chronic immune depression illnesses. Be aware that echinacea should not be used where auto-immune (over-stimulated) diseases are apparent, e.g. rheumatoid arthritis, lupus, multiple sclerosis, etc.

**The endangered herb, golden seal *(Hydrastis canadensis)* root and its substitute, barberry root bark *(Berberis vulgaris)*:** Golden seal is a wonderful immune herb, but it has been overused or often inappropriately used. Unfortunately it has been wantonly over-collected and pillaged in the wild, though it is still recommended for use in newly-published texts. It can, however, be propagated and grown and it is being commercially produced successfully in small quantities. Its inclusion in a few specific formulae is, therefore, admissible on a limited basis. Dr. Christopher taught me its myriad uses for conditions ranging from eye problems to typhoid, but if used for too long a period the gut and kidneys suffer.

Two important chemical constituents common to golden seal and barberry are berberine and hydrastine, therefore they can often be interchanged. Barberry's tonic activity on the gall-bladder and liver is supremely effective. Skin diseases are often alleviated, mainly due to this effectiveness on the liver. It makes an excellent tonic for the delicate, the weak and for children. The herbalist Christopher Hobbs reported that, when taken intravenously, barberry's anti-microbial effects are useful against a wide range of bacteria, fungi and protozoa – salmonella typhi, candida albicans, neissena, meningitidis, chlamydia and at least 15 more microbes. In fact, its action is much stronger than that of many commonly used antibiotics. One of its fascinating qualities is that it releases compounds that trigger an immune response, caused by increased blood supply to the spleen. It also activates macrophages and, in the laboratory, its anti-neoplastic abilities have been shown to inhibit tumour growth.

**Garlic** *(Allium sativum)*: the immune system's greatest friend: Fresh garlic, which is a stronger anti-fungal than Nystatin, has been proven to destroy viral infections such as measles, mumps, chickenpox, herpes simplex 1 and 2, herpes zoster, viral hepatitis, scarlet fever and rabies. It also kills many types of bacteria including streptococcus, staphylococcus, typhoid, diphtheria, cholera, bacterial dysentery (travellers' diarrhoea), tuberculosis and tetanus. It should be used daily to keep immune levels balanced. See the Chapter Four on 'Food and Nutrition' for further details.

**The sacred apple and the citrus family:** We have a beautiful British fruit of which it is said: 'an apple a day keeps the doctor away'. Apples should be organic and eaten whole, pips, core, flesh and skin, or made into fresh apple juice. The apple is a sacred and beautiful fruit and should be kept at the forefront of our fruit intake. It is a member of a particular category of plants containing nitrilosides, which naturally occur, mostly in the seeds, in more than twelve hundred plants, among the best-known of which are apple, apricot, cherry, linseed, peach and plum. The Hunzas, who are noted for their long lives (90 years and older) have been found to consume mineral-rich water and lots of organic fresh food, including apricot flesh and seeds, which are very rich in nitrilosides (B17). Similarly used, our homegrown apple could give us equally long and healthy lives.

Although not native to Britain, the beautiful family of plants known as citrus fruits are important additions to our diet in this country. In 1928, the Hungarian scientist, Szent Gyorgyi, isolated vitamin C from citrus and other sources. He knew that in 1757 a British doctor had prevented scurvy on board ships by using lime juice. Szent Gyorgyi later isolated bioflavonoids, which he called vitamin P. He blended vitamin C and P and named it Citrin. We now know this to be a prime antioxidant. In nature, vitamin P occurs naturally in plants.

Fresh lemon juice on salads, in spring water, added to herbal teas or to cooked food, is tasty and nutritious. It is able to cleanse the bloodstream and protect oxygen and is also rich in vitamin C. I also use limes, always keeping a stock of fresh limes and lemons, plus their dried, powdered versions. Try this treatment for viral infections: Collect the white pith of twelve organic lemons and put into the liquidiser along with a little peel and juice for taste. You can add some maple syrup if you like to counteract the sour flavour. Add enough spring water to loosen the mix and liquidise. This will produce a light, fluffy, frothy 'pudding'. It tastes delicious and really helps if you are suffering from cold sores, candida, 'flu or colds. The vitamin C and the antioxidant qualities of the vitamin P in the raw white pith help heal the system. It makes an excellent one-day cleanse, combined with other immuno-supporting herbs and teas.

Olive leaf (Olea europaea) is a very effective all round herb, not least for being of great assistance to the immune system and was used in 1927 to eradicate malaria in some areas. One of its chemical constituents seems to have particularly interested plant chemists who feel the 'calcium enolate' is largely responsible for 'killing' viruses, parasites and bacteria. In the case of a virus it is able to interfere with a number of key processes, thus inhibiting its spread, replication and nutrition. It will also very effectively disarm a wide range of fungi, parasites and bacteria.

There are literally hundreds of immune herbs. **Burdock root, oregano leaves, pine needles, pau d'arco bark and elderberries** are a small selection, capable of tackling a wide range of microbes, bacteria and viruses. We could also add chamomile flowers, which are capable of killing invasive bacteria such as salmonella which have evaded long-term multiple doses of strong antibiotics. But all herbs have their own special abilities and specific ways of disarming, which makes constant variety and the use of a number of immune herbs in any one formula very useful in this 21st century, post-antibiotic era.

## ESSENTIAL OILS

These are nature's antibiotics! Around 1910 it was discovered through a scientific experiment that the volatile oils from various plants were as strong as, if not stronger than, phenol, a much-used chemical antiseptic. These oils include garlic, angelica, lime, lemon and fennel. Lavender, oregano and rosemary are not far behind. Eucalyptus and thyme are not as strong but are, nevertheless, potent antiseptics. Australians use diluted eucalyptus oil wherever a European surgeon would use a non-plant antiseptic – for instance, to swab out surgical cavities.

Recent research has shown that tea tree essential oil is supremely effective against the scourge of antibiotic-resistant bacteria including staphylococcus aureus. These bacteria are becoming more common in hospitals where already vulnerable patients can easily pick up such opportunistic infections, and staff are unable to treat them. The resulting symptoms can range from debilitating to life-threatening. In tests, tea tree concentrations of between 0.2% and 2.0% of tea tree were added to cultures of these bacteria. The results indicated that as little as 0.25% to 0.5% killed the bacteria effectively. It makes a 10ml bottle sold quite inexpensively in health food shops look like a cheap and effective 'godsend'.

Pine tea, made from pine needles that are rich in essential oils, is a great antiviral aid. This is an old American Indian traditional remedy which has recently been discovered to be a prime antioxidant as well.

The use of essential oils can be part of keeping well and dealing with sickness. Oils can be added to the bath, used in the shower, put into shampoo and other hair and body treatments; added to toothpaste and mouth gargles, made into massage oils, added to foot and hand baths and used as fragrances.

Use an essential oil supplier who tests the oils, or has them tested using chromatography and other methods of analysis to ensure good quality oils, devoid of toxins. Making your own oils at home is perhaps the most desirable of all. Collect the plants, flowers, leaves or needles, liquidise them straight into olive oil and leave in the sun, shaking daily, for two weeks. An easy antimicrobial oil would be equal parts of pine needles, ecualyptus leaves and rosemary leaves.

## SOME COMMON IMMUNITY AILMENTS AND HOW TO HELP

### HELPING A FEVER

Fever is generally nature's way of getting rid of unwanted toxins, making it a healthy sign; the high temperature and consequent sweating burns and kills unwanted attackers. However, there are situations where it can be dangerous. Fevers in children and old people should be monitored, while in babies and those who are already chronically sick, good professional advice should be sought.

To help a fever in general, aim to keep your temperature up, but not too high – above 39°C (102°F) but below 40°C (104°F). Make sure the fever is 'wet' and not 'dry'. To keep the fever wet, drink hot, real fruit juices such as English apple juice with a stick of cinnamon and a pinch of pepper, or fresh lemon in hot water. Herb teas are ideal, too. Good herbal teas are yarrow leaf, red raspberry leaf, catnip leaf, peppermint leaf, elder flower and boneset herb. Drink as much as possible. Red raspberry leaf and boneset herb not only helps the sweating process but also provides calcium, which is lost in enormous amounts during sweating. These herbs also act to cleanse and clear the bloodstream and lymph system, which is a vital process. If you need a break from hot drinks, have sips of still distilled, filtered or mineral water, which must be at room temperature; you don't want to bring your temperature down.

Take 5–10 drops of echinacea root tincture hourly along with 5 drops of barberry root bark tincture. If the bowels have not opened recently, have an enema, because constipation can push a fever up very high. An enema in certain fever situations can actually save a life, being the only thing that will bring a dangerously high temperature of 41°C (106°F) or 42°C (107°F) down a few degrees. Ensure that the bowels keep moving.

If your temperature is too high, get into a bath at a temperature of 37°C (98.6°F) for approximately half an hour. If you feel low and exhausted, add ¹/₂ cup of cider vinegar, 2 tablespoons of Epsom salts and 5 drops of rosemary essential oil to your bath. Once you have dried off, use a skin brush, then go back to bed immediately and cover up well.

Use your thermometer frequently, to keep gauging how you're doing. Once you've broken the fever, have another bath; this time finishing with a cold shower. Change all night clothes, bed linen, etc. Keep drinking the fluids you drank during the fever to maintain the detoxification process and to build up the calcium you lost during the fever. This is a vital convalescent procedure. Also ensure that you consume appropriate liquid nutrients to maintain the healing process.

## GENERAL IMMUNITY FORMULAE

Immunity formulae will vary according to an individual's needs or chosen direction of the formula. Immune herbs will stimulate, disarm and destroy, while other herbs may be added to support different organs and systems, e.g. the liver, lymph system, bowel and circulatory system. Here are some suggestions:

Red clover flowers, pfaffia root, echinacea root, chamomile flowers, poke root, myrrh resin, neem leaf, barberry root bark, turkey rhubarb root, cayenne pod, mullein flowers, buplerum herb, red raspberry leaves, thuja herb, lobelia herb, pine needles, pau d'arco root bark, burdock root, liquorice rhizome and elder flowers and berries would make a good formula. However, using only one or two of these herbs would also do equally well and a selection must be made with a qualified herbalist in case some of the immune herbs should not be used at all or only for a short duration, e.g. poke root, and echinacea.

Take approximately 5ml of your chosen herb selection three times daily for ten days and then, with a two or four day break in between, for weeks, months or longer in some cases. Addition of tonic support may be needed for deep-seated chronic conditions.

If the problem is very exhausting, supportive nutrition and nurturing herbs will be vital, as they will tone and build while giving gentle energy to the nervous, digestive, hormonal and other systems. Such herbs might be:-

Slippery elm inner bark, Siberian ginseng root, dandelion root, burdock root, schizandra berries, rehmannia herb, elecampane root, skullcap herb, gentian root, nettle leaves, astragalus herb, saw palmetto berries, seaweeds, red raspberry leaves, marshmallow root, fenugreek seed, lobelia herb and Chinese liquorice rhizome.

The 'Essiac formula' is an old, yet still very effective, immunity formula that belonged originally to the Native American Indians, and contains: slippery elm inner bark, turkey rhubarb root, burdock root and sheep's sorrel herb. This formula takes into account some important basics, immune support, supportive tonic help and bowel and liver detoxification. It is also highly regarded as a preventative and as a treatment for cancer.

## HOME-MADE IMMUNE SUPPORTER AND FIGHTER – 'HOOCH'

This formula is a modern-day plague remedy, stimulating the blood whilst detoxifying.

Fill a jar ³/₄ full with equal parts of chopped fresh garlic, fresh chopped white onion (or the hottest available), freshly grated ginger root, chopped fresh horseradish if available and chopped cayenne peppers (the hottest available, such as African bird peppers). Then top up with organic apple cider vinegar and shake vigorously. Other additions can be mustard seeds and black pepper.

This formula benefits from being made on the new moon then strained on the full moon approximately 14 days later. Filter the mixture through muslin or a fine sieve and keep the liquid. However, leave some of the mixture unsieved and use it as a delicious hot relish with food. Keep in the refrigerator.

Dosage: 1–2+ sp (5–10mls) fluid ounce two or more times daily. Gargle and then swallow.

## BOOK LIST

*Book of Sound Therapy* by Olivea Dewhurst-Maddock (Gaia)
*Echinacea The Immune Herb* by Christopher Hobbs (Botanica Press)
*Echinacea* by Jill Rosemary Davies (Element Books)
*Ginseng: The Energy Herb* by Christopher Hobbs (Botanica Press)
*Siberian Ginseng* by Jill Rosemary Davies (Element Books)
*Laughter, The Best Medicine* by Robert Holden
*Olive Leaf Extract* by Dr Morten Walker (Kensington Health)

## RESOURCES

Robert Holden runs a series of laughter workshops in Britain, both on the NHS and at private health centres. For details, telephone: (0121) 5512932

EIGHT

# LIFE-STAGES

This chapter is a commentary on the natural development of the human body, with emphasis on those times when healthy growth and development may need extra care and attention – be it to ensure correct hormone balance or sufficient nourishment of certain organs and systems. All is aimed towards achieving a healthy and happy mind, spirit and body.

## CHILDHOOD

Children are the new generation and should therefore be given guidance, love, support and appropriate protection to enable them to develop into healthy and balanced adults. Children do not belong to parents but have their own unique lives; yet parents are fully responsible for the unfolding and nurturing of their development, some task!

One of the best gifts children can be given is that of good health. Good nutrition is the basis of good health; it is the fuel that builds and sustains the physical body and also influences the emotional development of children.

Calcium, vitamin C and magnesium are essential for growing children; therefore consider food sources for all of these like citrus fruit, walnuts, parsley and sunflower seeds. Superfood is pleasant tasting if made with fresh fruits and is full of essential nutrients. A daily cup of nettle leaves, dandelion root, chamomile flowers or hibiscus flower tea will also support children – in fact, any simple herb tea will be preferable to tea, coffee, squashes and fizzy drinks.

If you choose to bring your child up as a vegetarian you must ensure that you replace the nutrients which meat would have provided. Chapter Four gives fuller information on all aspects of food and nutrition.

### BABIES AND TODDLERS

When feeding babies and young toddlers it is always best to use a variety of home-made meals. Some nutritional and easy recipes follow:

### Breakfast

50% ground organic millet flakes (or cooked whole millet).
50% fresh fruit or vegetables – preferably organic, but definitely alkaline, like apple,

peach, banana, cauliflower, carrot, parsnip and courgette. With fruits, add powdered cinnamon, and with vegetables, add a pinch of powdered turmeric and a little finely chopped garlic.

Soak the millet overnight and gently cook through on a very low heat (sieve for very young babies). Add sieved or mashed fruit or vegetables and serve. If using vegetables, add finely chopped parsley for older babies which will provide useful iron and calcium. This meal provides protein, iron, magnesium, calcium, B vitamins and a range of other vitamins, minerals and trace elements.

### Rice and Seaweed Soother

1 cup cooked organic brown rice
$^1/_4$ cup pre-soaked dried seaweed (any variety e.g. purple dulse, bladderwrack or arame – there are so many kinds, so always vary your choice)
$^1/_2$ cup steamed chopped carrot
1 tsp arrowroot
$^1/_4$ tsp thyme leaves
$^1/_2$ clove garlic

Mix all the ingredients together in a liquidiser. Add a little spring water if the mixture needs moistening. For extra protein, which is a vital body-building component for growing babies, add either 2 chlorella tablets or 2 tsps of Superfood to the mixture whilst liquidising. Finally stir in a teaspoon or two of virgin olive oil before serving. This meal supports good, easy digestion and provides a rich variety of vital food values.

### Energy Meal

1 cup cooked quinoa
$^1/_4$ cup freshly sprouted seed, e.g. alfalfa or sunflower
1 tsp olive oil

Liquidise the quinoa with the sprouted seeds and olive oil.

This menu provides a good balance of protein, vitamins, minerals and trace elements, with the bonus of the raw sprouts giving plenty of raw energy.

### The White and Green Dish

1 cup mashed organic potato
$^1/_2$ cup mashed avocado
$^1/_4$ cup chopped fresh parsley
$^1/_2$ tsp dried marjoram (or 1 tsp fresh leaves)
$^1/_4$ tsp fennel seeds (or 1 tsp fresh fennel leaves)

Liquidise all the ingredients together for very young babies. Rich in protein and oils, this dish also contains a host of vital vitamins and minerals, while helping digestion considerably with the herbs.

## Fruit Delight

1 cup apple puree
$^1/_2$ cup prunes, mashed
$^1/_2$ cup vanilla stick, finely chopped – scrape out the inner flesh and add the paste.
$^1/_2$ tsp cinnamon powder

This recipe is excellent for digestion and slightly sluggish bowels. It is also easy to prepare. Add 1tsp of uncooked arrowroot if more help is needed with digestion (and correspondingly a little water to loosen the mixture). Apple is a very healthy food. 'An apple a day, keeps the doctor away'.

A company called Hipp Organic supplies a range of baby and toddler food based on organic ingredients which make an acceptable occasional alternative to home-made foods at this age. Hipp Organic stocks a wide range of foods, with an emphasis on diversity of flavour and texture. It believes that exposure to a variety of new foods will help babies and toddlers to develop a wider appreciation and encourage them to become more adventurous eaters as they grow up.

## CHILDREN

When preparing food for children make it appealing and fun. Occasionally, cover the table with many foods with different tastes, for example sliced raw carrot, olives, olive oil, garlic, raw mushrooms, cauliflower, sunflower seeds, carob pods and apple slices, then let them try each of them while you draw attention to the different flavours and colours. Children love to copy, so join in!

Children eat proportionally more food than adults. This is necessary because they are growing and, therefore, their metabolism is working at a much faster rate. They are also naturally more active than adults, leading to their using more calories, so it is always advisable to have nutritious snacks for them to eat, such as bananas, apples or pre-soaked dried fruits. In the summer you can make your own fruit juice ice-lollies.

**Banana rice milk shake** is a tasty and energising drink, which is ideal for children. To make, liquidise up to three bananas with $^1/_2$ cup of rice milk, soya milk, coconut milk or almond milk, 5 pollen grains and $^1/_4$ tsp powdered cinnamon.

Children, like adults, will show clear reactions to certain food-groups if they have allergies to them. They will also experience reactions if they are nutritionally deficient e.g. headaches, insomnia, a lack of appetite, constipation, diarrhoea, nausea and/or catarrh. Candida or a runny nose and general low health may all indicate possible nutritional problems with reactions or allergies, stemming from inadequate digestion, malabsorption or nutritional deficiency.

Avoid food colouring and additives in foods and limit the intake of sugar, especially 'hidden' sugars like those in cakes, pastries and chocolate. These can complicate and exacerbate conditions such as hyperactivity and attention deficit disorder.

Some 80% of children who have a combination of physical, intellectual and emotional difficulties are simply afflicted by food-related allergies or childhood candida.

These cause a range of symptoms including stomach, liver and bowel disorders, chronic fatigue, eczema, aggression and specific learning difficulties. Food allergy testing will help you identify foods that should be avoided, but a good rule of thumb is to initially avoid pesticide-ridden vegetables, steroid and hormone-fed meat, dairy products, and wheat products altogether. Some professionals believe this may be due to the observed trend that children's blood grouping is changing. Many are now type A or AB, rather than the usual type O of their grandparents. This means they have less hydrochloric acid in their stomach and this, in turn, produces allergies if mishandled. Over time the digestive capacity of the child can be built up by using herbs like meadowsweet herb, genetian root and slippery elm inner bark, with a range of intestinal flora foods. Eventually the child should be able to process a wider range of foods with little or no reaction.

Immunisation, the overuse of antibiotics and an increase in 'junk food' have radically altered the health of children and there are now visible reactions to these changes. Children will especially benefit from linseed oil and other essential fatty acids that will support neuro-transmitters, thus supporting the brain. (For more detailed information, refer to the section on 'The Nervous System' in Chapter Nine and the 'Dietary Advice' given in Chapter Four).

Zinc levels, so important for building up the immune system, are also often difficult to maintain in children because they use so much to grow with. To help calm and soothe children on all levels, whether they are overworked at school or generally hyperactive, use the following formula containing equal parts of: lemon balm leaves, vervain leaves, lavender herb, dandelion root, chamomile flowers, skullcap herb, lobelia herb, red clover flowers, catmint herb and Chinese liquorice rhizome.

## GENERAL CHILDHOOD ILLNESS

Children can be quick to get sick but equally quick to recover, and essentially they have the potential for greater resilience and strength if every illness is treated correctly. Those who are supported with herbs, baths, massage and good food and left to fight out their illnesses without antibiotics and invasive, suppressive medicines, will build up better long-term defences and consequently require less nursing in the long run. There is nothing better than parental care, home and bed to deal with sickness, and early, good support can keep the child out of both the doctor's surgery and the hospital. Having been involved in the parenting of four children, two from birth and two from the ages of 9 and 12, the latter now in their early 30s, I know it takes effort, input, patience and knowledge, but that the results are worth it.

First signs of illness can be anything from a lack of appetite to high or low facial colour with shivering or fever. A child can be restless, loud, angry or quiet, withdrawn, vulnerable, weepy and in need of holding (or being near you). Be alert to odd behaviour for that particular child. Very often they complain of headaches or nausea, or will simply need sleep at odd hours. Knowing when to call in professional help is a difficult decision to make, for we have fewer large family groups nowadays in which grandparents, aunts and so on can help and advise: but seek help if you feel that you need it.

**This list may help you to know when to ring for help:**
Prolonged vomiting and diarrhoea, convulsions, a temperature that fluctuates quickly
between hot and cold, blurred vision, drowsiness, headache after a bang on the head,
drifting in and out of consciousness during fever, turning pale or blue, shallow
breathing, eyes dull, sullen or glazed, can all be signs that you need prompt professional
help. In fact, you will probably feel it when something is really wrong, you will know
it by instinct – trust your instinct.

Giving lots of water but less food helps all illnesses. Children generally know what
is best for them in these situations, much as animals do. However, these gut instincts
are becoming blurred as natural healing skills in the home diminish and nutrition
loses its true value.

## SOME CHILDHOOD CONDITIONS

### Teething

This is a time when your baby should have as much calcium and magnesium as
possible. The teething pains will be greatly minimised if the new tooth can quickly
break through by having adequate energy resources to do so.

To give your baby calcium use 'tissue salts'; there is one specifically for teething
(available from many high street chemists and health food stores). Give nettle leaf
(and occasional pau d'arco inner bark tea) with honey (if needed) in a bottle as a
long-term measure. Short-term use of valerian rhizome and honey tea (seek dose
advice) will help the baby to sleep; it will also calm any fever and quickly supply large
amounts of assimilable calcium.

When all the child's available energy is going in one direction, digestion can
become upset. Where this happens, provided they are no longer being breast fed, give
young children in a feeder beaker, juices and Superfood. A little diarrhoea is to be
expected but, if there is constipation, use gentle laxative foods like prunes, and olive
oil. They should be encouraged to drink meadowsweet herb tea, three times daily
before meals. A formula to aid poor digestion would be equal amounts of: liquorice
rhizome, cinnamon sticks and fennel seed taken as a tincture or tea (with honey).

### Growing Pains

'Growing pains' can afflict toddlers, older children and adolescents, especially if they
have a poor diet. I have talked to many patients who remembered suffering weeks or
months of aching limbs; their parents had told them that growing pains were a
normal part of growing up.

What is actually happening is that the body is growing and stripping itself of the
materials it requires for growth. Normal childhood growth can induce pains if the diet
is not sufficiently balanced (see section on calcium in Chapter Four), but occasionally
massive growth spurts take the body by surprise. If this occurs, extra calcium and
magnesium must be given immediately by increasing the intake of herbs like boneset
and nettle. Nettle leaf tea should be drunk daily; boneset tincture can also be

given for a few days at a time only, until the pain has gone away and then for a little while longer. Carrot juice, home-made or shop bought, is also a good source of calcium. My children told immediately they got any aches; they will then have fresh carrot juice for a week, on top of their daily calcium and magnesium input.

Fever and muscle aches leach a large amount of nutrients from the body, not least calcium. If this is not replenished, what began as an acute and easily rectifiable ailment can become chronic, simply due to the lack of calcium in the body. Drinking milk at this point is not recommended as its neutralisation of digestive foods would make an already hampered digestive system work at an even lower level. Get them to drink nettle leaf tea to increase levels of calcium and magnesium and use rice milk, soya milk or other milk alternatives. Leg twitching during the night can indicate a need for calcium, magnesium and iron in children, in which case nettle or red raspberry leaf will help as they both contain large quantities of all these minerals.

**Fever**

When taking a child's temperature, remember that their higher rate of metabolism means that they can more safely sustain a higher temperature than an adult. Your first course of action should be to keep the child sponged down and ensure high fluid intake. If you are concerned about your child call in professional help. Normal body temperature is 96.8°-98.6°F (36°-37°C). A fever is said to exist if a temperature is over 100°F (37.8°C). You must call for help if the child's temperature reaches 104°F (39.3°C). You can take rectum, armpit, or, in older children, mouth temperatures. Rectal temperature readings are very reliable. Lay the young child or baby on your lap, tummy down, bottom up, and hold him or her down with one hand, allowing a small amount of movement. Lubricate the anus and slip the thermometer in as you hold the buttocks open. Insert at least one third to a half of the thermometer. Take a reading while it is still in place. Remove the thermometer and give the child a big cuddle. Refer to 'Treating a Fever' in Chapter Seven.

**Childhood Convalescence**

It is normal for a child to want to play the moment he or she feels better, but this stage must be handled carefully. If there has been a fever, much vital calcium, magnesium and other vitamins and minerals will have been lost. These must be replenished before the child is allowed to expend what little energy is left to the detriment of the body both in the short and long term.

- Begin with fresh organic carrot juice and Superfood, as good sources of vitamin A, B, iron, calcium, and more. They are easy to digest.
- Feed up on rich broths and soups containing root vegetables and pulses, whole-grains, stewed apple purèe and other easily digestible foods. Blessed thistle tea will return digestive enzymes to normal, but also include some pineapple and papaya to assist.
- Move slowly back to normal eating patterns, without rushing this transition, even if the child is very hungry.

- Give nettle or red raspberry tea as they are both rich in calcium, magnesium, iron and other nutrients.
- Massage the child frequently and use baths with essential oils.
- Keep the child stimulated with creative options that do not require excessive energy, but insist on rest periods.

## THE HORMONE ARRIVAL

Hormones prompt many of the next developmental stages in life. Adolescence is the period during which boys begin to become men and girls begin to become women. Girls start to menstruate, their bodies preparing for pregnancy, birth, motherhood and, eventually, the menopause. Boys' bodies begin to change shape, their voices 'break' and they begin to grow facial hair. Hormones drive all these changes.

Plants contain many hormones and have a full, rich history. Of the world's hundreds of hormone herbs there is still a vast amount of scientific research to be done but it is known that the same herb can often affect men and women in varying ways in different situations. They mostly contain saponins, which have a steroidal effect on the body, acting as building blocks which can be converted by the body into the exact requirements that are needed. Sometimes these hormonal herbs increase or decrease the output of the pituitary gland or hypothalamus, while others have a more broad spectrum effect on the entire endocrine system.

What follows is an appraisal of the current knowledge regarding the three main male and female hormones, about which science is constantly discovering more and enlightening revelations.

FUNCTIONS OF OESTROGEN, PROGESTERONE AND TESTOSTERONE IN THE BODY

### Oestrogen

- guides the young female foetus from babyhood to womanhood, partially explaining why girls behave like girls (such as playing nurturing games) and why eventually they grow breasts and develop higher voices and broader hips
- helps in the growth of the endometrial tissue that forms a 'nest' for a fertilised egg – it is the fertility hormone
- helps to relax blood vessel walls and aids circulation and tone in the genital tract. This relaxation causes cervical secretions that are inviting to the sperm
- helps to retain bone calcium
- needs to be balanced in order to prevent dramatic mood swings, painful cramping in menstruation and more problems in later womanhood. A joyful woman has balanced oestrogen
- levels increase after menstruation and ovulation, then decrease pre-menstrually, although this hormone is present throughout the whole cycle
- excessive production creates an imbalance in the production of a hormone called aldosterone and this, in turn, disturbs water balance in the body, resulting in swelling and tenderness of the breasts, stomach and ankles. Excessive oestrogen will

lower progesterone levels and cause a chemical imbalance in the brain, involving the hormones, adrenaline, serotonin and dopamine. It will also cause poor metabolism of some vitamins, minerals and fatty acids and will over-stimulate the body, causing paranoia, anxiety, palpitations, hot and cold sweats, shaking and lowered blood sugar

- deficiency interferes with the successful breakdown of trytophan and other mood-balancing and enhancing chemicals in the brain
- appears in great concentration, together with other steroid hormones, whenever the body is damaged by physical trauma, chemical action or illness, possibly serving as stimulants or catalysts for cellular growth and body repair
- encourages the development of male hormones in pubescent boys.

## Progesterone

- is the precursor of the other sex hormones, oestrogen and testosterone
- is the predominant hormone in the second phase of the menstrual cycle, acting to maintain any fertilised eggs
- mainly prepares for and supports pregnancy (in fact the word progesterone is derived from the Latin meaning 'supporting gestation'). Without it, spontaneous abortion can take place. It is vital for the survival of the embryo and foetus throughout gestation
- protects against breast fibrocysts and endometrial and breast cancers
- is a natural diuretic and can alleviate a pre-menstrual bloated feeling
- helps use fat for energy: fat is built by oestrogen, progesterone works to balance this
- is a natural anti-depressant – lack of it will bring on apathy, sluggishness and depression. However, an excessive amount of progesterone may cause depression, lack of concentration and weepiness
- helps thyroid action and resulting energy levels
- normalises blood clotting. If clots are seen menstrually, progesterone herbs will help
- helps normalise blood sugar levels; often pre-menstrual sugar cravings mean that there is too little progesterone available
- normalises zinc and copper levels, which are especially vital for the immune system.
- stimulates bone growth, which is vital for the development of children and to prevent osteoporosis in later life
- is the precursor of cortisone synthesis produced by the adrenal cortex, which is essential for sustaining the balance of the adrenal glands. This in turn directly supports the thyroid
- restores proper cell oxygen levels and therefore helps concentration and, in particular, mental agility.

## Testosterone

- is produced by the testes in the male body. The testes lie dormant throughout infancy and early childhood until the onset of puberty, at which time the male organs enlarge

- if levels are low during the development of the foetus, the testes will not descend properly, if at all. The development of sperm may also be adversely affected
- causes aggression which, when channelled correctly, is a major human survival instinct
- promotes hair growth on the face, abdomen, pubis, chest and armpits and increases larynx development, which results in the adult male voice becoming lower
- increases the protein content of muscles, bones and skin
- encourages the development of female hormones in pubescent girls.

## ADOLESCENCE

Every child is sensual to varying degrees but the arrival of sex hormones adds a different dimension to these earlier feelings. If you look around, you will observe that girls are usually a few years ahead of boys in developmental terms and in their emotional moods and feelings which are swayed by hormone changes. Nevertheless, boys catch up and have their own particular problems to deal with. Girls can begin to menstruate as early as eight to ten years old but it is more common around the age of twelve. With a stepdaughter, a stepson and two girls of my own, I have watched these hormonal developments and I'm happy to report that, with the use of good food, occasional herbs and other balancing modalities, a lot of what parents refer to as 'horrible hormone moods' can be partially (I do say partially!) alleviated and supported, making it easier for adolescents to step out of childhood and into adulthood.

It is essential that we remember that adolescents themselves do not enjoy their own body swings and emotional outbursts – or parental reactions. During adolescence, a great many new hormones are circulating in the system, dramatically affecting the whole energy of the body, moods and feelings. I feel that in cultures where the passage of maturing into adulthood was traditionally celebrated, this recognition of the transition may have served to create for adolescents a greater understanding of the immense challenges that lay before them. To publicly honour, respect and take note of this phase can only be beneficial, giving self-confidence, self-worth and a sense of responsibility which are all very empowering, especially when the going gets tough. Unacknowledged puberty can be a chaotic and anxious time in which nature's blossoming is left denied, instead of enjoyed and celebrated. Young men and women need to know they are special at this time. Denial of this passage can lead to many problems, including anorexia, bulimia and liver problems.

The liver has an important role for menstruating young women and for those who are not yet menstruating but are cyclic. The liver produces many of the sex-related hormones itself as well as processing others which are produced elsewhere in the body. Occasionally, and particularly pre-menstrually when progesterone is high, the liver becomes congested with excesses of hormones. Unable for one reason or another to deal with these, the liver becomes sluggish. Toxins accumulate as a result of this incapacitation and things can go from bad to worse. The liver is joyful if functioning properly and angry and depressed if overworked and under-functioning so, at key hormone times, it can become quite an emotional time bomb. The liver can also work in harmony or at cross purposes with the spleen and both are worth looking at together on a regular and frequent basis.

The kidneys must also function well and, along with the adrenal glands, may need to be supported in times of stress as weakness in these will adversely affect hormone production. In this case Siberian ginseng would help. A healthy bowel is also essential.

The endocrine or hormone system as a whole must be understood. Apart from the major hormones which have already been discussed, there are glands situated in key areas throughout the body which secrete very small amounts of other hormones, e.g. adrenals, thyroid, pancreas, ovaries and testes. Their healthy and balanced function is essential to adolescents as they dictate to a large extent this delicate transition from childhood to adulthood. It is often observed that the endocrine system is very similar to the Ayurvedic system of chakras, so yoga exercises, deep breathing and any other chakra-balancing exercises you may know of can help. Watching for the first showings of pubic and underarm hair and breast development will help mums, dads, daughters and sons tune in to what is going on and to be more alert to any uncomfortable mood swings which may be alleviated by foods, herbs and exercise. (For young women who are already menstruating read the section on menstruation for more ideas).

**Pau d'arco** (inner bark) from South America is a rainforest tree and influences both the liver and endocrine system. It can be safely taken over a period of time and is extremely rich in calcium, which is useful for growing bodies.

**Wild yam** (root) beneficially affects the liver, digestive system, adrenals, colon and the endocrine system. It is also a hormone precursor. It can be safely taken over a period of time by both sexes.

**Siberian ginseng** (root) and **Chinese liquorice** (rhizome) are major endocrine gland tonics and contain properties similar to adrenal cortical hormone; they will therefore help exhausted teenagers! They will also generally detoxify and support the liver and bloodstream.

**Dandelion** (root) and **burdock** (root) make a great team as liver cleansers, and the burdock really helps to get rid of teenage acne; both are supreme endocrine tonics. Teas made of these two herbs are excellent with a little liquorice to sweeten.

**Bladderwrack seaweed** can be useful to the thyroid in certain conditions and can really help with growth spurts or unexplained tiredness patches.

**Iron** intake is vital, especially for girls, but adolescence generally increases the need for this mineral. 'Florodix' (available at many health food stores and Boots) and nettle tea will generally provide sufficient quantities for their needs.

All teenagers should avoid tea and coffee because these damage hormone production, clog the liver and encourage problem skin. They also interrupt growth in children and adolescents, reducing the absorption of iron and calcium, both of which are vital for growing bodies. These much-used drinks can also cause hyperactivity.

Herbalist, James Green, author of *The Male Herbal*, is careful to point out that, in many ways, boys and girls, men and women are all quite similar. He explains that the prostate can be interpreted as a male uterus and, although it manifests no cyclic menstruation, it is dependent on the endocrine system. Some would say it could also be the counterpart to the breasts in the female. He points out that it is a nourishing organ and says that testicles are ovarian tissue that has dropped down. Certainly, when a male suffers a blow in the testicles, he says, much of the pain is felt in the vicinity of where the ovaries are located in a female's body. He goes on to draw similarities between vaginal and penis tissue and the 'hood' found on both the clitoris and the penis; and points out that the male scrotum and the female labia majora are of homologous tissue.

Men produce ten times more testosterone than women. This gives men their more muscular features, just as oestrogen produces the female curves. For the adolescent male these testosterone surges can be quite alarming and can be reflected in loud, reckless behaviour, which is often difficult to handle for them as well as those around them. Add to this a congested liver and the result can indeed be explosive. Alcohol reduces testosterone levels and may result in stunted masculine development. Just as for women, the endocrine system is very important to male adolescent evolution. Similarly, acne can be a problem for male teenagers and confidence levels can swing, but with good food and herbs this problem can be reduced. Good diet alleviates general growing pains and gives vital energy.

## ACNE TREATMENT FOR BOTH SEXES

- Avoid sugar, coffee, tea, drugs, alcohol, tobacco, junk food and food which is devoid of freshness and variety. Drink dandelion tea instead of coffee or tea. Drink plenty of water.
- Eat plenty of fresh fruit and raw olive oil.
- Evening primrose oil (Mega GLA) will help balance hormones.
- Use herbs for the liver and endocrine system: agnus castus berries is one suggestion (check with a herbalist) for young women and saw palmetto berries for young men. Milk thistle (liver) for both.
- Use a formula containing equal parts of: sarsaparilla root, nettle leaf, barberry root bark, burdock root, cleavers herb and saw palmetto berries for young men and agnus castus berries for young women.
- Face wash: Mix together 1 or 2mls each of the following: witch hazel, tea tree and sweet fennel essential oils, adding essential oil of geranium for women and essential oil of rosewood for men. Mix with 300mls of water. Shake before use, as the oils will float on top of the water during storage. Dab affected areas with cotton wool two or three times a day. The oils will clean and unclog, giving antibiotic-like protection to the skin.

## A Male Herb

A wonderful male herb that helps to balance the body is saw palmetto. This safely and efficiently tones and strengthens the male reproductive system, enhancing the male sex hormones when required. It also helps prostate enlargement, debilitation and infection and benefits bladder efficiency and the nervous system. (It is also very useful to women in many situations.) Dosage: 1tsp tincture, 3 times daily

## A Female Herb

For young women, even before menstruation has begun, there can be obvious cyclic patterns mirroring what will become full menstruation. For those already menstruating, pain and pre-menstrual mood swings can really be alarming. Hormone-balancing herbs can be overly strong for young women and careful dosages are therefore required. A good choice is agnus castus in the majority of cases as it helps to regulate the female gynaecological system. It is most frequently used for menstrual complaints in women (but also involuntary ejaculation in men). It works by normalising the secretions of the pituitary gland, hypothalmus and ovaries which then appropriately signal to balance the endocrine system.
Dosage: $1/2$ tsp tinctures, 3 times daily (build up to 1tsp, 3 times daily over 2 to 3 months).

## MENSTRUATION

Read the previous section on adolescence to remind yourself where and when this all begins. The effects of progesterone and oestrogen need to be understood. However, most of all, menstruation has to be seen as a natural occurrence whereby monthly weakness and vulnerability are clearly associated with the strength of women, especially their ability to procreate. Most women's views on menstruation are laid down in their early years, depending on the emotions surrounding it at the time. Our mothers, family and society create some part of this view. The rest is governed by our physical experiences, which may include discomfort and pain.

Women naturally feel more vulnerable, both pre-menstrually and during menstruation. The physical pains often associated with the pre-menstrual phase are often the most debilitating part of the menstrual cycle. The ability to help herself through these times using foods, diet, herbs and other natural methods is a real gift to any woman. Understanding of this needs to become more widespread as it could change many negative feelings and beliefs surrounding menstruation, and very real physical discomfort, which of course only dampens the joys of womanhood. Herbs really do excel when it comes to hormones and should be used more frequently.

Menstruation should not be painful; the blood should flow with ease, with no clots (clots tend to suggest an oestrogen excess) and should be brownish red rather than a bright red in colour; the latter indicating poor assimilation and possibly an excess of sugar. If the flow is dark red and stringy, excessive unassimilable proteins, especially meat and eggs, are likely to be the cause. The menses can last anything from a day or two to seven or more days, but between four and six is considered normal. After menstruation has finished you should feel uplifted as your hormonal balance changes again. Provided you have kept your iron and calcium levels up (blood loss lowers serum iron levels and calcium is lost in womb activity) with seaweeds, nettle leaf, pau d'arco inner bark, yellow dock root or red raspberry leaf tea, you should feel spirited, excited and at peace. Menstruation can be an enjoyable time for a woman, especially if the bleeding is not too heavy or painful and the emotions are not excessively haywire. From the beginning of pre-menstrual symptoms (anything from ten days before the period) to one or two days into menstruation, tension, anxiety, tearfulness, depression and even anger can build up, smoulder and erupt! Water retention can make you feel large and clumsy, while little upsets can become major issues. If this is the case, you need help from herbs, exercise and good diet. Some women can experience painful ovulation or even post-menstrual blues, but these can usually be helped and realigned so that symptoms are lessened or eradicated altogether.

## Some ideas to keep a healthily menstruating body:

- If you have water retention problems, sprinkle plenty of celery seeds on your food. Drink dandelion root tea. Hormone imbalance often produces the situation in the first place, especially excessive oestrogen with too little progesterone.
- Gamma linoleic acid (G.L.A) helps balance the female system. Take one capsule of blackcurrant seed oil or evening primrose oil a day. It can also help aching eyes, fuzzy head, bloating, fatigue and other pre-menstrual symptoms.
- If the adrenal glands and kidneys are not functioning correctly they will need to be built up using Siberian ginseng root among other herbs.
- Use relaxing essential oils for cleanliness; also to avoid cystitis and vaginal infections. Organic lavender, geranium and chamomile are wonderfully soothing and are 'in tune' with your hormones – add one or two drops to your bath water.
- Use plastic-free and chemical-free sanitary towels. Try to avoid using any kind of tampon, however chemical- and plastic-free it is. Tampons of all descriptions keep stale blood where it shouldn't be, even if they are changed every four hours. (Some women even experience life-threatening toxicity from using tampons – toxic shock syndrome.) There is also considerable speculation that pelvic inflammatory disease (P.I.D.) and endometriosis can arise from tampon use over the years.
- Wear cotton or silk pants and avoid sweaty nylon tights or other tight, airless clothing. Don't restrict your belly with tight skirts or trousers.
- Keep your circulatory system healthy; exercise and breathe deeply.
- Look after your nervous system and make sure magnesium and calcium levels are maintained (refer to Chapter Four). Take care of your immune system – echinacea may be enough to boost it for a few days if you feel low.
- The contraceptive pill will upset normal menstruation. There are, however, some circumstances in which this is preferable to the risk of pregnancy. Consult your doctor as some people are in higher risk health categories and are therefore unable to use the contraceptive pill. Ensure that you are fully briefed on the possible side-effects of the oral contraception that you are prescribed by your doctor.
- Don't plan exhausting work or social schedules around these times – stress disrupts the delicate balance of hormones. Think ahead and plan accordingly, giving yourself permission to take time off if you're able.

- The colours of menstrual blood are important. A good menstrual colour is reddish-brown.
- Avoid tea, coffee and alcohol. They are all known to disturb hormone balance, increasing sugar imbalances and congesting the liver. If you have sugar cravings, eat fruit or choose bitter and sour foods which will offset the craving for sweetness.
- Avoid high fat content foods, such as dairy products and meat, as these affect prostaglandin levels in the body. Avoid all hormone-fed meat, dairy produce and eggs, as these will also disrupt your hormone balance.
- Make up a tea which is specially good for pre-menstrual and menstrual time, containing dandelion (for liver health and water balance) along with red raspberry and nettles, both of which are rich in iron and calcium.
- General hormone balancers include blessed thistle herb, agnus castus herb, sarsaparilla root and red raspberry leaf.
- Liver health is important, therefore consider liver cleansing and supportive herbs.
- Bowel health is important (especially if you are generally constipated). Therefore bowel herbs and colon cleansing may be necessary (refer to 'The Colon' in Chapter Nine and 'The Three-Stage Colon Cleanse' in Chapter Six).
- For menstrual cramps, use equal parts of cramp bark and black cohosh. Also ensure that you have sufficient calcium and magnesium intake.

## INFERTILITY

For men and women, the current infertility figures are very distressing. Findings show that 25% of infertility cases now relate to men compared to 10% a few years ago. Much blame is laid on chemical pollution, including the wide use in British farming of organophosphate pesticides, along with dioxins in meat and dairy products and PCBs (polychlorinated biphenyls). However, good food and a few herbs can go a long way to redressing the balance.

For more detailed ideas on how to redress these imbalances, see the resource section at the end of this chapter for recommended books. Some hormone tests, for both sexes, are helpful, although they may not be able to pinpoint the exact problem in men. Be warned, however, of possible side-effects of some hormonal treatments. Patients of mine have told of cysts and fibroids developing and they're sure these are too coincidental in their appearance not to be the side-effect of the drugs used to stimulate egg production. The *Lancet* has published studies of ovarian cell tumours occurring in women undergoing fertility treatment. The scientific director of an infertility clinic at Nottingham University estimates that one cycle of fertility drugs may be the equivalent of up to two years' natural egg production.

Men should take male hormonal tonics like saw palmetto berries, damiana herb and squaw vine herb. Adaptogenic herbs like Siberian ginseng root will feed the adrenal glands, which are the masters of all hormones. Women should use female hormone balancers like agnus castus berries, squaw vine herb and false unicorn root. All the men and women I have worked with in this situation have needed a total health review, personal programmes of treatment and adaptogenic herbs, such as

114

Siberian ginseng. A whole body approach to natural healing is needed, involving proper diet, healthy function of the digestive system, the use of cleansing programmes, exercise and hydrotherapy.

- Nutritional support should focus on organic foods, thus avoiding synthetic hormones fed to animals and pesticides in plants, all of which can affect conception.
- Eat generally a wholesome diet, reducing dairy and wheat intake and increasing fruit and vegetables.
- Consume at least 3 litres of water daily.
- A whole-body approach to natural healing is required; especially ensure that your bowel is working well and your liver is working efficiently, rather than labouring under hormone imbalances which, in turn, affect the liver.
- Exercise will be important. Sitz baths will really help; see Chapter Five.

## PREGNANCY

Creating magic in our bodies is part of the miracle of life, pregnancy being a time of bliss, vulnerability, femininity, creativity and change.

It is a time to build and tone the body, to balance feeding oneself and the baby within, without over-burdening the heart, circulatory system and other organs with unwanted weight gain or any other condition. Before pregnancy is even entered into, it is wise to cleanse the colon, liver and kidneys (see Chapter Six), and to be consistently eating nutritious foods. This pattern should be established long before conception, if possible – even though pregnancy is not, of course, always planned!

Pregnancy is not the time to heavily cleanse and detoxify the system, although some minor cleansing work can be carried out with guidance and under supervision. However, good food, herbs, and a well-functioning colon are vital. Once the placenta has grown (by the third month) and, your baby has its own line of nutrition and detoxification processes, you should attempt only very minor cleansing programmes, guided by a professional. A suitable mini-cleanse could be aimed simply at decongesting the liver which has a tendency to become overworked, overheated and over-congested just by the pregnancy itself, with all the extra hormonal commitments it has to cope with. Likewise, the colon can become a bit sluggish, due to hormonal changes and the extra bulk of the baby filling up available space in that area. The kidneys, the home of female nurturing, need to be able to perform the important role of helping to detoxify waste.

I strongly advise reading Chapter Four, as the very best nutrition is vital whilst building another human being. Do not consume fish, meat and dairy products raised on synthetic hormones as these can complicate and unbalance the body's own carefully balanced hormones. Do not take stimulants like tea, coffee and alcohol and do not smoke: these will all disrupt, among other things, the baby's nervous system, sugar balances and circulatory system. (See 'Anaemia', Chapter Ten, for information on iron and folic acid.)

## DAILY HERBS FOR PREGNANCY

Herbs to help the colon – seek a practitioner's advice on this as some colon herbs will be too forceful, but constipation is more likely to manifest or get worse during pregnancy and must be treated. Increase your water intake, drink fresh fruit juices and eat linseed and psyllium husks.

Liver herbs are important – a simple daily choice is dandelion root, brewed as a 'coffee', for liver and kidney function. Wild yam root is generally considered to be a safe choice, working on the liver, bowel and digestion; it also helps with morning sickness. In wild yam there is a colon soother and a hormone balancer specifically used for pregnancy, which is gentle to the developing foetus.

Squaw vine herb is a wonderful uterine tonic and is indicated in pregnancy. Dr. Christopher reminds us that it is 'another legacy from the American Indians, who held it in high esteem as a uterine tonic to take during pregnancy which later helps with the birth'. It certainly helps many common difficulties.

It is good to remember that all herbs have specific actions but are also all high in natural vitamin, mineral and trace element sources which are very easily assimilated. However many are contraindicated, so seek professional advice on which ones to avoid. Nettles and chickweed are ideal choices. Any pregnant woman who feels she ought to rush to the vitamin and mineral counter at the chemists in order to do the best for the development of her baby should stop to consider that, if she has the time, her best source for these is essentially nature and her plants. The body finds natural sources easiest to assimilate, and these should come first, and the synthetic version second.

Iron, calcium and magnesium levels should be met by eating lots of seaweed or by taking kelp tablets and drinking three cups of strong nettle tea daily (for extra calcium sources, see Chapter Four). Folic acid and iron are often given to women at the onset of pregnancy or after the first three months. You will find excellent folic acid and iron sources in chlorella and algae. Floradix, a pre-made herbal iron drink, is also excellent. I would highly recommend that you take these, increasing the quantities as time goes by, although folic acid in particular is vital in the first trimester as it is important for healthy bone formation in the foetus.

For calming and feeding the nerves, and for relaxing after a tiring day, drink weak chamomile tea each evening.

## MORNING SICKNESS

### Herbs

Pregnant women have used a range of safe hormone balancing herbs during pregnancy to alleviate morning sickness, but only after consultation with a herbalist. Choices can include agnus castus berries, squaw vine herb, blessed thistle herb, wild yam root and dandelion root and leaves.

There are many herbs that should be avoided in pregnancy, especially during the first three months. This is the time when the foetus is most vulnerable as, having no placenta, the baby is defenceless against anything toxic. Herbs that are rich in alkaloids, or those used to induce menstruation, are among those to avoid. These include barberry root bark, poke root, blue and black cohosh root, nutmeg kernel, yarrow herb, angelica herb, motherwort herb, pennyroyal leaf, mistletoe leaf, cramp bark, male fern, sage leaf, wormwood herb, thuja leaf, false unicorn root (except in cases of threatened miscarriage), coltsfoot leaf and comfrey leaf. **Echinacea**, however, is a very useful herb to know about should you have an infection or virus while pregnant. As this is a complicated herb with many different dosages, seek guidance from a herbalist and avoid if you have an auto-immune imbalance.

The same rule applies to using essential oils. However, making your own rose and lavender oils by soaking rose petals and lavender flowers in a base oil of almond and wheatgerm for 24 hours in sunshine, would be safe and a lovely idea, producing a nourishing scented gift for your skin.

## Natural Healing

Take gentle, rhythmic exercise but do not overdo it. Extensive running, swimming and jogging should be reduced; aerobics could be replaced by yoga. Listen to what your body is telling you and work in tune with it.

Breathing is very important, and practising different breathing patterns will get you ready to use them to ease pain and steer labour when the time comes. Deep breathing in the belly during pregnancy provides extra oxygen for the baby and is very calming for it.

Give more time to relaxation and be creative. Notice colours or delightful sounds, and cut out shocking or upsetting television programmes, arguments, and stress. If stress does enter your life, talk to your baby in calming tones so as to form a close relationship. This helps to minimise trauma inside the womb and, later, outside it.

For individual problems like protein in the urine (this often means that B vitamins are low – particularly choline), high blood pressure (in this case cayenne pods and hawthorn herb should be used) or heartburn (this indicates that the liver is over-burdened and needs help), consult a practitioner.

### THREATENED MISCARRIAGE

If you have a history of miscarriage you would be well advised to carry out a serious health, nutritional and lifestyle check before getting pregnant again.

## Nutrition

Vitamin A and folic acid are very important for physically strengthening the 'hammock' of womb muscles designed to hold the baby. Consuming carrot juice, chlorella and Engervita yeast for B vitamins before and during the first trimester (first three months) will provide these. Folic acid helps form correct genetic blueprints thus reducing the likelihood of spontaneous abortion due to faulty combinations. Good sources of folic acid are chlorella, Engervita and Superfood.

## Herbs

Should bleeding occur, inform your practitioner and consider taking Dr. Christopher's formula which has been tried and tested the world over. I have used it in my own clinic for 15 years (and he for nearly 50 years). It consists of $^3/_4$ false unicorn root and $^1/_4$ lobelia herb, made into a tea by adding 1tsp. of the herbal mix to 1 cup of water. Drink $^1/_2$ cup of tea every $^1/_2$ hour until bleeding stops, then each waking hour for one day. Stay in bed. Subsequently take it three times a day for three weeks. If bleeding increases, instead of decreasing, inform your gynaecologist immediately. Dr. Christopher always told his pregnant patients that this formula would either keep the baby or help it depart effectively.

### MISCARRIAGE

Should this occur, seek professional advice immediately.

## Herbs for after a miscarriage

Herbal douches, vaginal cleansing suppositories, herbs to re-balance the sudden change of hormones and help to support the nerves, e.g. agnus castos berries, skullcap herb, passion flower and a little lobelia herb – which will all help you come to terms with the grief, loss and other emotions associated with miscarriage.

### SIX WEEKS BEFORE EXPECTED LABOUR

Dr. Christopher's formula prepares the whole body for labour. It should be taken six weeks before your due date and is designed to aid, and give elasticity to, the pelvic and vaginal areas, generally strengthening and toning the reproductive system specifically for delivery. I have known mums on their third or fourth baby take it for the first time and comment on how much quicker and easier it made things. Some maternity units and their midwives also know of the formula, and have been happy for their pregnant patients to be on it.

- The formula contains equal parts of squaw vine tuber, holy thistle herb, black cohosh root, pennyroyal leaf, false unicorn root, red raspberry leaf and lobelia herb.

### LABOUR

This should, ideally, be a relaxed affair. Whether you give birth at home or in hospital, you should take every possible means to feel as confident and 'at home' as possible. Special music, familiar pillows and nice smells can all help.

## Herbs

There are herbs that can be used to help a birth along, should it become apparent that intervention, such as forceps or a Caesarean section, may be needed. Yet it is important to let the body do its own thing as far as possible, so herbs should be used no less reluctantly than any other interventionist methods.

Blue cohosh root and pennyroyal leaf will both stimulate contractions, squaw vine herb and raspberry leaf will generally support the labour, while cramp bark will relieve any contractions that are too sharp or painful. Small amounts of herbs like chamomile flowers may be drunk or sipped during labour, to relax and help concentrate the breathing, though large amounts will relax the contractions too much. I prefer to keep things simple unless intervention, herbal or otherwise, is really necessary. One herb I would choose would be lobelia herb tincture smeared on the lips, because this herb will provide relaxation and stimulation as required.

## POST PARTUM – AFTER THE BIRTH

### Herbs

Pains after birth can be treated with a combination of cramp bark and lobelia herb. Nettle leaf tea will restore vitality, help mend torn or injured tissue and provide iron to compensate for lost blood. Should there have been a considerable haemorrhage, high and constant doses of nettle tea should be kept up. To stop the haemorrhage itself, take 1tsp of yarrow tincture every $^1/_2$ hour.

Equal parts of squaw vine tuber (hormone balancer), fennel seed (galactagogue), nettle leaf (calcium, magnesium and iron) and marshmallow root (calcium and galactagogue), will help balance you hormonally and provide a good supply of nutritious breast-milk for your baby. British women breast-feed their babies less than any other European women. A breast-fed baby is provided with vital life-long immunity factors as well as irreplaceable physical and emotional nourishment. It also helps form good brain cells. I have never seen herbs fail a mother who really wants to breast-feed. Fenugreek seed, fennel seed, marshmallow root and motherwort herb are classified as galactagogues and will all help provide an abundance of rich nutritious milk. Intake of plenty of water is important, but by also drinking plenty of these herbs as teas, your fluid intake will be up anyway.

Breast-feeding should start at delivery – the clear colostrum which comes at birth and lasts for the first two days is vital, immune-enhancing and nourishing food for the baby. Only stay in hospitals where you are encouraged to sleep all night with your baby and to feed the baby the colostrum. You should be allowed to feed as needed. If you feel very tired, look at the broader pick-me-up herbs such as Siberian ginseng root which is the primary choice, but also pfaffia root, schizandra berries, rehmannia root, astragalus herb, burdock root, red raspberry leaf, marshmallow root, fenugreek seed, liquorice rhizome and damiana herb if you feel particularly exhausted. You can also take evening primrose oil capsules. If you suspect that you may be anaemic it is important to treat this quickly.

## NUTRITION AND NATURAL HEALING

Plenty of rest is important while recuperating from labour and the nine months of pregnancy. You have to have the energy to care for and feed this new bundle of joy. Being constantly woken up in the night to feed can be very draining if there are not occasional blocks of time when you know you don't have to keep an eye or ear open, but can sink, instead, into a completely undisturbed sleep. Good food is, of course, vital, and, if you are looking for a good ready-prepared source, Superfood will be ideal. It may be that you need to seek some extra professional help here to find out how best to meet the nutritional needs of the two of you. But, as a general rule, look for calcium and iron sources to back up the nettle leaves and marshmallow root, do not forget to support your nervous system using herbs like vervain leaf and oat straw, and take Siberian ginseng root and a little Chinese liquorice as they will support the adrenal glands.

Practise pelvic floor exercises. You should have learned these first during pregnancy to make labour easier. They are also very useful throughout one's menstruating and lovemaking life. These exercises help maintain a healthy womb, along with bladder and rectal control. To do them, simply sit, stand or lie down – my midwife said, 'Do them while you're washing up!' – and squeeze your 'hammock' muscles as if you were trying to stop urination. Squeeze even harder, count to 12 slowly, then slowly relax again. Breathe evenly and naturally. Repeat the whole process ten times. A lot of women rush around too soon after birth. This makes it very difficult for the uterus to return to its right size and correct position, and may also lay the foundations for prolapse later in life. It is important to rest for at least ten days in order to allow this process to take place. During this time, these pelvic floor exercises are best done lying down. After six weeks, get the position of your uterus checked. If it is not in its correct position a professional should be able to realign it.

## POST-NATAL DEPRESSION

This is a sad fact of life especially in the West, but is also a condition where herbs can really help those women affected by it. Attention to the nervous system and adrenal glands is vital. However, all women need some kind of hormonal and nutritional re-balancing. The squaw vine tuber and some or all of the milk-producing herbs will generally be sufficient for most mothers and you could even add some agnus castus berries. An additional formula for post-natal depression is made up of equal parts of damiana herb and St. John's wort flower (the latter must only be used at the directive of a professional). Some women lose respect for their bodies by becoming violent or uncaring, and can become a danger to themselves. Alternatively, they may become depressed and uninterested in their new baby simply through suffering from post-natal depression. With the right herbs this condition can be quickly rectified. There must be an extra intake of calcium, magnesium and vitamin B (refer to Chapter Four for suggestions).

## THE MENOPAUSE

This is the third cycle for women, after puberty and the time of childbearing. It is The Moon Pause – the final long pause in the monthly moon cycles.

This life-stage conjures up different feelings for different women. Certainly, among the new generation of grandmothers, some interesting changes are taking place. Magazines are now full of women's talk on the menopause, and HRT is widely available, for good or bad. At least society is paying attention to what the menopause means. In the past, women were sometimes much more revered at menopausal age, with its potential wisdom. Just as frequently, however, their depression, hot flushes and other symptoms went unsuccoured as their fertility and sexuality diminished in the eyes of society, their partners and children. Just as with menstruation, the menopause was not discussed as it is now.

Potentially, therefore, we would seem to have it all now – HRT for those who want it, herbs for others, and a more aware society which, through understanding the power and femininity of women, is able to recognise the emotional changes taking place as being simply another step along the female path. The apparent loss of sexuality can be a severe blow for those who were largely driven by sexual prowess and appreciation. These emotional issues need to be addressed and helped if the woman isn't to end up feeling dowdy and worthless now that, in her eyes at least, her main role has diminished.

How graceful the menopause is, therefore, depends partly on how much we can express our pain and our physical changes, and partly on how we can emotionally view our new position in life. Again, in my experience with women, the ones who suffer most are those with stress in their lives. A disturbing marriage, sick or elderly parents and rowdy young adults still at home provide three of the most common stress patterns which can treble the incidence of hot flushes and other symptoms of the menopause. The role of the carer leaves little time for personal care or reflection.

Not all women will suffer. In fact, it is estimated that as few as 10% go through a really difficult menopause, with vaginal dryness, hot flushes, night sweats, depression and insomnia. The rest may encounter one or two of these symptoms without too much distress, while at least 20% will hardly notice any change at all. Statistically, in Britain, women go through the menopause at the average age of 47. However, some menopause much earlier. This can be due to illness, poor nutritional care, genetic tendencies (i.e. one's mother or grandmother did), or extreme stress. Some women don't reach their menopause until they are in their mid-fifties. On the whole, though, the tendency in the last five years or so, has been for women to become menopausal earlier – mirroring the pattern of women menstruating earlier.

The menopause is caused by a huge shift in hormonal patterning which can take place over several years. Eventually, the ovaries no longer release eggs and the opportunity for childbearing is over. However, the menopause can slowly start its journey even before menstruation shows any signs of decreasing, as a very gradual and gentle drop in oestrogen and progesterone occurs. Uncomfortable symptoms, if they occur at all, are due to the fact that the changes come in drops and rushes, similar to the sudden swings associated with puberty. Large amounts of hormones can suddenly be dumped into the bloodstream and emotional and physical swings can follow. No one really understands what causes hot flushes or sweats. However, the nerve centres are affected by blood flow, which triggers the familiar hot, prickly feeling. During the pre-menopausal stage, periods will become less frequent and scantier. Occasionally the opposite is true, sometimes resulting in flooding. This is often due to the body attempting to galvanise the ovaries into activity. Caucasian Western women are eight times more likely to suffer calcium loss than other women world-wide; therefore care must be taken to obtain enough calcium and magnesium. (See the 'Kidney' section in Chapter Nine and 'Food and Nutrition' advice in Chapter Four).

Other symptoms experienced can be as diverse as: heart palpitations, depression, more frequent vaginal infections, chronic night sweats, becoming nervous and anxious, irritability, anger, fatigue, aching joints, headaches, weight gain and mood swings.

## NUTRITION

A good diet will go a long way to stabilising hot flushes and other symptoms. Cut out or considerably reduce the amount of coffee, tea, alcohol, sugar and chocolate consumed; also foods with chemical and steroid additives.

Weight gain or loss is often associated with the menopause. Thinner women will not be as able to produce oestrogen as plumper women. Body fat helps to produce oestrogen, therefore eat well and keep to a healthy weight.

Increase your intake of whole grains e.g., rice, millet, oats, barley, quinoa, etc. In addition, eat plenty of fresh vegetables and fruit. Lots of sprouted seeds, tofu and other soya products will also help, along with fennel, garlic, fenugreek, rosemary, sage and bananas. All of these foods are rich in natural hormones. Take Superfood daily. If you wish, you can also take 1 tablespoon of bee pollen daily.

## HERBS

Herbs to help general menopausal symptoms are very diverse but here are just some: agnus castus berries, saw palmetto berries, vervain leaf, liquorice rhizome, dong quai root, astragalus herb, angelica root, yarrow herb, sage leaf, lobelia herb, hawthorn berries, dandelion root, black cohosh root, blue cohosh root, sarsaparilla root, hops strobile and wild yam root.

Herbs to help hot flushes, sweating and insomnia: false unicorn root, wild yam root, red clover flowers, sage leaf, and ladies mantle herb. Low blood sugar can also produce these symptoms so it would be worth looking into this.

Herbs to help calm the nervous system: hops strobile, wild lettuce leaves, oatstraw and pasque flower.

To promote sleep at night (beyond the sleeplessness which is associated with hot flushes and sweating): valerian rhizome and passion flower.

To help depression use false unicorn root and St. John's wort flowers.

Herbs to help adrenal glands weakened by stress and hot flushes include Siberian ginseng root, wild yam root and Chinese liquorice rhizome.

Make sure your calcium and magnesium intake is good.

Liver health is also always important with regard to the balanced and even flow of hormones and a liver cleanse is always helpful. Also drink dandelion coffee and put fresh dandelion leaves in salads. Consider milk thistle seed, buplerum herb and other liver herbs.

If you already have a heart problem or high blood pressure, seek professional advice on treating the two problems together. Take hawthorn leaves and berries and possibly motherwort herb.

Sometimes the immune system can become weakened with all this hormonal fluctuation; take echinacea root and Siberian ginseng root.

For vaginal dryness caused by decreased oestrogen take pfaffia root internally as it stores 'sisterol', which produces enough oestrogen to help the situation without producing an excess. It is also a very supportive herb that generally acts as an adaptogen and immune supporter. Diet and lifestyle adjustments will eventually balance enough to produce more lubrication. Meanwhile make a mix of slippery elm powder with aloe vera gel, and teaspoon it into the vagina while lying on your back. Always use a lubricant when making love – macadamia oil is very good, or use olive oil. Other oestrogenic herbs are hops strobile, red clover flowers, parsley leaves and fennel seeds.

If there are any deep-seated problems, it is advisable to cleanse both your liver and colon.

## NATURAL HEALING

Take up new pursuits and do other creative things with your life, perhaps painting, gardening or sewing. Indulge your life and your body. Soak in essential oil baths and listen to music. Take up meditation and tune in with your new dimensions. Enjoy your sexuality in its new maturity.

Exercise: do keep moving – this is vital for all organs and systems to work properly.

## HORMONE REPLACEMENT DRUGS

Finally, HRT can work for many women. However, unlike herbs that can eventually be discarded once the 'gap' has been bridged, when HRT is stopped symptoms may return with a vengeance. The day has only been put off! All the hormones used in HRT are synthetic and therefore do not have the natural 'cut out switches' available in herb hormone precursors. Even the so-called natural versions like 'Premarin' (made from urine collected from factory pregnant mares, kept in 'battery chicken'-like pens) can cause blood clots. For those prone to liver disease, thrombosis or heart disease, HRT carries the same risks as the contraceptive pill.

Progesterone cream is another alternative that is available on prescription. It is made from soya beans. Read Marylin Glenville's book, *Natural Alternatives to HRT,* for a valuable insight into this product. For many reasons, she does not advocate its use, although I know other natural healing therapists who do and who personally find it works well. Personally, I solely rely on herbs. A practitioner can help anyone who wants to slowly come off HRT, but the transition requires professional supervision to make it painless and easy. HRT side effects are numerous and I have seen many women presenting many alarming symptoms without realising that the HRT was to blame. These include weight gain, anger, aching joints, fluid retention, abdominal and leg cramps, migraine, loss of appetite, 'bingeing' and depression.

## THE ELDERLY

According to many sources, including the World Health Organisation, as time goes by we are going to have far more elderly people around who will not necessarily be in good or better health. Their prediction is that the number of cases of cancer and bowel diseases will dramatically increase.

As life expectancy extends, it is perhaps time to really grasp a good understanding of home self-healing methods. Anything that can ordinarily harm the body will simply continue to do so for longer, the older we get. So, whether it is the bowel congesting or the liver stagnating, the answer lies in learning about and implementing natural healing routines designed to cleanse and rejuvenate the body's organs. This may, at first sight, appear to be a tough option for the elderly who are perhaps more rigid or dogmatic in their approach to their lifestyles, as they justifiably relax into the evening of their lives. It certainly requires those noble elder status elements of wisdom, enlightenment, balance and courage in order to make these changes.

Nutrition will have a different focus, as digestion becomes less efficient and shopping for food and cooking becomes more tiring. Added to this is the fact that older people tend to eat less as they require fewer calories and protein to fuel their daily activities. For them, a combination of liquid foods balanced with fibre, good quality fruit and vegetables, juices, Superfood and some good quality and well-placed supplements would be ideal; making sure that what little food is eaten is of excellent quality and taste. Ensure that, every day, a salad including carrots, beets, cucumber and ginger is grated and added to dandelion leaves, lettuce and sorrel. Vary the range each day if you are able to. Now is the time to grow a few herbs like thyme, oregano, coriander and garlic and to use them to flavour each meal.

Some older people find that memory and brain agility begin to fail them, just at a time when memories are more delightful to recall and they have all the time in the world for crosswords and conversation. Gingko (which is already used in copious amounts by the elderly) will really help, as will other brain restoratives such as Siberian ginseng root, rosemary herb, gotu kola nut and prickly ash berries – refer to Parkinson's and Alzheimer's disease in Chapter Ten.

Brittle bones are an increasing problem as we grow older; some 200,000 hip fractures are reported each year in Britain and, likewise, cases of osteoporosis are increasing. Refer to 'Osteoporosis' in Chapter Ten.

The immune system must be lovingly cared for; so that colds, flu and other respiratory disorders and diseases do not have a chance to become established. Include herbs like garlic clove, burdock root and Siberian ginseng root daily in order to maintain your immune system. Use olive leaf and/or echinacea root if you should get an infection.

Take care of the liver and avoid accelerating tissue and cell degeneration through 'free radical' damage. Use olive oil wherever possible and consume lots of fresh fruits and vegetables to ensure that your body receives plenty of antioxidants.

Gentle but regular exercise is vital for this age group; in fact this is the time to increase the amount that you do, especially if you have the time available. If you are infirm, hydrotherapy and massage will be essential alternatives.

## BOOK LIST

*Herbal Healing for Women* by Rosemary Gladstar (Simon & Schuster)
*Male Herbal* by James Green (Crossing Press)
*Menopausal Years* by Susan Weed (Ash Tree Publishing)
*Natural Alternatives to HRT* by Marilyn Glenville (Kyle Cathie Ltd)
*Tao of Health and Longevity* by Daniel Reid (Simon & Schuster)
*Woman's Guide to Herbal Medicine* by Carol Rogers (Hamish Hamilton)

## RESOURCES

**Bio-care,** Lakeside, 180 Lifford Lane, Kings Norton, Birmingham, B30 3NT Tel: (0121) 433 3879

**Hipp Organic** – Organic Baby Food, Hipp Nutrition UK Ltd., 165 Main Street, New Greenham Park, Newbury, Berks, RG19 6HN

**Superfood** – Herbs, Hands, Healing, The Cabins, Station Warehouse, Station Road, Pulham Market, Norfolk IP21 4XF. Tel.: 01379 60820. Fax: 01379 60820.

# NINE

# BODY SYSTEMS

## THE DIGESTIVE SYSTEM

The digestive system runs from the mouth through to the rectum. In many ways it is the focal point of the body. It is our earthy centre. Whatever we eat, we must have the ability to absorb and make use of it. Most illnesses, from chronic disease such as cancer to many modern allergies, arise out of gastro-intestinal debility with a range of

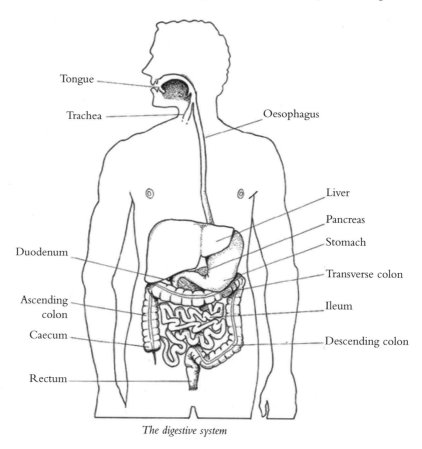

*The digestive system*

causal factors that include bacterial, fungal and viral overgrowth. One such condition is 'leaky gut' where the integrity of the stomach becomes thinned and 'leaky' like a colander. One survey has shown that the high incidence of asthma among children – and, no doubt, the whole spectrum of allergies – is caused by low hydrochloric acid levels, leading also to low levels of vitamin B12, B6 and magnesium. It is sobering to think that asthma, one of today's most common diseases, often, though not always, stems from the intestine. Note also that, if you are blood group A or B, you may have a tendancy towards low hydrochloric acid levels, resulting in poor digestive enzyme activity.

Meadowsweet, a Northern European herb, which grows in plentiful amounts in Britain, is capable of stimulating the cells in the stomach to produce hydrochloric acid and pepsinogen. It is also capable of treating over-acidity with tremendous results. There are many other herbs which can stimulate and support digestion in a variety of ways, not least the common culinary ones such as oregano, marjoram, fennel, coriander, basil, garlic and ginger. Additionally, drink meadowsweet, peppermint leaf, or chamomile flowers tea after eating. It may even be necessary to avoid herbs which could be too harsh on the stomach for some, like pau d'arco bark. Your stomach will generally tell you if herbs don't suit you, but do consult a herbalist.

## NUTRITION

Working out which foods suit you and can be processed efficiently by your body is a key factor in the upkeep of your digestive system and balanced health. As a general rule, you should avoid common food intolerances, vary and rotate foods and increase fibre intake via whole grains, vegetables and fruit. It may also be necessary to take probiotics occasionally. Pineapple, papaya and apple cider vinegar will help digestion, while slippery elm inner bark will soothe and protect if this is needed.

Good chewing is vital and you can check on how good you are at it by looking at your stools. If you are able to recognise much of your food then chew more! Even if you are desperately hungry, restrain yourself because your haste may easily backfire. In the short-term it may produce wind, and in the long-term poor assimilation and ill health, not to mention a backed-up bowel, resulting in constipation or diarrhoea. Take it slowly and chew.

Bad dental care and mouth problems can hamper your ability to chew well, so go regularly to the dentist, brush your teeth and take care of your mouth. Mouthwashes containing salt, oak bark, fennel seed and myrrh leaf are helpful for abscesses, receding gums and infection. They can be especially effective alongside regular brushing.

## NATURAL HEALING

Anything that helps the process of digestion will be useful. Start with sound sleep and exercise accompanied by cleansing programmes where necessary, especially of the colon and liver.

## THE COLON (BOWEL) OR THE LARGE INTESTINE

### The Journey

The colon digests foods that have not been digested in the small intestine. These and fully digested matter from the stomach need to pass through as quickly and efficiently as possible. The digested or undigested food passes from the small intestine via the ileum into the large intestine via a kind of flapping door called the ileocaecal valve. Often this valve doesn't open and close properly – rather like a non-operative 'kissing gate' – due to the colon being sluggish. Consequently, a toxic and decaying build-up of old food can accumulate in this area, making it, potentially, a prime site for general disease, parasitic infestations and, ultimately, digestive diseases including cancer.

This faecal matter then has to travel uphill through the ascending colon. It is never easy to work against gravity, so a strong and healthy peristaltic action is needed. The appendix plays a vital role in this process by secreting fluid which helps lubricate the faecal matter, reducing the possibility of it becoming 'stuck'. In this lubricating substance are antibacterial, anti-viral and fungal fighters, which are vital for the colon. The appendix has an important role in the immune system. The ascending colon is a common site for problems and cancers, along with more common diverticuli and herniations (pockets). Partially undigested food arriving from the small intestine, low-quality food, deficient bowel flora and candida can all contribute to problems. A lack of exercise, poor general circulation, tension, smoking, drugs and other factors, such as a diseased or imbalanced liver, can all create colon problems, especially in this area.

Next, there is a corner to navigate, the hepatic flexure. This can often be another problematic area. As matter passes through the bend it leaves residues, in much the same way as rivers leave silt as they meander through valleys. The debris left here can build up and create bulging and distortion. The faecal matter then continues its journey across to the transverse colon. The transverse colon can sag when elasticity has been lost, particularly when overburdened with faecal matter; through a prolapsed womb, or simply old age. The colon then goes downhill via a bend called the splenic flexure. Like the hepatic flexure this corner can be badly managed, resulting in faecal matter building up creating an area where dumping and ballooning occur. Once around the splenic flexure, the journey is downhill through the descending colon. Potentially, things should get easier at this point. Finally, it is on into the rectum. Without sounding relentlessly pessimistic, however, problems can and do arise here too!

This process can become a strain if the incoming foods are deficient in fibre, are over-processed or lack any built-in digestive properties and nutrients. Then the colon will not be able to process the materials it needs in order to function properly. As one of the major eliminative channels it is vitally important that it functions freely; something that will mirror good health in the entire body. Imagine old toxic, fouled faeces, poisoning your bloodstream, lymph system, brain, liver and more. The liver may eventually become exhausted and congested, the stomach may become disabled, resulting in over or under function, and the pancreas can inflame due to its inability to produce enough digestive enzymes. In short, the internal task force will generally be in trouble in a myriad of ways with resultant symptoms and diseases – all caused by general bowel toxicity.

An overwhelming number of people have colons that are overloaded and misshapen with old faecal matter. This can cause sagging and ballooning, distortions and constrictions where disease can lurk along with old glue-like partially-digested food which can often become stagnant, making it an ideal breeding ground for disease. In 1995, nearly 31,000 people in Britain were diagnosed with colon cancer, and 20,000 are estimated to die as a result. It is the third most common cancer, and could easily upgrade to second if our eating trends and accompanying lack of exercise continue. When combined with other colon diseases, it is already the second largest cause of death in Britain. When the colon starts to become clearer and cleaner, the symptoms of the disease begin to slowly ebb away, layer by layer. Remember, if you do not cleanse the colon, your other organs and systems will not be able to cleanse their wastes either and an auto-intoxication situation can easily arise.

Check with close relatives, especially older members of your family, for bowel problems. This way you will be able to see if your own tendencies might be hereditary. As always, prevention is the key.

## A Healthy Colon and What Can go Wrong

Dr. Bernard Jensen is a well-known herbalist in America and has written many books on the bowel. They are worth searching out, not least for the photographs he uses of autopsies showing the variety of distorted colon shapes found in the deceased. These distortions occurred due to old faecal matter piling up by the pound, creating pockets, narrowings, balloonings and so forth.

In these balloons, old faecal matter slowly becomes part of the bowel wall itself, hardening and impacting, layer upon layer; encouraging viruses, bacteria and fungi to take hold and thrive with opportunistic parasites also setting up home – all will drain the entire body of health and vigour. The ensuing strain on the colon walls also causes thinning and, where the wall has become too thin, fluid bowel matter can slowly seep into the rest of the body. It is not only toxins that can cause bowel problems. Positive microbes in the colon can become dangerously pathogenic if they escape from their regular environment.

Many common viruses and bacteria lurk in bowel pockets of both men and women. Candida is commonly found in the bowel pockets of women, in particular, and can often stubbornly proliferate due to the presence of parasites. Whenever ballooning occurs, narrowing before or after the affected area results, making it difficult for faecal matter to pass through. Very often it doesn't, and the faecal matter gets dumped into the existing balloon or pockets after attempts to negotiate the stricture have failed. What little faecal matter does get through is often very watery and thin and this is the form in which diarrhoea sometimes presents itself, especially if it comes after years of constipation.

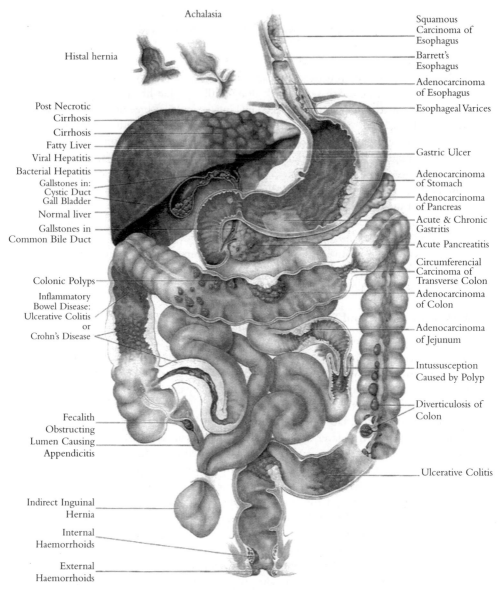

Achalasia

Histal hernia

Post Necrotic
Cirrhosis

Cirrhosis

Fatty Liver

Viral Hepatitis

Bacterial Hepatitis

Gallstones in:
Cystic Duct
Gall Bladder

Normal liver

Gallstones in
Common Bile Duct

Colonic Polyps

Inflammatory
Bowel Disease:
Ulcerative Colitis
or
Crohn's Disease

Fecalith
Obstructing
Lumen Causing
Appendicitis

Indirect Inguinal
Hernia

Internal
Haemorrhoids

External
Haemorrhoids

Squamous
Carcinoma of
Esophagus

Barrett's
Esophagus

Adenocarcinoma
of Esophagus

Esophageal Varices

Gastric Ulcer

Adenocarcinoma
of Stomach

Adenocarcinoma
of Pancreas

Acute & Chronic
Gastritis

Acute Pancreatitis

Circumferencial
Carcinoma of
Transverse Colon

Adenocarcinoma
of Colon

Adenocarcinoma
of Jejunum

Intussusception
Caused by Polyp

Diverticulosis of
Colon

Ulcerative Colitis

*Diseases of the digenstive system*

## How Often Should I Have a Bowel Movement?

One needs a bowel movement roughly two to three times a day, dependent on the daily food intake. You should eliminate four-fifths of your food intake over an eleven to nineteen hour period of time. Every 8 hours there is a peristaltic urge triggered by the gall-bladder. If a bowel movement is achieved upon waking at 7am, then the next one should be at approximately 3pm. Candida and other bowel flora imbalance can severely hamper peristalsis, much as liver and gall bladder dysfunction do. Many people find that having a meal triggers a bowel movement. This is because the filling of the stomach triggers the emptying of the colon. This idea to many people seems horrendous and ridiculous – they feel they don't want to give away that much! Nor do most of us check the amount of time that food takes to pass through. Try swallowing some sunflower seeds – the white seeds show up well against the other colours of the faecal matter and are a useful way to measure the amount of time food takes to pass through your system.

You need to look at your bowel movements if you are to begin a self-help programme. The ideal bowel movement should preferably float in the toilet bowl. Sinking suggests compaction, due to the faecal matter having spent too long in the bowel or being congested with mucus. Bowel movements should come out of the rectum effortlessly and break up slowly or remain only partially in light floating pieces. The colour should normally be lightish brown. However, green/browns will suggest you've eaten many green things recently, darker reds indicate, perhaps, that you've eaten beetroot and so on. But white and yellow movements could signify liver and gall-bladder problems. Look and think. They shouldn't be pungent, and there should be no wind, pain or foaming.

## Nutrition

Eat a diversity of food types, according to your individual needs. One of the most important things to remember is that all foods must be completely digested in order to successfully move through the colon. Consuming plenty of water and fibre will help enormously.

## Herbs

See Chapter Six for information on colon cleansing. Drinking Aloe vera will soothe, heal and help to repopulate bowel flora in all conditions.

Liver and kidney cleansing may also be beneficial.

## Natural Healing

Try keeping a footstool in the toilet. This is useful because we are really designed to squat when having a bowel movement – a position not encouraged by the design of most modern Western toilets. Using a footstool or a child's plastic stander will help align your body into a more natural position.

As with all bodily functions, the spinal column provides nerve supply and the lower vertebrae, if misaligned, will cause problems in the bowel. Therefore, consider a visit to an osteopath or chiropractor in order to make sure that your vertebrae aren't hindering the correct flow of impulses and fluids.

Massage will help, especially along the whole length of the intestine, where it will encourage and increase its vitality.

Self-massage can really help the bowel: always use circular movements, starting on your right side at the bottom of the stomach and moving up to just below your ribs, across to the other ribs and down to your genitals. Use a soft, light touch, until you get to know how deeply you can go. Eventually go as deeply as feels comfortable, stroking and kneading (like bread making). If you ever reach a painful spot, stop and hold your hand over the pain for a while till it ebbs away. For a relaxing oil, you could try diluted frankincense essential oil (5–7mls in 250mls of base oils). Other essential oils may be recommended for particular problems, but black pepper and camphor are two other general ones. You should also practise deep breathing exercises. Yoga will also be of great benefit, as some of the postures deal directly with internal massage.

## THE URINARY SYSTEM

The kidneys constantly regulate, distribute, sort and filter matter. Without this ability, the body cannot survive for long – it will become poisoned. To do this job properly, large amounts of water are required in a body that is itself composed of 70% water, at least 2 litres a day to prevent dehydration.

The kidneys also maintain the acid and alkali balance within the bloodstream. With an adequate intake of fluids a more alkaline state will prevail, which is the base of all good health.

The kidneys also have quite a few hormonal functions. They help to process calcium and magnesium. In women this is done in connection with oestrogen. The kidneys also help produce a hormone called renin that is vital for regulating blood pressure. Weak kidneys can sometimes be the root cause of blood pressure imbalances.

### NUTRITION

Too little salt can be as harmful to the kidneys as too much (sodium over-stores water). Choose and use a variety of salts from rock to sea-salt. Consume 2 to 4 litres of water daily according to your size and body weight. Drinking water, any water, is vital. Tap water is the least advisable, but even this with all its nitrates, chlorine and so on is better than no water. Next comes spring bottled water or filtered water. *Your Body's Many Cries For Water* by F. Batmanghelidj is an excellent book on the subject. (See also Chapter Four.)

Common foods and drinks such as tea, coffee, chocolate and, to a lesser extent, peanuts, rhubarb, tomatoes and spinach, contain oxalic acid which create more work for the kidneys. Some foods are strongly active on the kidneys and bladder and eating them in season can help maintain, cleanse and thus balance the kidneys and bladder, preventing stagnation, stone formation and infection. Asparagus, for instance, is useful in late spring as a means of doing this, but don't use it if your kidneys are known to be, or suspected to be, inflamed. Also avoid asparagus if you already feel exhausted and tired, as the diuretic effect could increase this feeling. Parsley and nori seaweed in salads, soups and stews provide a nice all-year-round addition, while blackberries, raspberries, cranberries, celery, water melon and watercress are more summer choices. Whole barley and sweet corn in soups and stews could then be used in the autumn and winter months. If you have inflamed, weakened kidneys make a soup of 70% courgettes and 30% potatoes. Carrots, lettuce and cabbage are also very helpful. Oxalic acid-rich foods must be avoided by those who are prone to kidney problems as they are known to help create kidney stones.

Drink barley water – refer to Chapter Four for the recipe.

## HERBS

It is important to note that some herbs are just as capable of exhausting the kidneys as synthetic diuretics available on prescription are. This is due to the forceful nature of their action and therefore they should only be used for specific purposes and only for a short period of time. A prime example would be horsetail herb. It is true that they don't leach potassium from the body because, like all plants except liquorice, they are rich in potassium and low in sodium, (usually by a ratio of 3:1), however, if used for long periods, their potent diuretic action on the kidneys will cause weakening and draining.

The safest herb, which cannot harm the kidneys yet helps shed excess water in the body, is dandelion. As Dr. Christopher so clearly puts it, 'it's the safest diuretic in the botanical kingdom.' It also has the ability to aid the work of the liver.

## NATURAL HEALING

Cold, damp, too little or too much water, wintry weather and fear can negate the effectiveness and balance of the kidneys. Your environment, lifestyle and the climate in which you live can all make a difference, depending on your body structure. The kidneys and the urinary system work hardest or stagnate in extremes of weather, either hot or cold. So, in winter, wrap up well and never let your kidneys become chilled. If your kidneys ever feel inflamed or you suffer from genito-urinary problems, applying a castor oil pack over them will bring instant relief, or wear a kidney scarf.

A summer kidney cleanse is often advisable – see Chapter Six.

## LIVER AND GALL-BLADDER FUNCTION

The liver is the largest organ in the body and one of the most important for overall health. It is situated under the lower right ribcage. The liver is capable of complete self-renewal at a faster rate than the rest of the body. Given this ability to restore itself via good foods, rest and herbs, its meaning, 'live' or 'life', is very apt. The liver makes and releases into the body an amazing amount of useful substances and sustains us in a myriad of vital ways. It also stores vitamins, minerals and sugars. A lack of these are due to a congested, poorly working and under-par liver, and can contribute to a huge number of conditions, including low blood sugar levels, diabetes, menstrual and other hormonal problems. The raw material for these chemical processes comes from our food. This is the key to keeping it healthy; it absorbs food via the intestine and then releases it into the body at the necessary rate.

The gall-bladder is a small organ attached to the underside of the liver. It is here that bile is condensed and stored until it is required, once it has been received from the liver. The job of the gall-bladder is to eject bile into the duodenum when food passes from the stomach into the intestine. Bile has many functions, and one of its uses is to help digest fats. It is also a natural laxative because it acts as the liver's own personal eliminatory channel.

The liver creates immune substances, and also purifies and filters the blood by neutralising poisons. During its many chemical reactions, it produces a great deal of heat that can warm the whole body. If the liver is pushed and overwhelmed with the work it needs to carry out, perhaps because of excessive hormonal demands or toxicity, it can become 'overheated'. This, in turn, will deleteriously affect other organs and systems. The liver also instigates some hormonal processes and inactivates others; it plays a major role in the pre-menstrual phase, menstruation, menopause and other endocrine times for women.

This cleansing, manufacturing and storage centre, through its influence on nutrient and energy supply as well as detoxification, has a direct link with the mind and its function. Emotionally, one can feel very depressed or even angry; sad, weepy and, at worst, jealous, if the liver is over-extended by one's daily input. Fortunately, the liver is also very capable of making us feel happy, joyful, balanced, sprightly and energised when it is functioning well. Such drastic differences are often plainly seen before and after a liver cleanse.

## NUTRITION

When the liver is sick, avoid fatty foods except for extra virgin olive oil, which is very good for the liver. Increase your intake of antioxidants as they protect the liver; foods like peppers, parsley, chlorella, algae, fresh vegetables and fruit juices, garlic, carrots, greens, citrus fruit and soaked or sprouted whole seeds all eaten raw or gently steamed. Choline (a B vitamin) is vital for the balanced use of cholesterol by the body; soya bean products are rich in this, so is vitamin C, lipoic acid and essential fatty acids found in olive oil. Keep your protein intake to an optimal 30–65g a day, as Westerners eat far too much protein, which disrupts liver enzyme activity. Eat foods that contain sulphur – for instance, garlic, leeks, chives and spring onions, as they decongest the liver. Keep your intake of refined sugar to a minimum. Eat lots of 'sour' food, such as lemon juice which is thought to initiate enzymatic releases that de-toxify the liver. Avoid cooked spices and test to see if raw ones are appropriate for you or not; listen to your body and take note of its reactions. Eat steamed rice and vegetables and organic wheat. Avoid drinking coffee, tea, and alcohol, in fact anything that stimulates, including heating spices like chillie.

By keeping the gall-bladder working properly, the liver can work less stressfully, thus relieving the bowel, the heart and the kidneys. Raw juices make good liver and gall-bladder cleansers; blend together 60% carrot juice, 30% beetroot juice and 10% cucumber or apple juice and drink 8 to 16 fluid ounces a couple of times a week. Dr. Christopher warns that those on large amounts of carrot juice can look as if they are suffering from carotene poisoning, developing an orange tint to their skin! However, he says reassuringly that this is just the liver clearing, when bile flows out in quantity and that normal skin colour will soon be restored. In my experience, before returning to normal, many patients have had a hard job calming down anxious friends and relatives about their skin colour, so before embarking on liver cleansing, it may be wise to give them due warning.

Grapes activate the liver to stimulate glycogenic and bile secretions. Ripe mango is invigorating and stimulates appetite. Rosemary is beneficial in cooking or salads, due to its bitter flavour. Radishes and their green leaves can be beneficially taken daily for jaundice. Drink a glass of tomato juice mixed with cayenne pepper if you suffer from a sluggish liver. Then turmeric – fresh or dried ground root added to food – is a prime Indian liver and gall-bladder cleanser (avoid if gallstones present). Globe artichokes contain cynarine, which promotes the flow of bile and stimulates liver cell regeneration.

Dizziness, eye problems and a flushed face could suggest a deficiency of liver enzymes – eat more dark green vegetables and cabbage.

## HERBS

Many liver herbs are bitter or sour; these act as a digestive stimulant. Some common and wild herbs in Britain and Europe are dandelion leaves, sorrel leaves, angelica root, watercress and wormwood herb and, in the kitchen, turmeric and lemon.

If the gall-bladder is actually inflamed, then gentle herbs will be needed like marshmallow root, dandelion root and leaves, gentian root, wild yam root, and chamomile flowers.

All the following herbs could be used to help the liver and gall-bladder, either by stimulating bile flow, or by helping to protect, cool and clear the liver; milk thistle seed, buplerum herb, artichoke globe, barberry root bark, wild yam root, burdock root, ginger rhizome, lobelia herb, mugwort herb, gentian root, dandelion root, olive leaves, turmeric rhizome, rosemary herb and peppermint leaves.

Chamomile flower tea, taken daily, helps digestion and liver function and re-plenishes bowel flora. It is ideal for calming children as well!

Herbs for the bowel, bloodstream and lymph systems can also be vital in order to assist the liver: mullein flowers, lobelia herb, burdock root and cascara sagrada aged bark.

Neck or breast lumps may point to a congested liver with insufficient blood and oxygen. Probably digestion is poor and in need of repair. Dredging the liver and toning digestion will greatly help. Use dandelion root, milk thistle seed and gentian root.

Weak tendons, ligaments and brittle nails can be a result of an over-stimulated sympathetic nervous system and overworked liver and gall-bladder. Eat lots of cabbage and broccoli and use burdock root, dandelion root, yellow dock root, barberry root bark and buplerum in teas or tinctures.

Liver-related skin disorders, such as acne and psoriasis, suggest that the liver and digestive system are usually in trouble! Milk thistle seed, dandelion root, barberry root bark and burdock root will all help. Performing a liver cleanse will also be of great benefit (see Chapter Six).

Digestive, spleen and liver imbalances are often mirrored in blood sugar problems and indigestion – use wild yam root, Siberian ginseng root, astragalus herb, liquorice rhizome, burdock root and dandelion root and leaves.

For the emotions of the liver – anger, sadness, emotional depression and frustration – use milk thistle seed, lavender herb, and dandelion root and leaves. Drink herb teas like mint, lavender and chamomile.

## NATURAL HEALING

Spring is a time when sap rises and trees and plants burst into new growth. Birds can also be heard joyfully singing their songs of love and wooing. In ancient medicine, the element 'wood' ruled the liver and gall-bladder. Spring cleanses are therefore traditionally based around liver cleansing. (See Chapter Six.) Additionally massage the liver area daily for 1 minute. Take daily hot and cold showers. Use castor oil packs over the liver if it is swollen (see castor oil packs, Chapter Two). Release anger and worry constructively so that they do not get stuck in the liver and gall-bladder; exercise will greatly help. Don't forget to drink plenty of water in order to flush out all extraneous toxins, hormones and other unwanted congestive elements.

## THE REPRODUCTIVE SYSTEM

Without hormones, the whole intricate network of our beings would cease to exist, not just sexually and reproductively but in a more widely functioning sense. As hormones surge through the bloodstream they continuously send vital instructions to all parts of the body. In fact the origin of the word describing this active and constant transmission comes from the Greek for hormone meaning 'to excite'.

We all seem to know about testosterone, oestrogen and progesterone – hormones that have a particular influence over our gynecological systems. But there are many more hormones – fifty located by science so far – influencing many aspects of our metabolism.

Women have a very complex reproductive system. Consequently, a great deal of their daily energy is drawn towards its production and upkeep, from monthly menstruation through to childbirth, breast-feeding and menopause. The end result of this is that women are statistically three times more immunally vulnerable than men are. They constantly need to tend their bodies in a way that is not so vital for men. Men and women store hormones, semen and other vital essences needed not only for their sexual and reproductive lives but also for general vitality and strength, especially of their immune systems. Therefore they must be nourished and rested accordingly.

## NUTRITION

Avoid foods that contain synthetic hormones and steroids, such as dairy products and meat. It also helps to avoid 'fast' foods wrapped in plastics that contain synthetic hormones. Stop, or drastically reduce your tea and coffee intake because they disrupt hormone regulation. Eat a generally diverse, wholesome and, if possible, organic diet.

For more detailed dietary advice refer to Chapter Four.

## HERBS

A young American engineer called Galen Hieronymus, with Dr. Ruth Drown and some others, collaborated at length to make a machine that detected what appeared to be the plant equivalent of the seven human endocrine glands: pineal, thymus, pituitary, adrenals, thyroid, ovaries and prostate. Plants are rich in hormones and, unlike their chemical counterparts, are subtle in their interaction in human beings. They can switch on and off, go to where they are needed and generally act in a responsive way. Plants and trees need hormones for exactly the same reasons we do, and the wealth of hormones found in plant life is incredible and highly effective for its varying properties and usage. Whether for tempering adolescence, balancing menstruation, aiding fertility, helping the menopause, supporting the prostate or balancing an oestrogen dominance in the case of some cancers, plants have the rainbow of hormone and hormone precursors necessary. These are known as phytosterols and are capable of enabling their human recipients to create their own hormones from them. Between 4,000 and 5,000 plant species are believed to contain hormones. Among them, sarsaparilla root, dong quai root and saw palmetto berries are just three herbs commonly used to tone, regulate and balance the endocrine system in men and women.

## NATURAL HEALING

To keep both male and female hormones healthy, we must eat well, exercise, be happy and breathe properly. Deep breathing stimulates vital hormone secretions, while sitz baths encourage an increase in circulation to the womb, ovaries and prostate. Take hot and cold showers, as they will benefit the entire endocrine system. Massage with geranium and ylang ylang essential oil in a suitable base oil (for more general information see pages 107–123, 'Life Stages'). Colon, liver and kidney cleanses will all be beneficial. (See Chapter Six.)

## THE THYROID

The thyroid is part of the endocrine system and is found in the front of the neck, either side of the Adam's apple. Its main job is to produce the hormones Thyroxine T4 (75%) and L-Thyronine T3 (25%), but it also stores iodine and, should the correctly balanced amounts change, problems will occur.

A common reason for thyroxine output problems is when the adrenal glands and/or the pituitary gland and hypothalmus are unbalanced and unable to correctly stimulate the thyroid. The thyroid gland is the body's internal thermostat and the hormones it provides are in charge of this job. If it fails, the body can initially over-burn calories, and then under-burn calories.

The two major dysfunctions of the thyroid are hypothyroidism (underproduction of the thyroid hormone) and hyperthyroidism (overproduction of the thyroid hormone). Energy is low for both conditions and frequent illness can occur from the resulting impaired immune function.

There are thyroid self-help tests where temperature-taking can assess under-active conditions. Your basal body temperature can be determined by placing an old-fashioned mercury thermometer under your arm for 10 minutes first thing as you wake in the morning. For women, this is best taken during the menstruation week. Plot your temperature on a chart in order to determine your average trend. It would naturally fluctuate but be around 97.4°-98°C. Low basal temperature readings (below 94.4°C) over a month could indicate not only an under-active thyroid but also low adrenal function, so it is always advisable to take your results to a GP or nutritionist to get them further analysed. Refer to Chapter Ten ('Under-active Thyroid') for symptoms. There are also thyroid blood tests that can ascertain overly high thyroid problems, when the strini hormone (TSH) levels are too high.

An overburdened or overheated liver is known to affect thyroid function, so liver foods and herbs will often help. Liver conditions often occur during pregnancy, leaving many women with short-term or long-term deficiencies which, if left untreated, may become chronic. It is, therefore, important to support the liver and adrenals in order to assist the thyroid, but of course the entire endocrine system.

## NUTRITION

Refer to 'Over-active' and 'Under-active Thyroid' in Chapter Ten.

## HERBS

Refer to 'Over-active' and 'Under-active Thyroid' in Chapter Ten for appropriate choices of herbs and include Siberian ginseng root and, occasionally, echinacea root. All endocrine and liver herbs will indirectly and directly support the thyroid, like dandelion root, barberry root bark, milk thistle seed and agnus castus berries.

## NATURAL HEALING

Castor oil packs (see Chapter Two) placed over the thyroid can help to regulate its function. Hot and cold showers will encourage circulation to the area. Take exercise and practise deep breathing. You will need to cleanse the colon, liver and kidneys (see Chapter Six).

## THE PANCREAS

The pancreas is mainly concerned with secreting digestive enzymes in order to break down protein, carbohydrates and fats present in the duodenum. It neutralises the acids issuing from the stomach. It is key to the overall balanced functioning of digestion in the body and therefore an extremely important organ with all the digestion based diseases and disorders.

The health of the pancreas relies upon a well-functioning stomach, spleen, liver and gall-bladder and the entire endocrine system. The pancreas produces two hormones required to control and balance the body's glucose and fatty acid levels. One of its jobs is to release insulin, which reduces glucose production in the liver. When the body's blood sugar levels rise, they affect the production of glucagon which increases glucose production. The pancreas regulates blood sugar and its health dictates the balance of sugar levels. Many people, especially women, have low blood sugar levels. In these cases, pancreatic health must be at the forefront of a support programme.

Oestrogen is found in large quantities in the growing foetus. By the eighth week, however, it dissipates when the foetal pancreas begins to function. The pancreas continues to be a key part in total gastro-intestinal well-being and, like all digestive enzymatic activity, needs to be well-balanced. Pancreas imbalance can create future chronic diseases and can be an aspect of cancer.

## NUTRITION

Refer to the section on digestive system foods, using the full spectrum of flavours from neutral to bitter. Eat seaweeds and garlic, both of which help to normalise blood sugar. Garlic does this by stimulating the pancreas to produce sufficient insulin. Poor pancreas function often goes hand in hand with low or high blood sugar levels and, therefore, the pancreas needs support and stimulation. The plant stevia helps to balance blood sugar and safely stimulates the pancreas while providing a sweet flavour (500 times sweeter than sugar). Other supportive foods are fenugreek seed and leaf and sweet root vegetables like yams, while one of the best fruits is kiwi. Generally, eat little and often (six meals a day) as this helps to support blood sugar levels. Be sure to eat some protein-rich foods in order to stabilise sugar levels. Liver health via food cleanses will, in turn, greatly assist pancreatic function. Excessive alcohol harms the pancreas and liver and can give rise to pancreatitis.

## HERBS

Consume 2 or 3 garlic cloves a day, fenugreek seed and Chinese liquorice rhizome along with burdock root, Siberian ginseng root, schizandra berries and astragalus herb. Add wild yam root because it helps normalise blood sugar levels. Liver and colon cleanses will be vital (pay particular attention to any colon congestion around the splenic flexure which can press on the spleen and pancreas).

## NATURAL HEALING

Take hot and cold showers but if you feel fatigued or experience symptoms of low blood sugar e.g. lightheadedness and dizziness, concentrate more on cold than hot.

## THE SPLEEN

The health of the spleen relies upon good stomach and pancreatic balance because it is part of the supporting tissue of the stomach. This supporting tissue means that the spleen plays a valuable part in the digestive function. In Chinese medicine the spleen and liver have a special relationship – again related to digestion. Many traditional

139

models of medicine place the main emphasis on its digestive importance, its job being to extract nutrition and, therefore, energy from food. The spleen transforms our food, changing the impure to the pure. The spleen is also a major immune component, so when the role of the spleen is hampered, its immune function becomes restrained. It loses its force and this is often accompanied by chronic fatigue. Digestion also becomes badly impaired. You may experience pain upon eating, bloating, wind, constipation and/or diarrhoea and weight loss. Support of the entire endocrine system is vital.

## NUTRITION

Seaweeds, vegetable juices and Superfoods made up as energy drinks are ideal as they require very little digestion. A few examples are algae, wheat grass and seaweed. Otherwise, use foods for the pancreas, as stated. Slow cooking of foods helps aid digestion. Excessive worry or obsessive behaviour can overburden the digestive process.

N.B. For those who are chronically ill, e.g. those suffering from cancer, an excess of raw foods which are usually vital for the healing process can produce a deficiency in the spleen and hamper the immune system. Therefore let the practitioner keep an eye the behaviour of the spleen – an acupuncturist can do this by feeling the pulse.

## HERBS

Those herbs that are supportive to the pancreas are also appropriate here, along with herbs like echinacea root (as long as auto-immune problems are not present) and burdock root to support the immune system.

## NATURAL HEALING

See liver and colon cleanses and general advice for the pancreas.

# THE ADRENAL GLANDS

These are found just above each of the kidneys and are, in effect, part and parcel of kidney function. When our adrenals are low and exhausted our whole being becomes depressed in a variety of ways. Severe mental dysfunction can be attributed to their depletion and many diseases and conditions, from allergies to chronic illness, can have their roots in adrenal dysfunction. Their depletion can either be inherited or produced by other factors.

One group of hormones produced by the adrenals helps to build, fuel and regulate growth and repair within the body. These hormones also work to control and instigate inflammation, which is vital when infection or tissue damage is apparent. They are known as natural 'steroids'.

Another group of hormones produced in the adrenal glands acts to maintain the balance of potassium and salt (sodium) ratio, helping to inhibit loss of salt and water through the kidneys. This is important because 'waterlogged' tissue strains the heart.

Finally, the adrenal cortex glands produce sex hormones. It is their individual balance that creates the differing biological genders.

The adrenal medulla, the other section of the adrenal glands, is associated with the 'flight or fight' response, and is really part of the nervous system. Varying amounts of adrenaline are released into the bloodstream, circulating and preparing the body to react to particular situations. Should this adrenaline reaction become a constant stress 'norm' the body will become exhausted, and digestive problems (digestion is temporarily shelved during this response) will manifest themselves, along with other problems. Adrenaline reaction is a useful response in cases of genuine danger, increased breathing patterns and varying responses to allergens. Unfortunately the body can often become trigger-happy and, apart from being subjected to physical toll, may produce confused emotions – for instance, anxiety and paranoia may occur. Exhaustion, depression and the potential for acute or chronic diseases of the digestive system, pancreas, spleen, liver, thyroid and colon could ensue. Blood sugar levels will also be badly affected. Entire endocrine support will be vital.

## NUTRITION

Food and physical focus should be similar to those recommended for hypoglycaemia and diabetes (Chapter Ten).

For the adrenal medulla, all foods for the nervous system can very often help, particularly oats.

## HERBS

Plant hormone precursors are invaluable for feeding exhausted or trigger-happy (that is, under-active or over-active) adrenals. They are wild yam root, Chinese liquorice rhizome and Siberian ginseng root. Marshmallow, astragalus and codonopsis root, and schizandra berries also provide bed-rock tonic support. Take chamomile flower and skullcap herb tea at bedtime. Drink one cup of parsley herb tea a day.

## NATURAL HEALING

The advice which applies to the kidneys is also applicable to the adrenal glands. On the whole, the body requires appropriate exercise and rest. 'Burning the candle at both ends' should be avoided. Good sleeping habits are vital as well as catnapping which can be a very useful habit to develop as it conserves and restores energy.

## THE CIRCULATORY SYSTEM

Heart attacks (or 'episodes') and circulatory disorders are often a 'disease of the knife and fork' (a key phrase often used by natural healer, Richard Schulze). It may not have been our own 'knife and fork', it may have been our parents' – but diet is, nevertheless, very frequently the cause. Although in America cholestrol conscious diets are having a positive effect. If we were to give heart and circulatory fatalities as much attention as we do AIDS, or even cancer, we would be faced with the reality of examining what the British and other nationalities eat. Most people don't want to look at this or to change their habits, so the high death rate continues. We create problems for our children and our children's children by passing on our bad habits via our genes, creating burdened circulatory systems at birth which, according to surgeons, are giving rise to heart problems in younger and younger people. Women are four times as likely to succumb to general circulatory disorders as men (in Britain), though actual heart episodes are higher in men.

Dr. Christopher healed hundreds of people with minor heart problems and circulatory diseases in the 1930s using natural healing methods. Now angiograms and CAT scans are able to prove the value of this kind of work to other medical professionals, showing that through diet, herbs and changes in lifestyle, coronary plaque in the arteries can be greatly reduced, thus ultimately making surgery unnecessary.

The heart, to all poets, painters, spiritual guides and those who really know, is the key to emotional well-being. 'Open' your heart and you will feel loving, caring, compassionate and at peace with life. Should your general disposition be low, your nervous system stretched, or should you feel depressed or angry, your heart will be affected. In many ways, the heart and the way we feel, or rather how the mind feels, are interconnected. Singing, chanting, movement, dance, meditation and food can all 'open' and get to the 'heart' of the matter.

In Oriental traditions, the small intestine is connected with the heart. This 'partnership' gives the male role to digestion (small intestine) and the female role to the heart, the rhythmic, perpetual beat. If one side of the partnership is disharmonious, then its partner will feel it.

There are, of course, many drugs for these conditions. Drugs to prevent spasm, to dilate arteries, to strengthen heart beat, to drive out excess water and salt, to block beta cell receptors, to slow down clotting processes, to help decrease cholesterol levels – but all carry deleterious side-effects, especially if they are used for long periods of time. It would be much better to avoid them if at all possible. Sometimes they provide first aid measures but finding alternatives is really worthwhile.

## NUTRITION

The Chinese teach us that bitter foods are very supportive and strengthening to both the small intestine and the heart and, in our present sugar-oriented society, I think this is an ever more important point to remember.

Avoid eating excessive amounts of meat, in order to lower cholesterol levels and homocysterine levels. High homocysterine levels cause plaque to build up in the arteries. Folic acid and other B vitamins will greatly help lower cholesterol and homocysterine levels.

Fats should be avoided in general, while saturated fats, found in meat, should never be used. Moreover, when you are shopping, read all the labels on the foodstuffs you buy and, whenever you see oil or fats mentioned, consider that product undesirable. Olive oil, low heated (not above 90°F) or used raw, is the safest oil to use, along with flax seed oil which is also rich in Omega 3 and fatty acids. Be sure to use a cold-pressed, oxygen-free source, supplied in special light and oxygen-excluded containers (available from Higher Nature).

Salt is good as long as you use the good-quality. If possible, hand-harvested, sun and wind-dried variety, such as Celtic salt. These salts have the correct balance of minerals and naturally tend to be lower in sodium. Used sparingly in cooked food, they are acceptable. Raw food does not need extra salt flavouring, but explore the use of herbs and spices which often negate the need for salt. Consider using coriander seeds, bay, thyme and fennel leaves.

Avoid alcohol as it increases the strain on the circulatory system and heart, breaking open veins and expanding the arteries. It also increases free radical damage and oxidation. Oxidation is what happens when something is over-exposed to oxygen. Like a piece of rubber when it gets older, it goes hard, loses its elasticity and will finally crack or sag.

Basic positive foods include beetroot (the colour of blood). Taken raw, juiced or cooked, it will clear, cool and strengthen the blood and heart. Use it mixed with apple or carrot if the taste seems too intense. Onions and garlic are master cleansers and coolers of the heart and whole system. Whole wheat (the whole organic grain of wheat) is another good heart strengthener. It will also help to cool and clear the blood, easing any inflammation. You can sprout the grains and eat the grass with salads – a preferable choice for the many who need to avoid cracked wheat. Following a mainly juice-oriented vegan eating programme for just 1 month can go a long way to normalising blood pressure and removing cholesterol build-ups. Use plenty of garlic (three to six cloves a day). You should also add plenty of medium to hot raw cayenne. As a guide, take a minimum of 1 small teaspoon per day, but 2 teaspoons per day would be better and 9 tsps would be excellent (but check with your stomach)!

Most fruits are rich in salicylate and this plant constituent helps to keep the blood from becoming sticky and clumping together to form dangerous clots, so eat plenty of bilberries, lemons, oranges, peaches, prunes, figs, grapefruit, rhubarb, cherries, melons, nectarines, plums, apples and pineapple, always eating the skins (except, of course, those of melons, pineapples and grapefruit). The inner skins (pith) of lemons, grapefruit and oranges are an excellent source of riboflavinoids (vitamin P) which really strengthen the veins, arteries and capillary walls. All the above fruits are also rich in vitamin C and will aid the structure and elasticity of the veins. Vitamin C also protects arteries from oxidation and diminishes the growth of plaque on the vessel walls. Most fresh fruit and vegetables are rich in antioxidants that keep all cellular structure healthy and functioning as required. In modern life we are becoming more than ever deficient in vitamin C. This is because stress and pollution rob us of this vital vitamin which we are not capable of making for ourselves. If you have cold extremities, add raw black pepper or ginger to the fruits to add fire and warmth for yourself. Meadowsweet herb and white willow bark are rich in salicylate, which is helpful for digestion and aids the whole small intestine and heart partnership.

Cholesterol is a vital part of cell membrane structure. It is needed for bile form-ation, hormone production and vitamin D synthesis and is transported from the intestine to the liver in order to perform these functions. Any excess that cannot be metabolised will be deposited in the linings of the arteries. Cholesterol-like particles called lipoproteins can cause the growth of plaque, which gradually builds up to an extent where it constricts blood flow. Vitamin C helps to reduce the risk of these lipoproteins binding to the wall of the artery. The amino acid lysine also helps enormously as it 'reverses' the plaque build-up.

A cholesterol test kit available from High Street pharmacies will give you a quick guide to your cholesterol count, or you can ask your GP for a test. Always do the test before you eat in the morning. If it is high, here are some ways to help reduce it:

- Eat a generally good and balanced diet (see Chapter Four), and make sure that you have enough vitamin E. Avoid eating sweet pastries, cakes, savoury snacks and any other foods of this kind.
- Eat plenty of lightly steamed green vegetables, green salads and Superfood as you need higher levels of vitamin C, potassium, magnesium to maintain the vascular system in general.
- Increase fresh garlic intake (also onions, leeks and chives).
- Take blackcurrant or evening primrose oil capsules (GLA) as they help the metabolism rid the body of cholesterol. Gamma Linoleic acid (GLA capsules) are rich in Omega 3 and 6, which are two essential fatty acids for this job.
- Eat oats and oat-based foods.
- Eat pineapple and pawpaw, which will cool and calm the liver and gall-bladder while also addressing the problems of platelet stickiness.
- Make sure you have good vital stomach and bowel flora, as acidophilus and other beneficial bacteria lower cholesterol levels.
- Check your thyroid function through a blood and temperature test (see Chapter Eight).
- Refer to 'Angina' in Chapter Ten for extra dietary advice.

## HERBS

Apart from garlic and cayenne, hawthorn is perhaps the most important single herb to use in healing the circulatory system. It is a 'heart' food capable of protecting, buffering and repairing the heart muscle. You can make hawthorn teas and hawthorn syrup. Collect your own hawthorn leaves and blossom in the spring and berries in the autumn when they are bright red. Research has shown that hawthorn adheres to the heart cells, making them absorb oxygen more efficiently thus preventing a heart attack. It can equally well restore those who have sustained a heart attack or 'episode' and miraculously remove palpitations and 'murmurs'. It does this particularly by buffering beta cell receptors and is a more sophisticated version of the drug beta-blockers as it is also able to 'unblock' as required. Hawthorn is also an antioxidant, being rich in a chemical called flavonoids, which is useful for de-plaquing the circulatory system. If you are taking hawthorn leaves, flowers and berries and you do have a heart episode, your body will repair itself three times more quickly than usual.

Dandelion root, made as coffee, aids the dispersal of water retention, which can be a problem with heart and vascular blockages – swollen ankles are often a sign of water retention. Repairing and cleansing the vascular system via diet and herbs will drastically alter this waterlogged situation as the blood slowly begins to move more and more freely around the body.

Cayenne which has already been mentioned under the section on nutrition, is a wonderful herb for any heart and circulatory disorders, just like garlic and both should be used daily to thin cholesterol and maintain blood pressure; they can both be taken as tinctures or capsules.

It is as vital for the bloodstream to be clean as it is for it to be rich in iron and uncongested with plaque. Should the blood constantly carry infection, debris and toxins (often from a constipated bowel) the whole body will feel sick and depleted. Red clover is particularly good at cleaning the bloodstream due to its chemistry di-coumeral, which is capable of stopping the production and function of vitamin K (Vitamin K helps to clot blood). The overall result is thinner blood, which allows better, less inhibited circulation. Nettle leaves, liquorice rhizome, burdock root, dandelion root and leaves, plantain leaf, sarsaparilla root, prickly ash berry, yellow dock root, barberry root bark and garlic clove are also prime blood cleansers, while burdock root has the added advantage of being able to deal with high cholesterol levels. Lime tree flowers can help de-plaque the system and at the same time calm the nerves and heart. Motherwort also needs a mention as a useful heart herb, its Latin name showing how useful it has been for centuries – *Leonorus cardiacus.*

A clean bowel is essential for clean blood. Look at the 'Three-Stage Herbal Colon Cleanse' in Chapter Six in order properly to clean the bloodstream. The liver should also be cleansed.

## NATURAL HEALING

Cleanse and cool the blood, taking care of general circulation, liver, gall-bladder, stomach and bowels via cleanses.

A little sweating (through hot showers, baths, saunas and exercise), as long as it's not exhausting or too heated, is beneficial as cholesterol can be sweated out through the skin.

Smoking will similarly stress and inhibit the body, therefore DO NOT SMOKE. Smoking accounts for a large proportion of cases of heart failure and circulatory diseases (see the respiratory system).

Exercise is vital, particularly with reference to the heart. It should be taken daily and carefully paced. At some point during the day, ideally after a period of gentle exercise, push the heart to rapid beat for five minutes; this will really make it pump and flex. If you experience heart pains, stop immediately and take a few drops of lobelia to relax the muscles including the heart and remove the associated pain. Then tell your health professional.

Hydrotherapy will greatly help the heart and circulatory system; adjust the temperature of the water according to your individual strength and tolerance. Train your body gradually over a period of time to tolerate the extremes of hot and cold, which will be extremely beneficial.

A castor oil pack placed over the sternum is excellent (see Chapter Two); make one the size of a washing-up bowl and place it slightly towards the heart side. A compress made from ginger, cayenne and mustard powders will also help. It can be a great relief to the circulatory system because it gets the blood moving. Increase the strength of the herbs according to your own strength and use once or twice daily.

Massage and meditation will enhance the circulatory process. Essential oils of hyssop or ylang ylang are particularly good to be either massaged in or added to the bath.

## THE RESPIRATORY SYSTEM

Modern society truly underestimates breathing and its key role in the well-being of our bodies. Older cultures and societies understood the role of breath much more than we do. They used it as emotional and physical nourishment for the body.

A freely and fully breathing body is healthier and better equipped with natural defences against negative effects including pollution, infection and nutritional deficiencies. One of the most potent ways of stimulating the lymph system, thus aiding the immune system, is by deep yogic breathing.

Yogic breathing and other breathing techniques devised and practised in other parts of the world have been used for centuries to allay hunger, heal sick bodies, balance strong emotions and to explore different states of consciousness. Anybody at any time can explore breathing this way; it is an attainable goal. What usually happens to our breathing is that we forget it and generally get so mixed up with our emotions that we literally stifle, repress and contort its healing potential and daily life-giving properties.

After our first breath as babies, we generally continue for roughly the next three years breathing deeply into our bellies, expanding and pushing our diaphragms and filling our lungs. Around the age of two to three years old this pattern changes as the ego asserts itself more. A colourful range of more advanced emotions come into play and breathing moves from the round cherubim belly up into the chest during the day, returning at night time to the more relaxed belly area. Practising and remembering how a baby breathes can be a tool for life, helping emotionally and physically at any time where there is stress or strong emotion (or indeed coughs and asthma). (See Chapter Five.)

Whatever age you are, when threatened, your breathing may become rapid, uneven, shallow and jerky, and when panic takes over breathing can collapse altogether. A reaction to emotion – any emotion, good or bad – generally tends to be breathing that is shallower and higher in the chest. Negative emotion usually creates an added restriction in the belly area and even a temporary paralysis of the air sacs in the lungs, creating a kind of physical and emotional suffocation. Relaxed breathing and a calm feeling always come from the belly. Laughter comes from the belly and is one of the most potent lung healers of all.

In Chinese medicine the lungs are said to be the 'female' side of the partnership with the 'male' colon. As with everything in this universe, upset one side of a partnership and the other will be in imbalance. If the lungs are not working well the colon will falter, and constipation, diarrhoea and other symptoms can easily develop.

## NUTRITION

Avoid dairy and wheat products if you have respiratory problems; the excessive mucus production caused in your body when these are eaten will clog and inhibit proper lung, sinus and other related mucous membrane function. Nutritional deficiencies also affect the respiratory system; low hydrochloric acid levels in the stomach and a lack of zinc and magnesium are often found in those people who suffer from respiratory diseases, so eat cabbage and garlic. Garlic should be eaten on a daily basis to create and then maintain digestive equilibrium. Other important minerals which will assist respiration are those for immune system function and include selenium, vitamin C and vitamin A.

## HERBS

Lobelia is a key herb to help alleviate and relax overburdened lung function. The lung herb, lobelia, helps release mucus congestion, relax and open the tiny air sacs filling the lungs, making oxygen replenish easier. However, an overdose will make you vomit. Ancient laws have victimised this plant and modern governing laws still restrict its access and dose, but if used sensibly it is a wonderful and very useful plant. Seek advice from a herbal practitioner. Other useful herbs include horehound herb, garlic clove, raw chilli pods, horseradish root and mustard seed.

## NATURAL HEALING

Adopt and practise a programme of belly breathing (see Chapter Five).

Exercise and explore hot and cold showers which are essential for circulation and lung air exchange.

Colon cleanses will help maintain the health of the lungs.

Saunas, if taken for short periods of time alternating with cold showers, will be beneficial to lung health. Avoid if pregnant, weak or elderly.

Essential oils can really help breathing and different ones will produce a wide range of effects. Eucalyptus and camphor will clear and open the lungs and the majority of people will find this mixture most effective. Some asthma sufferers, however, may find it makes things worse. In these cases use essential oils like frankincense and mandarin that will calm and regulate the breathing.

**Smoking**: Nicotine affects the central nervous system, particularly numbing autonomic ganglion blockers, which is partly why it's addictive. However, nicotine and the herb lobelia are similar in some ways (it contains lobeline which is similar to nicotine, both of which raise serotonin levels in the brain), so for anyone wishing to give up smoking, the lobeline-rich plant lobelia would be an ideal substitute, with no side-effects except thoroughly positive ones. When you stop smoking, bowel function is often affected, as it is a stimulant and laxative. You may feel sleepier with less stimulation and, if this presents a problem, use the herb prickly ash berries which will almost instantly bring oxygen to the brain. Cigarettes inhibit the circulatory system; they force the heart to beat faster and create a constant oxygen deficit in doing so, because the carbon monoxide from cigarettes releases oxygen from the bloodstream. One cigarette creates a six-hour reduction of blood supply to the hands and feet. With this in mind, healing of wounds, internal and external, is inevitably slowed down, and so too are all the vital functions of oxygen and blood. Blood sugar levels are also severely affected by tobacco, creating low blood sugar, as a result.

**Smoking Herbs**: You may compromise by smoking herbal cigarettes, but any plant material will contain smoke and tar which both clogs and inhibits the bloodstream and lymph system. Short-term choices could be red clover flowers, honeysuckle flowers, mullein leaf, elecampane root, American ephedra herb and lobelia herb.

## THE NERVOUS SYSTEM

This system affects both our emotional and physical well-being. Without feeding and sustaining it with a positive lifestyle and nutritious foods, we can feel stressed and emotionally unstable, and exhibit a range of ill-health patterns, from epilepsy, shingles, insomnia, hyperactivity and poor memory to learning problems.

There are two principal divisions of the nervous system:

Central Nervous System (CNS) which includes the brain and spinal cord and the Peripheral Nervous System (PNS) which includes the cranial and spinal nerves.

Our nervous system is similar to the electricity network of our homes, our nerve fluid acting like the electric current. When the nerve endings get worn down and the protective covering is no longer in place, these naked nerve endings spark and leap like live wires, and we feel as frazzled as they look. In fact, excessive electrical charge does build up in the body during the course of each day if we predominantly live on concrete and are constantly exposed to synthetic materials such as nylon carpets, man-made shoes, and so on. The cure for this is to ground and earth ourselves, just as all electrical systems need to be earthed. The famous remedy of walking barefoot when feeling hyper-nervy, unable to sleep, unstable or 'nerved-out' really does work and many a patient has found relief and benefit by a bare-footed night foray into the back garden!

### NUTRITION

Nerve foods that actually repair and feed the nervous system are non-active yeast flakes, spirulina and whole-grains, particularly organic oats and wheat germ, which are very rich in vitamin B. Vitamin B is vital because the immune system 'eats up' the acetylcholine receptors which are neuro-transmitters and B vitamins are able to remake them. Spirulina and non-active yeast flakes enter the bloodstream very quickly, need little to no digestion and quickly make these vital components. Soya foods naturally containing lecithin, which is an excellent nerve-building food. Celery, courgettes, avocados, lettuce, carrots, and pumpkin are supreme nerve foods and can be juiced, steamed or used raw in salads. Almonds and sesame seeds are rich in calcium and will feed the nervous system. Kitchen herbs and spices such as mint, rose petals, marjoram, rosemary, basil and aniseed will also help.

148

Daily nerve food suggestions would include: 1$^1/_2$ litres of carrot juice, avocado and cos lettuce soup, 2 cups of soaked oats with 12 almonds, 1tbsp sesame seeds and $^1/_2$ tbsp wheatgerm with added cinnamon powder, honey, pollen grains and lemon juice to flavour.

Vitamins and minerals and other components connected to the well-being of the nervous system are essential fatty acids, calcium, potassium, phosphorus, sodium, all B vitamins and vitamin D, magnesium and chloride. Foods rich in phosphorus are vital as a partner to calcium for bone and teeth formation; they are cabbage, bilberries and pumpkin seeds. Avoid tea and alcohol as it stops thiamin (a B vitamin) assimilation that is vital for the nervous system.

Drink plenty of water as it helps the body in many ways, not least to balance the correct functioning of the entire nervous system and it greatly helps elimination on all levels.

## HERBS

Herbs that specifically help the nervous system will also tone and aid the whole body. Circulatory, respiratory, digestive, glandular, reproductive and skin problems could all benefit from the nourishing treatment of the nervous system. This explains why nerve herbs are found so often in many other formulas. Nervous system herbs have an array of effects according to the type of action required. For instance, with depression, one would use nerve stimulants, nerve foods and nerve tonics, but not nerve sedatives, whereas with insomnia, one might choose nerve sedatives, nerve relaxants and nerve tonics. Depending on any prescribed drugs being taken, nerve stimulants may also be appropriate in the short term. Adaptogen herbs that help us to adapt to situations by supporting and encouraging equilibrium, which may well also feed the adrenal glands, are also important when looking at the whole body and its response to stress.

Nerve herbs are nutritionally rich in particular vitamins, minerals, trace elements and other components which help feed and connect the body in a better way; for instance valerian rhizome, pau d'arco inner bark, cramp bark, nettle leaves, Irish moss and wood betony herb, all of which are extremely rich in calcium and magnesium, apart from their other supportive chemistry. Plantain leaf and linseeds are rich in choline, which plays an important part in neurotransmitter pathways. Another herb that helps these pathways is St. John's wort flowers which, as a stimulant and relaxant, helps to produce 'happy chemistry' by producing serotonin in the brain. Siberian ginseng also helps neurotransmission in the brain and this particular plant can be given to anybody quite safely, unlike St. John's wort which has some contra-indications which must be taken into account. Below are some herb categories which can be combined as needed.

**Nerve Tonics** strengthen and feed the nervous system, restoring the tissues and cells to good condition. One such repair can be to the myelin sheath covering nerve endings which can become worn away and produce breakdowns and stress. Once encouraged to re-grow, the whole network of the nervous system can be made to efficiently interact.

149

Nerve tonics that help are skullcap herb, schizandra berries, vervain leaves and wood betony herb. Skullcap and schizandra are perhaps the best choices and should be taken for at least 4 to 6 months. Skullcap takes times to build up and then needs time to consolidate and repair. However, initial effects will be noticed within a week or less – skullcap is also a nerve sedative and will help with nervous tension, sleeplessness, seizures, epilepsy, drug withdrawal and much more. A good food nerve nutritive, similar to nerve tonics, would be oats, which nourish, balance and stabilise.

**Nerve Relaxants** are herbs that quickly calm the person to a state where the body and mind become relaxed. Chamomile flowers are a familiar herb for this purpose, ideal for babies, children, adults and the elderly alike. Lime blossom flowers are taken on an everyday basis in France for headaches, migraine or simply to soothe away a fraught day. In the USA, they use Californian poppy flowers in a similar way. Other herbs include hops strobile (a very British option), black cohosh root, vervain leaves, wood betony herb, cramp bark, lavender herb, passionflower, St. John's wort flowers, and skullcap herb. Wild yam is a digestive nervine, relaxing muscle fibres, soothing the nerves and providing pain relief for the bowel, stomach, gall-bladder and uterus. Valerian rhizome is a very strong herbal relaxant and is useful if all else has failed. But please note that it should only be used for a few weeks, during the initial crisis, otherwise it can become overly sedative. Other food nerve relaxants include non-active yeast flakes and spirulina.

**Nerve Sedatives** are the strongest form of nerve relaxants and are illegal in Britain, although legally used by herbalists in some countries. They are opium poppy and marijuana. Opium is very strong as it contains codeine and morphine. Both are traditionally used in the treatment of multiple sclerosis M.S. (although, with M.S., nerve sedatives can sometimes be replaced by nerve stimulants), cancer and AIDS. Marijuana has recently gained popularity for its medicinal benefits as a pain reducer but, as with any herb, correct dosage is important. In the case of this herb, excesses can cause paranoia, hyperventilation and panic attacks. Pain relief herbs like corydalis tuber and poppy leaf or resin can be tried, along with willow bark and/or cramp bark.

**Nerve Stimulants** are traditionally the least-used nervines, and are probably under-used in diseases where there are neurological breakdowns, like M.S., muscular dystrophy and myasthenia gravis. They are an absolutely invaluable category of nervine herbs as they directly stimulate nervous tissue. A famous one is kola nut. Common daily nerve stimulants like tea and coffee are, of course, completely overused and therefore lose their potential as useful herbs on these occasions. Guarana is a popular nerve stimulant; it contains three times the amount of caffeine as coffee, and was used to keep jungle hunters alert in South America. A herb for more daily usage, which is ideal in times of great stress, especially around exam times, is rosemary, which wakens the brain and also acts as a nerve relaxant and calmer. Prickly ash really moves the blood and has an almost instantly recognisable effect on a fuddled brain! Kava and coca leaves are other nerve stimulants used amongst traditional peoples around the world. Cayenne pepper, as well as being a nerve stimulant, will

150

also aid circulation and blood supply. So we have many choices. Among the safest are rosemary herb, peppermint leaves or cayenne pod but, for stimulating yet calming effects, rosemary is the best. Other fine nerve stimulants are oat seed and straw, and skullcap herb. Whenever you use nerve stimulants you must also take in a lot of B vitamins to replace those that the nerve stimulation uses. (Foodwise, blue/green algae is an excellent nerve stimulant). This whole category of nerve stimulant herbs is useful in treating neuro-stimulation addictions like cocaine and amphetamines.

**Lobelia – the Peacemaker**: Lobelia fits into all of the above-mentioned categories and was traditionally smoked in the peace pipe by native American Indians. The herbalist Dr. Christopher called it the peacemaker of all formulae and the 'thinking herb', due to its amphoteric action. He put it into almost every formula for two very good reasons – firstly, so that all the other herbs in the formulae could be directed to where they were most needed (called 'amphoteric'), and secondly because usually when people are sick, for whatever reason, their nervous systems need equilibrium. I have personally seen lobelia deal with a wide number of situations; I try never to be without it, having seen it work more quickly and effectively than the drug Neurofen for chronic menstrual cramps and for calming and supporting those coming off anti-depressants and many many more instances. It is, however, a restricted Section 12 herb and has limitations on usage, but just a few drops of tincture go a very long way.

## NATURAL HEALING

Rest is vitally important for the nervous system and this comes best of all in the form of sleep. Going to bed early enough improves the quality of sleep; indeed sleep taken between the hours of 10pm and 2am is reckoned to actually double its value in terms of quality. Meditation will repair, calm and bring peace to the day, so give this simple practice daily time if you can. Just sitting under a tree concentrating on or being aware of your breathing for 10 minutes has a tremendous impact. Those who travel, work and generally lead a high-intensity life need to guard their resources and prevent 'burning the candle at both ends'; catnapping can help to achieve this. For those with insomnia, it is important to use hydrotherapy and other natural healing routines, including internal cleansing, in order to stimulate the body and thereafter produce sleep. This is especially wise if you rely on sleeping tablets and could well help you finally to do without them.

Our nerves are dependent on blood and circulation for proper function, therefore maintain a good blood supply via exercise and hot and cold showers.

Saunas and cold showers create a beautifully relaxed state.

Skin brushing will stimulate the nerve endings and is a great rejuvenator, especially to those who are low, depressed and sluggish.

Creativity through, for example, dancing, painting, singing or writing are all important expressions of our emotions, and the nervous system will thrive when pursuing them with pleasure and in a relaxed manner.

Massage: try using nerve sedative and nerve stimulant essential oils as appropriate.

In times of extreme nervous stress, use equal parts of skullcap herb, black cohosh root and lobelia herb powders to make a poultice. Place it over the head, neck and down the entire length of the spine. For a more instant version, simply put lobelia tincture over these areas.

Add a few drops of chamomile, frankincense or geranium essential oil to your bath – or a couple of chamomile tea bags. A very good sedative is hop essential oil. This is useful for insomniacs and it is well worth the high price you'll need to pay for this essential oil. Lavender is another (and much cheaper!) soothing essential oil, and is suitable for children and most skin types.

Liver and colon cleanses will be vital for the good health of the nervous system. These alone have seen particularly overwhelming situations radically improve.

## THE SKIN

The skin is the outer covering of the body, protecting us from external influences, such as toxins, infections, dirt, light, heat and cold. It is our external immune system and eco-barrier.

Skin is also a very important excretory organ when it is functioning properly. It helps us rid ourselves of a quarter of our waste products. If the skin is inhibited by eczema, psoriasis or other conditions, this function will only partially be carried out. Should the skin be under-functioning the lungs, kidneys, bowel, liver and bloodstream will have to deal with the burden. When skin is unable to excrete, these organs will, in turn, feel the strain. It must be remembered, however, that these organs and systems could be the cause of skin problems, their own dysfunction giving rise to a stagnated skin.

Touching your own and other people's skin can be a truly sensuous experience; there's nothing more gorgeous, for instance, than a baby's skin. We touch, feel and exchange both emotionally and physically, sharing our feelings, thoughts and love with our skin. This emotional connection can be seen even more clearly when we note that, as unborn babies, our skin is developed from nervous tissue type cells. Skin diseases can be the result of internal, emotional upset and, accordingly, a loving touch can heal and mend like nothing else.

### NUTRITION

Avoid foods that are not typically digested efficiently, or that you know you are allergic to – e.g. dairy and wheat products. Reactions to foods can be reflected through the health of your skin, so keep an eye on your food intake and observe your skin's reactions. Skin needs essential fatty acids and water in order to maintain its good health, visually and otherwise.

### HERBS

Many herbs are useful but those that clear the blood and lymph systems will be of particular value. Blood cleansers (alteratives) are red clover flowers and burdock root, while lymph system herbs (lymphatics) like mullein flowers and the much stronger poke root will clear obstructions. Anti-microbial herbs such as chamomile flowers and echinacea root will help re-balance any micro-organism overgrowth. Diaphoretic and sudorific herbs will help you sweat; yarrow herb, for instance, which induces perspiration, cleanses directly through the skin.

## NATURAL HEALING

Never use chemical deodorants, they clog the skin and destroy natural bacteria. Use essential oil-based products and wash frequently. Try crystal stones (available in health food stores) as deodorants.

Make sure all the eliminative organs are working, so that the skin is not burdened. Explore colon, liver and kidney cleanses – refer to Chapter Six.

Avoid conventional washing powders, cleaning equipment, washing-up liquid and so on. Instead, research eco-friendly and body friendly products. Propyl alcohol, PCB and other toxic ingredients should not be used in your household and bathroom cleaners.

Do not wear man-made fibres. The skin needs to breathe, and nylon and synthetic fibres create temperature extremes, putting undue strain on the skin thermometer and immune responses. Use cotton, silk or wool – wear these at bedtime or sleep naked, if it is warm enough. Use cotton sheets and preferably an all-cotton mattress – a futon. Air futons and natural-fibre duvets by hanging over windowsills on sunny days. Leave futon matresses rolled up one day a week, to re-fluff and aerate.

A little sun is fine, but protect from excessive exposure so that drying-out does not occur and natural oils are not lost. Paler skin, which does not contain sufficient pigment for safe exposure to the sun, will, of course, need more protection than darker shades. Jojoba oil is a natural protective; with a sun protection factor of 16 making it ideal for many adults with medium to darker pigment skin. Those with very pale skin, children and babies, will need more strongly protective sunscreens. Go up to a factor 35 or 50 depending on the strength of the sun. With 'at risk' skins, covering with a sun cream on exposed skin from April to October in Britain will be important.

Drink plenty of water to allow the skin to excrete and function correctly.

Make contact with your body via your skin, through massage and barefoot walking on the earth or sand.

Low body temperature can affect skin problems so create more body heat via exercise. Take care of your adrenal glands and thyroid in case your low body temperature is a result of imbalance there – in which case, use cayenne pepper.

Swim in lakes, streams or the sea, if clean, but chlorinated pools, if possible; if not, clean off the chlorine by bathing afterwards with lavender essential oil. Hot and cold showers are vital; problem skin often becomes overheated and a cold shower or bath can bring instant relief.

Balance the drying effects of central heating by placing bowls of water containing essential oils next to hot spots in the room.

Exercise to promote good circulation and to ensure that lymph and lungs are moving.

Dog hairs, cat hairs, fleas, ticks, household dust and pollen are irritants and can provoke skin irritations. If afflicted, remember to support the immune system, cleanse the colon, liver and kidneys and get the lungs to work better. You must not lose sight of internal processes, even when there are external causes or outcomes.

## THE MUSCULAR AND SKELETAL SYSTEM

The skeleton is the support structure of the body. Muscles and ligaments interconnect and work together facilitating the movement of the bones. As we become older (and as Western society lives to a greater age), brittle bones will become an increasing problem. Therefore finding ways to maintain and support bone health will become more important.

### NUTRITION

The well-being of our muscles, bones, tissues and joints doesn't just depend on how much we 'wear and tear' or stagnate them in daily walking, running, lifting, bending, sitting or lying. It also relies on our internal health and the food we use to create and support this moving structure. Sugar, sweet drinks, processed foods, tea and coffee will strip magnesium, calcium and vitamin C from the body. All of these elements are vital for the formation and repair of bone, muscle, cartilage and synovial fluid. Magnesium, calcium and vitamin C can be found in dark greens, seaweeds and whole grains and should be eaten daily. Also note that iron is vital to structural well-being. Night twitching can be a result of a lack of iron, so the nettles and red raspberry leaves used for calcium requirements will also provide copious and assimilable amounts of iron. Vitamins A, E, B6 and B complex and zinc are all important for the synthesis and maintenance of good structure. Ensure that you eat foods that are rich in zinc and the above vitamins, such as red peppers, whole-grains, pumpkin seeds and carrots (see Chapter Four for more). Essential fatty acids and water are also vitally important lubricants.

For post-menopausal women, kidney health and ensuing oestrogen and progesterone levels should be maintained in order to guard against osteoporosis and brittle bone disease.

For serious injury, stop all food immediately and switch to Superfood, juices and herb teas in order to allow the healing process to begin quickly.

### HERBS

Use lobelia herb tincture both internally and externally for muscle strains (see page 170 on Lobelia), broken bones and the like; it will quickly relieve the associated spasms and pain. Pau d'arco inner bark, oatstraw and nettle leaves, which are rich in both calcium and magnesium, make ideal choices, while skullcap herb and peppermint leaves, rich in zinc, will give general support to the muscular, skeletal and nervous system. Echinacea root, and the zinc herbs above, along with vitamin C, will help the immune system fight any breaks, strains or bone porosity. Elasticity and mobility can be a problem with diseases like osteo-arthritis or simply old age. Devil's claw root and angelica root (angelica archangelica {British} and angelica sinensis {Chinese}) will greatly help here. So will pau d'arco inner bark and black cohosh root. Turmeric rhizome and the herb boswellia soothe joints and muscles – both can be used internally and externally for pain relief.

Boneset herb is a favourite herb of mine. Perhaps one of the nicest accounts of its bone-mending abilities is to be found in Tom Brown's book, *Guide to Wild, Edible and Medicinal Plants*. He tells us that he broke his hand quite badly and was informed by his doctor that it would take 6 to 8 weeks in a cast to mend. A native Indian healer helped him. He pointed to the boneset plant, showing him the new little leaves at the top which grew separately and then the lower leaves which grew together, almost as one. 'That,' he said, 'is what the boneset will do for your hand!' Tom drank a tea made from the fresh, larger leaves twice a day for the first week. During the second week he cut down to half a cup, twice a day. He felt an almost immediate difference, a kind of tingling feeling, as if the knitting process had started, while the dull ache and pain also went away and the swelling subsided overnight. If it weren't for the likes of Dr. Christopher and Tom Brown and their links with the wise and knowledgeable native American Indian healers, no one would be using boneset for healing bones. Scientific analysis can find no reason why boneset should heal bones, but it obviously does! My personal knowledge of boneset also goes back years and I have many stories of bones that have mended very quickly. In addition, I have noticed in our family (which is not disposed to bone-breaking) how quickly it delivers calcium to the body. Weak, broken and torn nails can be made into strong ones and growing pains can subside in hours. Comfrey leaf used to be a favourite herb in Europe for mending bones, but its recent public ban for general internal use has meant that it is not possible to use this plant in this way any more. However, it can be used externally and it is very effective as a bone-mending poultice or ointment when used in this way.

## NATURAL HEALING

Much benefit can be derived from practitioners who are able to manipulate, massage and cajole muscles, bones and joints into correct positions. These include osteopaths, chiropractors, masseurs and many other kinds of body workers, from acupuncturists and physiotherapists to yoga teachers. This sort of work is sometimes vital for the well-being of external functions but also for the proper working of all organs and systems and the neurological pathways, radiating from the entire length of the spine, that service them. In fact, the well-being of the spine alone is crucial, and much is rightly made of this in yoga. It provides an ideal way to service and tune one's framework and internal organs at the same time.

A home poultice made from turmeric rhizome is a handy kitchen option for treating injuries such as bruises, fracture, swellings and sprains. Mix enough powder with a little hot water to make a thick paste that will stay in place and apply to the affected area. St. John's wort flower oil is another wonderful herb for bruises, sprains and general injuries; it deals with the pain of pinched and damaged nerves.

155

Cold temperatures are important when swelling and pain is acute. Once they have subsided, continue treatment using hot and cold compresses, showers and poultices.

For muscular and skeletal damage, such as broken bones, torn ligaments, damaged muscles and weakly-structured joints, use Dr. Christopher's Bone, Flesh and Cartilage formula internally and externally. It is invaluable used as a tea or made into a paste or ointment. For a soothing, numbing and supportive massage oil, use Dr. Schulze's Deep Tissue Oil. (See Chapter Eleven for details of both of these treatments.)

When an injury feels as though it is starting to mend, start gentle exercise to strengthen the muscles. Begin with armchair exercises or gentle movement in the bath, then graduate to swimming, walking and body work in the gymnasium.

## BOOK LIST

*Guide to Wild, Edible and Medicinal Plants* by Tom Brown (Berkley)
*School of Natural Healing* by Dr. John Christopher (Christopher Publications)
*Tissue Cleansing through Bowel Management* by Bernard Jensen (Bernard Jensen International)

## RESOURCES

Supplier of water distillation units: **The Wholistic Research Company**, Bright Haven, Robin's Lane, Lolworth, Cambridge, CB3 8HH. Tel: 01954 781 074

Kelp tablets, chlorella tablets etc., silk kidney scarf: **Dr. Shamin Daya.** Tel: 0171 580 7537

**Higher Nature**, The Nutrition Centre, Burwash Common, East Sussex, TN19 7OX. Tel: 01435 882 880

# TEN

# DISEASES

When treating any illness holistically, you need to employ more than just one or two therapies in order to treat the whole person. It goes without saying that herbs will form a major part of any suggestions, and that their incredible range of plant constituents will be instrumental in honing, healing and revitalising. Good food and drink are vital requirements because these are the daily input upon which the body thrives. Regular internal whole body cleansing is also important, especially as we get older. Just as a car needs regular servicing, so do we. Seasonal food cleanses can be an excellent way to achieve this. If you are sick, you must take appropriate steps, according to the severity of the problem.

It is important to ensure that all your organs and systems are working freely and effectively so, one by one, they will need special support, nourishing, aligning and cleansing. Massage provides a loving touch and encourages blood and lymph flow, all of which will help organs to pump, squeeze and relax more efficiently. Acupuncture can tune, direct, stimulate or placate organs and systems – an acupuncture pulse-taking gives a good idea of exactly what needs attention. Iridology can also provide health assessment, giving clues to one's constitution, strengths and weaknesses.

If any part of your spinal column is damaged (it may be eroded, a disc may be trapped, the hips may be out of alignment) any resulting misalignment can affect other organs, from bowel function to menstruation, liver function or digestion.

N.B. There are many herbs suitable for treating diseases; however, there are too many to list for each disease. Therefore, a small selection of the most suitable herbs is given.

In the A–Z of Diseases and Treatments on the following pages:
✿   refers to diet
❦   refers to herbs
◆   refers to natural healing.

### Caution

*In general, this chapter does not specify exact doses for herbs or herbal formulae, neither have the contraindications of herbs been included as they are numerous and specific, those pregnant being in the highest category to avoid certain herbs. A list of contra-indications and a dosage guide is available from The Selfheal School (for address, see Schools and Colleges in Useful Addresses). Consult your GP and a qualified herbalist for all treatment.*

# AN A–Z OF DISEASES AND TREATMENTS

## ANAEMIA

If the body does not have high-quality blood containing enough iron, oxygen and other nutrients, the body cannot sustain itself. Iron-deficiency very often does not show up on tests for anaemia, as it is possible to have normal haemoglobin levels and still be deficient in iron. Symptoms include pale ridged nails, brittle, wiry hair, constant fatigue, a sore tongue and cracks at the corners of the mouth, poor general growth, a weak appetite in children, a weakened immune system, which leaves one open to infection. The individual can feel tired and low. For a quick haemoglobin test, look at the inner palm of your hand. Look at the lines – are these pale or even white or are they a good pink to red? Pale or white will indicate low levels of haemoglobin. Women will be most likely to suffer from this due to menstruation, so the above symptoms should be watched for and a good daily diet ensured. An average iron loss at menses is 15-30mg. Pregnant women need 130mg daily, coupled with relatively high amounts of folic acid; in the region of 700mg. This is best obtained from food and herbs because 'Pregaday' and other iron/folic acid pills frequently cause zinc deficiency. This deficiency can cause a host of problems just as with iron and folic acid deficiency. It should be noted that supplements of synthetic ferrous iron from the GP and chemist have a tendency to constipate and are often unable to be assimilated. Natural iron sources are able to burn up toxic wastes in the body, flushing the poisons out. Vegetarians are often low in iron.

- ✿ Foods rich in iron and vitamin C help the absorption of iron from food. These include cherries, blackcurrants, apricots, grapes and bananas, beetroot, globe artichokes, red kidney beans, watercress, black strap molasses and carrots.
- ✿ Tea and coffee drinking is very disruptive to iron absorption.
- ༀ Dock root, chickweed herb, mullein flower and pennyroyal leaf are rich in iron.
- ༀ I have used nettle leaf and red raspberry leaf tea with carrot and beetroot juice for patients who have been told they need a blood transfusion to save their life, but refuse to have one, owing to their religious beliefs. In one case, days into the herb treatment, anxious hospital staff carried out tests and evaluated the patient physically, especially for pallor and energy. They were pleasantly surprised at the outcome and eventually discharged the patient after convalescence with no major concerns.
- ༀ People with low copper levels often have lower iron levels; take skullcap herb.

## APPENDICITIS AND RUMBLING APPENDIX

This is acute inflammation of the appendix which, if left untreated, can result in a rupture causing peritonitis. Symptoms can include stomach ache, intense, sharp pain on the right hand side, or tenderness to the right and below the navel, which is increased by pressure and movement. There may also be nausea, constipation, rapid pulse, vomiting and slight fever (100°F–102°F). It is most commonly caused by faecal impaction in which the faeces have become compressed and immobile due to a faulty bowel. Occasionally foreign objects like buttons and safety pins are to blame.

158

## For a Rumbling Appendix

✿ A mono juice fast (apple, grape or carrot), with a glass of prune and lemon juice in the morning for two or three days. Ease into a wholefood (mucus-less) diet, starting with potassium broths, sweet fruits and steamed vegetables. Build up to raw vegetables, grains and legumes. For children: try one or two days of liquids – including juice and potassium broth and puréed vegetable soups.

✿ Drink plenty of water at room temperature.

ॐ Once the attack has subsided, take a tincture made from equal parts of: marshmallow root, slippery elm inner bark, liquorice rhizome, chamomile flowers and barberry root bark. Dandelion leaves and root, as a tea or chewed, will help.

ॐ Take herbs suggested in Formula B ('Three-Stage Colon Cleanse' – Chapter Six), to ensure the bowel is moving. Subsequently, for the next two to three days, take one tsp each of wild yam root and echinacea root, four times a day, and 3 tsp slippery elm inner bark mashed into a ripe banana, twice daily.

♦ Massage the abdomen with ginger essential oil or make a fresh hot ginger compress. Massage the abdomen and feet each night with the ginger mix. Castor oil packs will also bring relief.

♦ Take hot and cold showers.

♦ Childhood rumbling appendix is said to be associated with the fear of life. Night-time is a prime time for this to flare up, as with other illnesses. Place pillows and blankets snugly around the child at bedtime. Then put a few drops of lavender and sage essential oils on the pillow, or the plants themselves, placed at the head can help calm fears. Talking with children about recurring dreams and nightmares may also help this affliction.

## For Acute Appendicitis

♦ Ring for an ambulance or your GP. They can take a long time to arrive, the following procedure will help.

♦ Use a hot ginger compress over the area for pain relief or a castor oil pack.

ॐ If no help is at hand, then stop food immediately and quickly administer a hot enema of chickweed herb, catnip herb, spearmint leaf or wild yam root, or just plain boiled water if nothing else is at hand. This treatment may have to be repeated several times until the worst symptoms have subsided. At the same time, put compresses of the above herbs over the area.

♦ Use ginger packs and the hot and cold treatment, or a castor oil pack.

ARTERIOSCLEROSIS AND ATHEROSCLEROSIS

Both these conditions involve hardening of the artery walls. The arterial walls lose their elasticity and also become blocked with debris. This debris can consist of yellowish/white clumps called plaque which is made up of cells, connective tissue and large quantities of fat. At the same time the arteries absorb calcium from the bloodstream, resulting in their becoming gritty, hard and narrowed, much like old encrusted pipes in ancient house plumbing. This calcium debris produces arteriosclerosis. The flow of blood is restricted by the plaque which has dangerous implications. This process of artery encrustation isn't exclusively the province of the old. A much-quoted study of soldiers killed in the Korean war showed that nearly three-quarters of these young men already had some arteriosclerosis in their coronary vessels.

- Read up on Calcium Balance in Chapter Four.
- ✿ Take beetroot and grapefruit juice with cider vinegar to dissolve deposits.
- ✿ Refer to the dietary advice for angina, and stop all alcohol and sugar intake.
- ❧ Garlic cloves and burdock root will help to dissolve fatty deposits.
- ❧ A good combination of herbs to help with calcium removal are: 3 parts hydrangea root, 2 parts turmeric rhizome, 2 parts gravel root, 2 parts parsley herb, 2 parts marshmallow root, 1 part liquorice rhizome, 1 part dandelion root, 1 part ginger rhizome, 1 part Siberian ginseng root, 1 part buckwheat herb and 1 part ginkgo leaf, while general heart herbs for maintenance would be hawthorn leaf, berries and flowers and ginkgo leaf tea.
- ❧ Inhale and massage with rosemary, eucalyptus and juniper essential oils.
- ◆ Stop smoking.
- ◆ Refer to 'Cholesterol Care' (Chapter Four)

## ARTHRITIS AND RHEUMATISM

There are several types of arthritis and rheumatism.

Arthritis is the inflammation of one or more joints, causing stiffness, swelling, pain and a reduction in mobility. Osteo-arthritis is the most common form, occurring in those over 40 years of age and causing a degeneration of cartilage, muscles, ligaments and joints. Rheumatoid arthritis and juvenile arthritis are much less common forms and are auto-immune diseases. The body wrongly identifies the lubricating fluid in the joints as 'foreign' matter producing an immune response which in turn induces an inflamatory response coupled with the destruction of, or damage to the joints by the immune system itself.

The whole subject of arthritis in its various forms is complex. Sometimes bacterial, fungal or viral infections of the joints are to blame.

Here are some general tips:

- ✿ Drink plenty of water to lubricate the system.
- ✿ Eat plenty of garlic.
- ✿ Cut out dairy products, red meats, salt and sugar.
- ✿ Do not eat any foods from the Solanaceae family e.g. potatoes, peppers and aubergines, as they interfere with muscle enzymes.
- ✿ Avoid oxalic acid-rich foods as they make matters worse. Avoid tea, coffee, wine, spinach, rhubarb, tomatoes, gooseberries, oranges, strawberries, black and red-currants. However, some of these may eventually be re-introduced without incurring pain and inflammation.
- ✿ Use juice cleanses and Superfood. Use lots of pineapple in each of these; it will help reduce inflammation.

✪ Take apple cider vinegar on a regular basis as it works on a similar principle to lemon juice.

◆ Take essential fatty acids in the form of GLA capsules, as they will help any inflammation.

◆ Perform liver, kidney and colon cleanses.

⚭ For excessive inflammation and to help mobility use 3 parts Siberian ginseng root, 2 parts wild yam root, 2 parts devil's claw herb and 1 part plantain leaf.

⚭ For general help, use St. John's wort flowers, meadowsweet herb, marshmallow root, astragalus herb, liquorice rhizome, garlic clove, burdock root and red clover flowers.

⚭ To aid sleep consider the short-term use of valerian root, and drink chamomile flower tea.

◆ If overweight, start a serious weight-loss programme, as this will relieve joint strain.

◆ If there is a lot of conflict and disharmony, or emotional friction and pain in your day-to- day life, try to ease this.

◆ Exercise is vitally important, but build up slowly; do not overdo it.

◆ Take hot and cold showers to relieve stiffness and promote healing. Saunas will give similar relief, always finish with cold water.

◆ Massage St. John's wort flower oil or Boswellia herb ointment into the afflicted area and then apply a bag of frozen peas.

◆ Use a warming oil of ginger, chilli, lavender and rosemary, if circulation is poor and you feel cold, stiff and achy. Dr. Richard Schulze's Deep Tissue Repair Oil is supreme – see Chapter Eleven. Avoid if the area is highly inflamed.

◆ Add to your bath 1 cup of Epsom salts, 2 cups of apple cider vinegar, together with St. John's wort and lavender flowers tied in a muslin bag.

◆ Use warm-to-cool castor oil packs on inflamed areas overnight.

## ASTHMA

This is a lung condition. During an attack, spasms cause the lung muscles to constrict and the resulting lack of air flow causes coughing, wheezing and gasping. It can develop due to irritants such as pollution, fur or house dust and mites. Strong emotions and/or lifestyle and diet can produce tension, congestion and immune breakdown. However, research suggests that 80% of asthmatic children have insufficient hydrochloric acid levels, showing that poor digestion and assimilation may lie at the bottom of this allergy. Low hydrochloric acid levels leave the person/child open to fungal and other infections, with other allergies also being a possible outcome.

✪ Follow a mucus-free diet (see Chapter Four).

✪ Look at digestion, absorption and gut flora levels.

✪ Include 1–3 cloves of garlic in your diet daily.

⚭ If in spasm, use a few drops of lobelia herb tincture. It breaks the spasm, reduces shock, and feeds the nerves while gently and safely opening up the air sacs.

⚭ Use meadowsweet on a daily basis to help establish sufficient or balanced amounts of hydrochloric acid and pepsin. Also use apple cider vinegar.

⬧ Cleansing programmes will help, especially of the bowel.

✿ For the anxiety and tension preceding the spasms, which make breathing difficult, take daily teas, capsules or tinctures of chamomile flowers, hop strobile, skullcap herb (in the long-term, for excellent results), lime tree flowers (which must be fresh as old stock is dangerous), vervain herb, wood betony herb and lavender herb.

✿ A herbalist may wish to prescribe valerian root in the short-term. This helps to quickly break the tension and usually gives much-needed sleep. However, this herb does not actually feed the nervous system as other herbs do.

✿ Cayenne pepper capsules and raw chilli will increase circulation.

✿ Take Siberian ginseng root, pfaffia root and/or pau d'arco bark which will feed badly exhausted adrenals, giving long-term support and, at the same time, will act like hydrocortisone, helping to reduce any inflammation.

✿ Immune herbs to help fight infection and bolster your immune system include pau d'arco bark and echinacea root.

✿ General lung herbs include mullein herb, horehound herb, lobelia herb and eucalyptus root as tea or tinctures.

⬧ Practise breathing exercises

⬧ Take exercise.

⬧ Useful essential oils for baths, inhaling and massage are cubeb, eucalyptus, peppermint and tea tree, which open up the bronchi and help to rid them of any attendant infection.

⬧ Use chest poultices based on essential oils and mustard – these are very warming. A drawing compress could be made from a base of 2 parts bentonite clay and 2 parts slippery elm with 1 part poke root, 1 part mullein flower, 1 part garlic clove and 1 part red clover flowers – put all the dried herb powders into a liquidiser with warmed castor oil and mix. Daub on to the chest and back. This will relieve the chest from a build-up of mucus and, in some severe cases, blood clots from bleeding lung tissue.

⬧ Hot and cold showers over the chest will open it up – especially if they are combined with a few drops of lobelia herb tincture before and after.

## Athlete's Foot

This is a fungal infection that thrives in damp conditions, living on the dead skin cells of the feet, especially between the toes.

✿ Follow all the general advice for candida, including the dietary advice.

❦ Drink pau d'arco bark decoction.

⬧ Whenever possible wear only cotton or silk socks. Otherwise wear natural fibre shoes.

⬧ At night soak your feet for 20 mins in: 1 tbsp walnut inner hull tincture or decoction, 10 drops tea tree essential oil, 2 tsps cider vinegar, 1 litre of hot water in a foot bucket or basin, then use cold water to rinse.

⬧ Avoid swimming pools and changing your socks or walking barefoot in public areas.

ॐ Dust feet with equal parts of the following finely sieved powders: neem leaf, lavender herb, chickweed herb, garlic clove and walnut leaves and fruit.

## BOILS

Boils are pus-filled nodules caused by staphylococcus bacteria infection. Found generally on the buttocks, face, neck or under the arms, they are very painful and often contagious. Children and adolescents are commonly affected. Boils need both internal and external treatment. They are a sign of toxicity and low immunity leading to bacterial overload. You need to work on the immune system, lymph system, bloodstream and any elimination channels, which may be causing or contributing to the situation.

✿ Avoid most beverages and drink plenty of water with fresh lemon juice.
ॐ Use a formula of nettle leaves, burdock root, echinacea root and barberry root bark.
◆ Home remedies include placing baked onions and pummeled raw white cabbage leaves over the boil.
ॐ Use eczema herbs as an ointment.
◆ Use a drawing poultice: $^{1}/_{2}$ cup bentonite clay, apple cider vinegar (enough to make a paste), 2 drops tea tree essential oil, 2 drops lavender essential oil, $^{1}/_{2}$ mashed clove of garlic.

## BRAIN CLARITY

Forgetfulness can sometimes come with old age or simply be a result of stress and overwork.

✿ Drink plenty of water.
✿ The brain uses a lot of essential fatty amino acids. Superfood contains them and a glass taken morning and afternoon can keep your brain alert and blood sugar levels up.
ॐ Use a combination of 3 parts prickly ash bark, 2 parts gingko leaf, 1 part rosemary herb, 1 part gotu kola nut and 1 part lobelia herb as a tincture or tea.
ॐ Keep your vascular system clear of plaque, be it composed of calcium or fatty deposits, as this clogs and slows circulation, hampering the thinking process. A lack of blood flow, oxygen and nutrients to the brain can have disastrous results and toxaemia will add to this as the body deposits toxic substances in the brain.
◆ Liver and bowel cleanses can do much to encourage brain clarity and alleviate forgetfulness.
◆ Exercise is vital for proper brain function and oxygenation.

## BREAST LUMPS – CYSTS, FIBROIDS AND MASTITIS

We are taught to feel around our breasts after each menstruation to see if anything lumpy can be found. If lumps are moveable, and come and go with the period, then, we are told, they are generally nothing to worry about. However, if they are solid, but not particularly, if at all, painful, and do not come and go with menstruation, you should seek further help.

Breast tissue is fatty and is intended to produce milk for babies. The breasts change shape and content throughout our lives, according to levels, during the cycle, of the hormones oestrogen and progesterone. It is these hormone fluctuations that can cause swelling and water retention, pain and even fibrocystic lumps that painfully lollop around the breasts. This generally occurs pre-menstrually, settling down with the onset of menstruation; however, pregnancy and the menopause can also make breast lumps decrease. It must be remembered that most lumps are benign (i.e. non-malignant) and that many thousands of women – almost one in three – have them at some stage.

## For non-cancerous conditions:

- ✿ Avoid tea and coffee, as the caffeine they contain is oestrogenic and will encourage unwanted cell growth.
- ✿ Drink plenty of water daily.
- ✿ Eat soya-based foods – especially tofu.
- ✿ Take chlorella tablets and/or Superfood.
- ✿ Follow the dietary and cleansing programme suggestions for endometriosis and for ovarian cysts and uterine fibroids.
- ∿ Take evening primrose oil or some other source of mega GLA daily.
- ∿ Throughout the month use herbs to strengthen liver function, balance the hormones and maintain the lymph and immune system. A good formula would be equal parts of squaw vine herb, agnus castus berries, milk thistle seeds, olive leaves and mullein flowers.
- ∿ After this, pre-menstrual (more progestogenic) herbs will help – see 'The Hormone Arrival' in Chapter Eight.
- ∿ Drink dandelion root coffee – 3 cups daily, as it will alleviate water retention. If it is excessive, add corn silk and other kidney herbs.
- ◆ Exercise which stimulates the circulation and gives greater energy will help – e.g. power walking, dancing and cycling.
- ◆ Warmed poultices from powdered herbs can be used in extreme situations: 2 parts slippery elm inner bark and 1 part each of bentonite clay, poke root, cayenne pepper, fresh garlic puree and charcoal crushed into a powder and moistened with castor oil. Apply this at night-time and leave on.
- ◆ Take hot and cold showers, especially over the breasts.

## BRONCHITIS

Acute bronchitis is an infection of the bronchi. Chronic bronchitis is caused by frequent irritation of the lungs due to cigarette smoke, pollutants, cold damp weather or tissue damage from old infections and can be caused in part by the excessive mucus build-up in the lungs. Symptoms include pain in the chest, coughing, fever, chills and sore throat.

- Refer to 'Coughs', 'Sinusitis' and 'The Respiratory System' (Chapter Nine).
- ✿ Remove wheat and dairy products from your diet. Depending on the severity of your bronchitis, get professional help to tailor your diet beyond these general suggestions.
- ∾ Mullein flowers help to reduce mucus and soothe inflammation. Add a little eucalyptus leaf and drink as a strong tea, three times daily (Ratio 3:1).
- ∾ Take a few drops of lobelia herb tincture every few hours.
- ∾ Other herbs to use include poke root, cleavers herb, pau d'arco bark, elecampane herb, lichen species, fennel leaf and seed, pine needles, thuja leaf and echinacea root.
- ∾ Additionally, Iceland moss and Siberian ginseng root are anti-mucus and anti-viral and they will help to generally support the body.
- ◆ Use essential oils of eucalyptus, turpineless lavender, peppermint, rosemary and cubeb in the bath, for massage, or inhaled.

## BURSITIS

This is a condition in which the small water-filled cushions between the tendons and bones in various places on the body – especially the knees, elbow joints, hips and shoulders – become inflamed. It can be caused by an accident, wear and tear, a tendency to arthritis or rheumatism, allergies or even calcium deposits.

- ∾ Helpful anti-inflammatory herbs include pau d'arco bark, devils claw root and dong quai root.
- ✿ Should the problem become chronic, adopt the same dietary programme as for arthritis and rheumatism.
- ◆ A compress using St. John's wort flower oil and a hot castor oil pack, followed by a cold shower and cold packs can bring relief.
- ◆ Stop or limit the activity that aggravates the inflammation and pain.

## CANDIDA AND ORAL THRUSH

This parasitic, yeast-like fungal infection is something that virtually every woman (an estimated one in three) has had or will have at some time in her life. Men frequently harbour it too, but without being so aware of it as women. Increasingly children are becoming prone, sometimes from birth, or after vaccination, especially the triple or multiple ones when they are very young, where the immune system is vulnerable and easily overwhelmed. Antibiotic usage also lowers the immune system and thus invites fungal infestation. Parasitic invasion often goes hand in hand with it; especially flat worms called flukes, introduced via pets and/or undercooked meat etc.

Low hydrochloric acid levels and general poor digestive powers are very often a strong causal factor in candida. Candida can occur anywhere in the body and is frequently found in the mouth, stomach, bowel, vagina or anus. But it is by its very nature a problem, infesting the entire body. It thrives in damp, humid conditions. Disease and hormonal changes in the body e.g. during pregnancy, can instigate an imbalance in the gut and bowel flora, allowing the fungus to proliferate. Visits to countries with very different standards of hygiene can also instigate its appearance. Very often, allergic reactions to foods are simply a sign that candida is present.

The symptoms include weight gain that will not shift (whatever the diet or denial), low blood sugar, alcohol intolerance, constipation or diarrhoea, PMT, depression, bloating, wind, fatigue, irritable bowel, joint swelling and pain, itching and heat in the hands and feet, reddish pink blotches of varying sizes on the face, trunk, hands, legs, feet or abdomen; anal itching and athlete's foot, fungal nail infections, night sweats, kidney and bladder infections and pains across the chest, mimicking angina.

✿ Weak digestion will cause chronic candida, so refer to dietary advice for correct digestion.

☙ Avoid the apple cider vinegar normally suggested for poor digestion and low hydrochloric acid levels. Instead, take daily meadowsweet herb, gentian rhizome and others.

✿ Consume nothing that contains antibiotics – meat and fish do most of the time. Choose organic meat and fish.

✿ Eat organic vegetables and fruit.

✿ Cut out alcohol, tea, coffee, carbonated drinks and tobacco.

✿ Eat no fruit or sugar for a period of at least two weeks. Then have occasional fruit, but no fruit juice initially because the concentration of sugar is attractive to candida fungus. Avoid fruit concentrates and frozen juices. Instead, drink fresh lemon juice in plenty of water – 2 to 4 litres daily.

✿ Consider leaky gut and other digestive weakness as it may be the initial root cause, and/or liver, bowel congestion, constipation – and treat accordingly.

✿ Eat food with plenty of uncooked, cool spices and herbs. Do not eat cooked chillies or other 'hot' foods. The heat will attract candida fungus.

✿ Cut out all yeasty or fermented foods i.e. mushrooms, Marmite and other yeast-based spreads and sauces. However, practitioners in Germany and recent trials in Britain have shown that shitake mushrooms actually help eradicate candida.

✿ Avoid all refined carbohydrates – that is, any processed junk food.

✿ Eat only whole grains and raw foods – grains, vegetables, seeds and nuts.

♦ Take the probiotic Nature's Biotics (available from Springfield Pharmacy), which will establish gut flora and kill parasites. You can also consider using aloe vera to repopulate the bowel with beneficial bacteria, capable of overpowering the fungus. Vegetable caprylic acid and lactobacillus salivarius can be extremely useful. These are available from Bio-care (See 'Resources' at the end of this chapter).

♦ Avoid tinctures because of their alcohol content. However, pouring boiling water over the tinctures and leaving them to stand for five minutes removes 98% of the alcohol. They will then be acceptable to use.

♦ 'The Three-Stage Herbal Colon Cleanse' and the worming programme (Chapter Six) are very much designed to help eliminate candida as it commonly infests the large intestine. (You may also consider 'High Enemas', see Chapter Six). Continued use of barberry root bark for bowel maintenance will be vital after the cleanse. If you are pregnant do not attempt the colon cleanse; consult a herbalist and on their suggestion use instead bowel capsules based on barberry root bark with an additional supplement for candida from Bio-care – see 'Resources' section at the end of this chapter for contact number.

♦ Perform a mild liver cleanse.

◐ Use 2 parts valerian root, 1 part chamomile flower and 1 part passion flower if sleep is a problem. Daytime nervines may also be required (see 'Nervous System' in Chapter Nine).

◐ Take 2 parts squaw vine root, 2 parts agnus castus berries and 1 part red raspberry leaves to balance the hormones. Add 2 parts Siberian ginseng root as an overall tonic, especially for adrenal and thyroid restoration.

◐ The use of the pre-menstrual herbs will help mood swings and emotions that are aggravated by candida at this time of the month!

◐ Take immune strengtheners: olive leaf, echinacea root, and, particularly, pau d'arco bark. Drink two cupfuls of the pau d'arco as a decoction once a day. (If you have 'leaky gut' then pau d'arco can aggravate – cease using it if this is the case).

◐ Include three to four whole cloves of garlic daily, in addition to that which is added to cooked food. Treat it as a medicine rather than a food source. It will decrease the levels of fungus.

◐ Grapefruit extract is also very useful, just a few daily drops will go a long way to eliminating candida.

♦ Highly diluted tea tree oil can be used to treat external fungus, but be careful to dilute it thoroughly because, if used neat or overly strong, it can cause deep, angry flesh burns. Use 5mls tea tree oil to 250mls of safflower and olive oil.

♦ Use neat lavender oil on fungus. It may tingle or even feel like burning, but it will not actually cause harm.

♦ Use candida pessaries. (See Chapter Three.)

♦ Have a daily bath with a few drops of lavender essential oil.

♦ If possible avoid oral contraceptives as they can upset the micro-organism balance in the body. Ensure that you use alternative contraception.

♦ Saunas help – but it's vital to have long, cold showers during and after the sauna, otherwise the warm, damp atmosphere will encourage fungal growth.

♦ Take hot and cold showers – always finish with cold water. Never go to bed straight after a hot bath, only after a cold shower.

♦ Get plenty of sleep and use cotton sheets. Under-bedding and quilts should also be of natural fibres as these breathe, allowing moisture to escape, and will prevent incubating the fungus further.

## CHICKENPOX

This is a highly contagious viral infection which starts with a headache, tiredness and fever. The glands around the neck will probably be swollen and some spots may be apparent on the body, face, scalp or mouth. The spotting period can last for ten days and then the scabs should fall off.

The worst thing a child can do is pick the spots. Get the child to wear gloves to prevent scratching and picking, especially at night; however, regular application of herbal powders to the affected areas will often dispel any itching.

☼ Keep the child on light foods – fruit, juices, vegetable juices, soups, etc. As Dr. Christopher always said, chickenpox thrives in a medium of excessive mucus – remove this and the virus finds it hard to survive.

∾ Use echinacea root tincture with red raspberry leaf, yarrow leaf or boneset leaf tea – sweeten with honey.

∾ Use equal parts of chamomile flower and skullcap herb to calm and soothe the child. Take as a tincture with honey added or as a tea.

∾ 3 parts burdock root and 1 part echinacea root will help flush the skin through. A composite, sweetened tincture of all these is probably the easiest method of administration, given five or six times daily – seek advice on dose.

● Two warm baths a day, with a few drops of lavender essential oil added to the water, will relax the mind and cool the skin.

● After the bath, dust down with lavender herb and marigold flower powder. If available use neem leaf powder.

● Use only cotton next to the skin and only breathable clothing or bedding over this, if necessary.

## CROHN'S DISEASE

This normally affects the small intestine, but any section of the digestive tract can be affected. Inflammation and ulcers occur and, upon healing, slowly cause a narrowing of the digestive tract. The inflammation may be a result of bacteria, due to viral infection, or allergic reactions which may be caused by dietary problems, environmental influences, drugs, or unbalanced enzyme secretions, rendering digestion incomplete. Usually the liver, pancreas and stomach are equally involved and need treatment. Other recent theories suggest that it is an RNA and DNA abnormality, a genetic and hereditary pattern. Symptoms include abdominal pain which can be excruciating, diarrhoea and symptoms similar to those found in appendicitis and fever. Abnormal weight loss can also be a factor, as can depression. A diet rich in nutritious, mild foods with herbs that fight infection and rebuild the intestinal tract will help.

☼ Drink plenty of water. Begin with a three-day carrot juice fast, juicing a bit of garlic and ginger with the carrots, and chlorophyll or algae powders and barley sprouts for 3-7 days, or drink Superfood as it contains all of the powders listed.

☼ After the carrot juice fasting, add salads (with olive oil and cider vinegar), plus fermented or cultured foods. Eat only mild fruit (very ripe papayas, bananas, mangos and steamed pineapple), and raw and steamed vegetables, such as yams and squashes – but avoid sulphurous vegetables like broccoli and cabbage.

☼ Do not use whole-grains or other fibrous foods until after the fourth week of this programme.

☼ Drink a potassium broth once or twice a day and eat all fruit and vegetables as a separate course.

☼ Avoid hot or strong spices in cooking, eat the cooler, raw ones.

☼ Use fenugreek seed, cinnamon sticks, a little nutmeg, dill, cumin, coriander, basil, parsley, thyme, marjoram and garlic frequently in cooking.

☼ Avoid dairy products, processed foods, chocolate, sugar, alcohol, tea and coffee.

☼ Avoid harsh fibrous foods such as nuts and seeds, unless they are well-soaked, freshly ground or sprouted.

☼ A diet rich in nutritious, mild foods with herbs that fight infection and rebuild the gastro-intestinal tract will help.

⚘ Women should take up to 1000mg of GLA (evening primrose oil) per day – this helps to rebalance the system.

⚘ Use acidophilus and drink aloe vera juice and apple cider vinegar to restore colon flora balance.

⚘ Take Siberian ginseng root – it is a fine general tonic.

⚘ Use 2 or 3 tsp of: 2 parts slippery elm inner bark, and 1 part each of marshmallow root, plantain leaf, comfrey leaf and wild yam root powders. Mash into a ripe banana or mix with water to soothe the bowel, take 2 or 3 times daily.

⚘ Use plenty of garlic clove, barberry root bark and echinacea root to fight infection.

⚘ Drink plenty of meadowsweet herb, fennel seed, chamomile flowers or peppermint leaf tea.

⚘ Make sure the colon is functioning correctly by using gentle herbs e.g. barberry root bark and rhubarb root. If you are suffering from diarrhoea then refer to the appropriate section in this chapter for treatment.

♦ If you are in severe pain, drink aloe vera juice or administer aloe gel as an enema for immediate cooling and soothing relief. You will need a 'high enema', (see Chapter Six). For those with painful ulcers in the mouth and throat, use as a gargle – swallow after gargling.

## Coeliac Disease

This is an intolerance to gluten (mainly found in wheat and wheat products). More specifically, the allergy is to gliadin, a protein found in gluten. The condition manifests itself as uncomfortable bloating, wind and diarrhoea, caused by chronic inflammation. A specialist will need to confirm this classification by testing for gliadin intolerance.

• Follow treatment for colitis.

☼ There is plenty to enjoy – whole-grains like brown rice, quinoa, buckwheat and millet, all of which have a greatly reduced gluten content. A gluten-free recipe book will give you further insight.

⚘ Herbal astringents may be necessary if the diarrhoea is persistent. Include yarrow herb tea with grains of bentonite clay if diarrhoea is persistently watery.

⚘ Herbal demulcents that will soothe and heal may be needed depending on the severity of the inflammation, but this can be individually gauged. Mash up some slippery elm inner bark and arrowroot into a ripe banana, or simply add to cold water and drink.

## COLD SORES – HERPES SIMPLEX

This is a very common problem and a sister to herpes zoster and chickenpox. It can remain latent in the body for years but stress, other infections, strong sunshine, hormone swings, bad diet, constipation and many other conditions can trigger it off.

○ Vitamins B, C and A and zinc must be included in your food programme: Use equal parts of carrot juice and lemon juice, including its white pith. Eat whole-grain rice with spirulina, chlorella and other algae seaweeds or Superfood and Engervita for B vitamin.
○ Avoid arginine-rich foods which include wheat products, carob, chocolate, animal gelatine, coconut, oats, peanuts and soya beans.
○ Avoid coffee, alcohol, sugar, fried foods and hot cooked spices, as these will worsen the attack.
○ The chemical lysine helps and is found in all fruits and vegetables, especially beans and bean sprouts.
∾ Immune herbs and immuno tonics will be vital to support the body generally: olive leaf, echinacea root, pau d'arco bark and Siberian ginseng root.
◆ Work on all the elimination channels – at some point you will need to perform liver, kidney and colon cleanses.
◆ Nervous system support is often necessary here (see Chapter Nine).
◆ Get plenty of rest.
◆ Put organic honey and turmeric rhizome on the cold sore during the weeping stage. Use a lavender and tea tree essential oil rub and continue use for three days after the sore has visibly gone.
◆ Saunas are helpful and encourage the cold sore to come out, peak and die down.

## COLITIS

This is inflammation of a section or sections of the colon, mostly in the mucus membranes. It is a very common problem, and is perhaps the most common of all bowel complaints. It appears to pre-empt many other diseases like ulcerative colitis, which can ensue when ulcers develop due to chronic inflammation. It can be caused by intense stress, anxiety or fear or by bacteria, especially if antibiotics have been overused. The nervous system and adrenals need support if stress is a factor; but the food you eat also has a large influence on this disease.

○ No coffee, alcohol, tea, milk or cheese should be consumed.
○ No cooked spices should be eaten; the cooler, raw spices and culinary herbs like thyme and marjoram should be used instead.
○ Fibrous foods should be avoided at this point. Instead try fruit purées (always cook with stones, pips and skins and then sieve), vegetable purées, liquidised soups and generally soft steamed or baked foods. Continue until the inflammation has subsided.

☼ Often six small meals a day will be easier to digest than three larger ones.

☼ Eat plenty of garlic in food and let it do the main work on bowel putrefaction for you.

ॐ Use equal parts of: marshmallow root, cramp bark, lobelia herb, barberry root bark, wild yam root and red clover flowers to help soothe and relax any spasms and reduce the inflammation.

ॐ Drink meadowsweet herb tea for bouts of diarrhoea and to establish balanced hydrochloric acid and pepsin levels. Chinese liquorice rhizome tea would also help any constipation (in this condition the two often alternate).

ॐ Use the herbs recommended for diverticulitis along with bayberry as a blood cleanser, because it will help the colon wall regain elasticity and encourage peristalsis.

ॐ Blessed thistle herb tea helps reduce excessive mucus production and stimulates digestion. Dr. Christopher also pointed out that it improves the tone, structure and elasticity of the bowel walls, as well as aiding detoxification.

## CONSTIPATION

The results of constipation are far-reaching – not only does it distort the colon and build up toxins but the thyroid can also become under-active due to the entire metabolism slowing down. The liver and, in particular, the gall-bladder can become stagnant and diseased. The stomach and pancreas can also suffer and even the kidneys can become alarmingly involved. Brain function becomes clearer and sharper with a clean colon. Conversely a congested colon can produce all kinds of memory and brain function problems. Skin eruptions, swollen glands, general fatigue, a consistently and increasingly inoperative immune system are some of the possible effects of constipation. The body will become more and more intolerant to specific foods as general toxicity builds up. The whole emotional pattern becomes depressed, tense, angry and, of course, uptight! As with many things, due to the complexity of their hormones, women tend to suffer much more from constipation than men do. The female abdominal structure has a part to play in this as well. Check that you do not have candida as this can cause constipation. Surgery, where cut tissue grows into scar tissue, or a malfunctioning colon caused by adhesions where the walls of the colon are growing together, may initially cause constipation. So always consider these factors. Tumours and cancers cause blockages, but so does ballooning. A good bowel programme can give you some answers as to where the difficulties lie if conventional diagnosis is inconclusive.

• Look at the 'Colon' sections in Chapters Six and Nine.

• Correct any lack of nerve nourishment (available through food and herbs) especially paying attention to magnesium and calcium.

☼ A low-fibre diet will hamper natural peristalsis; so eat plenty of raw foods and whole-grains.

☼ Mucus-forming, binding foods such as eggs, cheese, potato starch and other starches, like white bread, custard and pasta must be avoided because they gum up the colon.

○ Raw food with plenty of fibre is very helpful.

○ Take plenty of beneficial flora-rich foods: make rejuvelac (see Chapter Four) and eat sauerkraut.

○ Plant proteins and fats, for example nuts and avocado, are important and should form part of your generally balanced diet.

○ Drink plenty to enable the bowel to move properly. Urination following a bowel movement signals that the bowel is completely empty. Two litres of fluid, mostly water, a day is a minimum requirement for good bowel movements. Always drink a half pint of water and fresh lemon juice first thing in the morning.

○ Soups made from whole grain organic wheat with lots of onions, garlic, black pepper and raw chillies will help.

ॐ Every day bowel management with herbs will be helpful. We have talked about the use of strong herbs to get the bowel working and about the softer bowel herbs, like barberry root bark, in Chapter Nine and 'The Three-Stage Herbal Colon Cleanse' featured in Chapter Six. Your bowel may be in need of a combination of these from time to time – even with a good diet and plenty of drinking water and exercise. Often, constipated people become worse when they are sick, while others may get diarrhoea when they are fasting, nervous or excited. So use both these types of formulas and recognise the interchangeability of the two. You need to find a balance that will work for you.

♦ Always go to the toilet when you need to, and if possible use a foot stool to keep the bowel at a more natural height – more like squatting.

♦ Avoid excessive worry.

♦ Do not sit a lot. Take regular exercise, especially if you are elderly. Ensure that a regular walk is included in your daily routine. Cycling and riding are both excellent for massaging the bowel.

♦ Hot and cold showers especially over the colon.

♦ Do not use drug laxatives.

♦ Drugs, whether GP-given or ones like heroin and opium, often over-stimulate or completely freeze peristalsis. Antibiotics can kill off beneficial flora, causing constipation. Even small doses of antibiotics can set the pattern for years of constipation.

## COUGHS

This is, in the main, an important reflex action provoked by various irritations in order to expel mucus. However, the reflex also works when there is nothing to expel, due to irritation of the mucus membrane.

○ If it is a dry, hacking cough with little mucus and sweating, then consume a lot of raw fruits and juices.

○ If there is a lot of mucus and congestion, avoid cold fruits and juices and use more warming foods like garlic and onion soups.

○ Take plenty of fluids – especially water and fresh lemon juice – and go directly to bed.

✿ Herbalist Dr. Richard Schulze has a wonderful kitchen home remedy for coughs and colds, and this alone can do the job. See Chapter Seven for the recipe ('Hooch'). Take between 2 and 10tsp up to five times daily, gargle with it and then swallow.

୶ As a preventative measure in winter, drink home-made elderberry and elder flower syrup. It encourages perspiration and provides valuable vitamins and minerals. (Refer to Chapter Three.) Take 1tsp at a time: 3–6 times daily.

୶ A tincture or syrup can also be made with wild cherry, myrrh resin, barberry root bark, liquorice rhizome, lobelia herb, poke root, cayenne pepper, and marshmallow root: this will promote the healthy removal of mucus and encourage productive coughing, while helping the lungs expand and the immune system to strengthen.

୶ Use mullein flowers, plantain herb and red clover flower tea, while other useful traditional herbs that can be excellent are horehound herb, elecampane herb and yarrow herb.

୶ For a prolonged, deep-seated cough take Siberian ginseng root for tonic, support and recovery.

◆ Soaking one's feet in a bucket of hot water with mustard powder added to it is a great way of heating and sweating the body, but the individual must be naturally strong. Then, massage an oil mix of eucalyptus into the chest and soles of the feet – already hot and yellow from the mustard!

◆ A sprinkling of eucalyptus on pillows and sheets is very helpful.

## CYSTITIS AND PROSTITIS

These very painful bacterial bladder infections create a scalding pain before, during and after urination. They also urge the bladder to constantly try and empty, even if there is no more urine left to expel. The urine may be cloudy and have an unpleasant odour. Cystitis is a commonly known problem to women, partly due to their shorter urethra and its closeness to the rectum, making cross infection more likely. A variety of spinal non-alignments can have an effect here, therefore a visit to a chiropractor could be worthwhile. Candida often goes hand in hand with cystitis and helping one often helps the other. Men also get cystitis and then the prostate needs to be examined.

✿ Avoid highly acidic food and drinks (coffee, tea, alcohol, chocolate); instead drink lots of alkaline fluids, like fresh lemon juice in spring water. (For acid/alkaline foods see Chapter Four.)

✿ Put 3 tsp of apple cider vinegar into a little apple juice and drink four times daily.

✿ Drink home-made barley water (see Chapter Four for recipe).

✿ Drink unsweetened cranberry juice or a drink made from dried cranberries soaked in water overnight. Do not drink supermarket cranberry drinks, as they tend to be loaded with undesirable additives.

✿ Raw foods and juices are alkaline, so concentrate on these; they will also strengthen your overall immune system if you are not a 'cold' type of person and underweight. If you have problems with excess roughage because of bowel problems, consult a natural healer for alternative suggestions.

✿ To help fight the bacterial infection, include garlic and thyme in your cooking.

❧ Every two hours drink a tea containing equal amounts of yarrow leaves, dandelion root, cleavers leaves and marshmallow root. Should there be blood in the urine, add corn silks because this will encourage rapid water release as well as soothing the inflammation and consequent bleeding. An equal part of juniper berries will help disinfect the area and act as a diuretic.

❧ Take olive leaf, echinacea root tincture for ten days and turmeric rhizome for three or four days, depending on the severity of the cystitis. In the case of prostitis, add saw palmetto berries.

🌢 Have regular baths and showers to keep yourself clean. Apple cider vinegar in the bath water will help, plus a few drops of any or all of the following: cedar wood, eucalyptus, bergamot, lavender or juniper essential oils. Don't stay in the bath too long, keep the water warm rather than hot.

🌢 Wear a long skirt or baggy trousers and no underwear if possible. Alternatively wear loose-fitting cotton or silk underwear. Avoid tight constricting clothing made from man-made fibres.

🌢 Make sure your bowels are moving at least two or three times daily because your carefully selected fluid intake will disinfect and cleanse the bacteria from the system. However, if these harmful toxins are left to stay in the system too long, re-infection will occur and healing will be a slow process.

🌢 Avoid being cold and chilled, take time for yourself to heal and spend time in bed if possible with natural fibre bedding.

## DANDRUFF

Dandruff is commonly caused by an imbalance in the oil secreting glands or by a slight fungal infection, so check that you haven't got candida or oral thrush. If there is a hormone or endocrine imbalance then this may also cause dandruff.

✿ No coffee, tea, sugar and junk food should be consumed.

✿ Switch to a wholefood diet.

✿ Eat plenty of garlic, olive oil, cider vinegar and lemon juice – whole-grains, fruit and vegetables.

❧ Consider hormone balancing and anti-fungal herbs.

🌢 A hair water made with ylang ylang, rosemary, sage, thyme and tea tree essential oils will help, or make your own rosemary water with 250mls spring water to 5mls of rosemary essential oil; use apple cider vinegar and water as a rinsing agent.

## DEPRESSION

This subject is too diverse to discuss here, but some general tips include:

✿ Eat healthily, drink plenty of water (especially if you are not using drugs to help with your depression) and increase your intake of zinc doses, for instance, pumpkin seeds.

ᨰ Support the adrenal glands with herbs, as they are often exhausted in this condition. Ask a qualified herbalist if St. John's wort tincture would be suitable.
🌢 Liver and colon cleansing will help.
🌢 Exercise often.

## DERMATITIS

This literally means inflammation of the skin. This inflammation can be due to an infection, or an allergic reaction, caused either by direct contact (as with some metals or animal hair) or through external factors – sunlight, perfumes and paints. Atopic dermatitis is hereditary in an allergy sense and dermatitis herpetiformis is a very itchy type associated with intestinal problems and disorders triggered by dairy products and wheat etc. Another type of dermatitis, caused by a malfunction of the sebaceous glands, causes greasy skin. The vitamins B6 and B2 are vital and a lack of them can cause dermatitis. With all forms of dermatitis, attention to the adrenal glands, nervous system, immune system and all the eliminative channels, especially the liver and colon, are vital.

✿ Follow a one or two-day fast on papayas or ripe bananas, with the help of a practitioner. Continue with large proportions of raw foods including lots of garlic.
✿ Eat whole-grains, non-active yeast flakes like Engervita and B vitamins, as found in seaweeds.
✿ Include virgin olive oil in the daily diet and use linseed seeds or capsules.
✿ Eat plenty of seeds, nuts, sprouted seeds and beans, and sometimes cooked beans and seeds.
ᨰ Take evening primrose oil (Mega GLA) capsules.
ᨰ Use blood cleansing herbs. Try 3 parts burdock root, 2 parts red clover flowers and 1 part dandelion root.
🌢 Liver and bowel cleanses and detoxification programmes are helpful. See Chapter Six.
🌢 Dr. Christopher often got patients to wash in a decoction of equal parts of burdock root, chickweed herb and marshmallow root which soothes. Alternatively, sponge yourself down using a mixture of plantain leaf and chickweed herb.
• See psoriasis and eczema for further herbal information.

## DIABETES

This affects over 1% of people in the West. In America, the land of sugar and junk food, it is the direct cause of 1 in 7 deaths. Diabetes manifests when the body fails to regulate the metabolism of glucose via a pancreatic hormone. If the pancreas is unable to produce enough glucose, or if the body is simply unable to process that which is present, then other organs – primarily the thyroid, adrenal and pituitary glands – will become involved leading to their eventual decline. In some cases, diseases or dysfunction of these glands can actually result in diabetes. If there is a history of diabetes in your family, it is advisable to take preventative action through childhood and on into adulthood.

Those who have diabetes before the age of 25 are classed as juvenile diabetics and it is believed that auto-immune factors may be involved. After the age of 40 it is classified as late-onset diabetes. Conventional treatment of the problem involves daily insulin injections. However, those with less severe diabetes can measure their urine periodically and use tablets to control their blood sugar levels. If you suffer from hypoglycaemia, then be aware that it is possible that this may develop into diabetes, if it becomes severe.

High blood glucose levels (with glucose-starved cells) can lead to weight loss, thirst, and an increase in the amount of urine passed each day. If untreated, the person will begin to feel weak and can eventually pass out or even fall into a coma. Trauma, stress and shock can push a person into late onset diabetes.

✪ Three to six large cloves of garlic per day would be a minimum requirement. It balances the amount of sugar in the blood by producing more insulin.

✪ Eating enough of the right things at the right time is important in the control of diabetes. At no time should the person ever fast. Diabetes is all about maintaining correct carbohydrate metabolism. Food should be high in fibre and complex carbohydrates with the correct protein levels to balance the carbohydrate ratio.

✪ No tea, coffee, alcohol or fruit juices.

✪ All sugars are to be totally avoided. Use instead rice syrup in minute quantities, barley malt, unrefined cane juice and stevia herb. Very occasionally you can use small amounts of raw unheated honey. Also avoid fructose, dextrose and molasses.

✪ Nourishing 'earthy' foods will be invaluable – but make sure you choose the right ones: seaweeds and wholegrains like rice, millet, quinoa, oats and barley are all good. Avoid all processed grains. Try the sweeter vegetables like Jerusalem artichokes, pumpkins, burdock root, onion and parsnips. Avoid potatoes, yams and carrots.

✪ Avoid bread but, if necessary, eat rye bread.

✪ Six small and easily digestible meals a day may be better than three large ones.

✪ Oats are rich in many vitamins and minerals and are generally very nourishing. They can slow the rate of sugar metabolism, thus aiding the work of the pancreas. Organic oats are best, they can be soaked overnight in spring water and cinnamon powder and eaten for breakfast.

✪ Seaweeds, especially hijiki, normalise blood sugar levels. Cook them with wholegrains and add to salads and soups.

✪ Drink one cup of home-made barley water daily (see recipe, Chapter Four).

✪ At least one or two apples per day are the best fruit for diabetics. Wild fruits, like blackberries, bilberries, quince and pomegranate, with their naturally sharp and bitter flavours, are also suitable. Do not drink fruit in their juiced forms, the sugar content will be too high.

✪ Other suitable fruits are pears, grapefruit, grapes (in small quantities) and bananas. Bananas are known to lower blood sugar levels, but only use over-ripe (nearly black) ones and only have two or three a week.

✪ Dried figs, dates, raisins and other dried fruits are best avoided by diabetics, due to their high sugar content. If they are eaten they must be soaked for at least 12 hours.

❖ Cut down on or cut out meat, especially red meat. Use vegetable protein sources instead (see Chapter Four). Avoid milk and cheese.

❖ Drinks containing nettles and alfalfa, among others, are invaluable, giving almost instantaneous energy and providing good nourishment between meals. Or, drink Superfood.

❖ Zinc levels must be maintained.

❖ All vegetables, raw and steamed, are helpful, particularly those that are opposite to sweet in taste, i.e. sour and bitter like chicory, dandelion leaves, artichokes and olives.

• Ideally, individual patients should seek more detailed advice from their own health practitioners, in order to address their particular needs, be they overweight, underweight or have any other important, different traits.

ॐ Fenugreek seed and burdock root both contain a substance called inulin which is very close to insulin. Make strong teas (simmered for twenty minutes) of these and drink one to three cups daily.

ॐ Meadowsweet herb tea or tincture will balance and heal digestive problems.

ॐ Individual herbal advice should be sought, but herbs like dandelion root, fenugreek seeds (1 month on, 1 month off), Siberian ginseng root, garlic bulb, cayenne peppers, juniper berries, wild yam root, burdock root and barberry root bark all help balance insulin levels.

ॐ Numerous other herbs are capable of beneficially activating the pancreas. Cascara sagrada is one example and has long been recognised by conventional medicine as being highly useful. All endocrine herbs will be invaluable and individual tailoring for the recipient will be required by a professional.

◆ Liver and colon cleanses and herbs will be necessary. (See Chapter Six.)

◆ Hot and cold showers.

◆ Juniper essential oil in bath water or added to a massage oil.

◆ If the pancreas is swollen, try hot castor oil packs. (See Chapter Three.)

◆ Stress and shock (both in the past and present) are an emotional factor in diabetes and such situations should be avoided by major lifestyle changes if necessary. Work on enjoyable exercise, relaxation and meditation.

## DIARRHOEA

Occasional diarrhoea lasting only two or three days is usually the result of an infection; it is nature's way of expelling the offending bacteria (or whatever) from the body. Because of this, the diarrhoea shouldn't be suppressed with drugs as people so often wish to. The body needs to rid itself of these digestive poisons as quickly as possible. If it lasts a long time the body will become weakened and if this happens the body will eventually exhaust itself through dehydration in its efforts to keep cleansing itself. If diarrhoea lasts longer than three days and recurs between bouts of constipation, then it may well be advisable to talk to a natural healer or GP about the possibility of having irritable bowel, colitis, coeliac disease or a worm infestation. Refer to the relevant sections in this chapter. If diarrhoea is affecting babies, small children or the very elderly, then special care must be taken. It should be closely monitored if it continues for longer than twenty-four hours, to prevent dehydration. Teething also causes diarrhoea.

## For Occasional Diarrhoea

✧ Make barley water (see Chapter Four).
✧ If you are able to, eat chopped garlic cloves, dipped in honey, to help with administration.
◆ Take acidophilus capsules to help the bowel flora, or home-made rejuvelac if no acidophilus is available.
❧ Raspberry leaf tea, meadowsweet leaf tea and slippery elm inner bark powders, mashed into a ripe banana will help slow down the diarrhoea and provide nutrition. Arrowroot could replace the slippery elm inner bark. Should all the latter not be readily available, try grated apples which have been left to turn brown.
❧ Take 2 parts echinacea root, 1 part chamomile flowers and 1 part barberry root bark or turmeric rhizome as a tincture to help fight infection if there is any present.

## For Babies

❧ Chamomile flower tea and home-made barley water (see Chapter Four), given by bottle or feeder mug, will help diarrhoea. If the baby is not too young, you can also try other ideas mentioned to help diarrhoea.
❧ For very severe bouts take oak bark or yarrow leaf tea as their astringent qualities will help. Alternatively, use very small amounts of bentonite clay. This should only be done with professional help, as it is very strong.

## Herbs for a Fragile Colon, e.g. for those who Suffer from Regular Diarrhoea

❧ Feeding and soothing herbs: use 3 parts slippery elm inner bark, together with 1 part of each of the following powdered herbs: chamomile flower, marshmallow root, liquorice root and peppermint leaf. Add 1–3 tsp of this mixture to a mashed ripe banana with the powder 3 times daily.
❧ Other useful herbs are: red raspberry leaves, cramp bark, meadowsweet herb, marshmallow root, yellow dock root, wild yam root, marigold flowers and turkey rhubarb root.
◆ Massage – very soft movements are vital. Use essential oils of cubeb, chamomile, geranium and lavender. You could also put them on an oil cloth and place under a hot water bottle over the area.

## DIVERTICULITIS

This is a condition where the mucus membranes have consistently remained so inflamed that pockets have developed in the bowel wall. Should these pockets grow larger they will become increasingly capable of catching the passing and occasionally sluggish faecal matter. These wastes will build up in the pockets which will then become toxic, through bacteria breeding and increasing. This can lead to inflamed areas which very often bleed. It is usually this point of chronic inflammation that produces pain, bloating and blood loss – all noticeable warnings that help must be sought.

✿ Any fibrous indigestible pieces of food, particularly raw skins of fruits and vegetables or their seeds, can easily set off intense pain and, although the problem has usually started through a lack of raw fibrous and unrefined food in the diet, this is not the time to introduce it.

✿ Nutritious baby food must be adopted – try cooking apples stewed in spring water with their skins, seeds and core, with cinnamon and a pinch of nutmeg. Sieve the pulp and eat a bowl of this apple purée daily with a tsp each of arrowroot, slippery elm and marshmallow root stirred in, with an added tsp of cinnamon. Honey may be added for taste. Continue until the inflammation, bleeding and pain subside.

✿ Gently inch into more raw foods. Buy a juicer – juicing fruits and vegetables will give first-class nutrition and aid easy digestion. Superfood is another option and is perhaps the easiest method of providing an instant, nutritious meal.

✿ When the colon has started to heal itself, try steaming your vegetables. Also try small amounts of very finely grated, de-skinned carrots and beetroot as an initial means of introducing raw foods. Make vegetable purées in the liquidiser, but leave the skins on.

✿ After a few weeks, rice and all the other whole-grains can be tried, but chewing has to become a must, so that all food arrives in the colon well mushed and changed beyond recognition of its earlier fibre content!

✿ Following the initial introduction of the apple purée mixture detailed above, continue with the following recommended regime as the new diet unfolds:

✿ Drink alfalfa tea and Superfood daily to support and replace vital vitamins and minerals.

ᦰ Drink aloe gel daily to soothe and heal.

ᦰ Take equal parts of echinacea root for immune support and pau d'arco bark tincture for viral and fungal build-up or choose olive leaf for all situations.

ᦰ A daily supportive herb would be Siberian ginseng root.

ᦰ Use 2 parts slippery elm inner bark, 1 part marshmallow root, 1 part chamomile flowers, 1 part peppermint leaf and ½ part liquorice rhizome powders, made into a smooth paste with water or mashed into a banana. Take 2 to 3 tsp daily; this will help soothe, heal and re-grow the damaged tissue.

◆ Colon cleansing and support will be required.

◆ For acute pain, use sitz baths and castor oil packs.

## DUODENAL ULCERS

These ulcers can often occur when the valve which controls the release of parts of the stomach contents into the duodenum gets a little stuck, thus allowing too much acid into an alkaline area, causing inflammation, pain and eventually ulcers. The cause of the 'stuck' valve is very often nerve-related, with stress being a large contributing factor.

- See Gastric Ulcers.
- ✿ Drink plenty of water. Dr Shamim Daya (a GP, herbalist and nutritionist) believes that drinking enough daily water is one of the simplest and best treatments for duodenal ulcers.
- ✺ Add a percentage of astringent herbs like bayberry or cranesbill to your everyday diet. Also include soothing ones like meadowsweet herb, marshmallow root, aloe vera and slippery elm bark.
- ✺ Treat the nerves. Use chamomile flower tea. Take 5 drops of lobelia herb tincture at high stress times – up to ten times a day. Valerian rhizome and passion flower will be invaluable to quickly calm and promote a peaceful, easy sleep. Take 1 tsp of skullcap herb, three times a day, for three to four months as well.
- ◆ Practise deep-breathing.
- ◆ Take walks, practise yoga or dance.
- ◆ Use relaxing essential oils in the bath.
- ◆ Watch funny, non-serious television programmes.

## Ear Infections

These lead to the ear canal becoming inflamed and swollen. Ear infections are common in babies and children. Common causes are food allergies, especially to dairy products, bacterial invasion of the ear, or a build-up of ear wax.

- ✿ Avoid wheat, dairy products and sugar if possible and investigate any other food allergies.
- ✺ Ear infections are best dealt with by using Dr. Christopher's 'B & B Ear Formula' (See Chapter Eleven) This formula helps to clear the actual infection as well as the lymph system and sinuses. Always warm the formula to body temperature before use. Mastoiditis, which is caused by an abscess or boil in the middle ear, can also be treated with this formula, as can ringing in the ears.
- ◆ Avoid swimming during an infection.

## Eczema

This may make the skin hot or cold, dry or suppurating. Each type must be treated accordingly and, depending on its severity, may require more individual and specialised help. It can be caused by food allergies and is likely to indicate inefficient digestion, particularly low levels of hydrochloric acid and pepsin, and a sluggish liver. Stress will exacerbate the problem, as will a delicate nervous system.

- Refer to dermatitis and psoriasis.
- ✿ Cold, scaly skin will be best helped by keeping to an eating programme of slow-cooked, warming foods, including grains and root vegetables and containing additional warming ingredients such as cinnamon.
- ✿ Wheat and dairy foods are common problem foods, but ensure that the soya foods and soya milk you substitute do not cause allergic reactions.
- ✿ Drink lots of water daily.

✿ Linseed oil (rich in Omega 3) is a good supplement; also use evening primrose oil (Mega GLA), for Omega 6.

✿ Oxalic acid foods can also cause disturbances, so be aware of sources such as tomatoes, oranges, gooseberries, strawberries and rhubarb.

✿ Use olive oil in cooking and raw on salads, the latter with apple cider vinegar; both of which are good for the skin.

∾ Immune and nervous system herbs will be important – olive leaf, echinacea root, Siberian ginseng root, skullcap herb and a little lobelia herb.

∾ Digestive herbs like meadowsweet herb, blessed thistle herb and aloe vera juice will be vital.

∾ Blood cleansing herbs. Use 2 parts burdock root, 1 part red clover flower and 1 part dandelion root.

♦ Use eczema ointment. (See Chapter Eleven.)

♦ Liver, bowel and stomach all need attention in terms of function, cleansing and support.

## Infantile eczema

• Sometimes, babies are born with eczema – in which case, the mother, if she is breast-feeding, must be treated.

∾ Very small amounts of simple herbs like burdock root and meadowsweet herb can be put into a bottle and given to the baby separately, if the baby can drink from one. If not, then the mother should drink the tea 2 or 3 times daily.·

♦ De-stressing by dancing, exercising and meditating is ideal.

## ENDOMETRIOSIS

Endometrial cells line the wall of the uterus and build up each month until being shed at the time of menstruation. Endometriosis is when this lining produces small nests of stray cells which are transported out of the womb and into the fallopian tubes, bladder, ovaries and elsewhere – sometimes even reaching as far as the lungs. The tissue still behaves as if it were in the womb and continues to fluctuate with the cyclic hormonal changes. Wherever these stray cells settle, they will bleed monthly, coinciding with the menstrual cycle. This blood collects and stagnates, causing toxic build-ups which eventually become inflamed and develop into blood-filled cysts (chocolate cysts). There is, of course, a great deal of pain associated with this condition. The cause of endometriosis is unknown, but poor hygiene, the use of man-made fibres in underwear, repeated infections including P.I.D., dirty surgical implements, dirty hands and fingers, tampons, retained placenta and all manner of outside poisoning sources create infections. Sluggish periods with inadequate emptying of the womb each month could also be a possibility. However, endometrial cells have been found in young girls, which does suggest a genetic link. While the causes of endometriosis are not really understood, recent information suggests that a poorly functioning immune system might, in part, be responsible. If the immune system is not functioning properly, any invasive straying cells, which should be instantaneously killed off, are not. Instead they travel through the bloodstream or lymph system and are deposited in other organs, e.g. the lungs.

If this disorder is caught early on, many positive steps can be taken, but treatment must be very committed and consistent. Orthodox methods of surgery and drugs can be used, but male steroid drugs like Danazol, which prevent a woman from menstruating, have alarming side-effects. Many patients feel very depressed on it, and an increasing number of GP's prefer not to use it. As in pregnancy (another suggested 'cure' for endometriosis) it is designed to work by giving the body a chance to stop menstruating. Another treatment consists of giving synthetic progesterone, but this does not suit all women or even help the situation.

Symptoms can include pelvic pain – especially around ovulation and menstruation – irregular or excessive menstrual bleeding, backache (lower back especially), painful lovemaking, infertility, discomfort in the stomach, small intestine and large intestine, painful urination, prolonged menstrual bleeding, and constipation and diarrhoea in fluctuation.

## Areas that should be Considered when Treating this are

✿ Maintain a good diet of whole-grains, vegetables and plenty of citrus fruit. Include Superfood.

✿ Avoid meats, dairy products and eggs which have been produced on synthetic hormones.

✿ Avoid coffee, tea and chocolate, as they also produce extra oestrogen. Avoid alcohol because it harms the liver, which must remain healthy.

~ For excessive bleeding use equal parts of yarrow herb and alfalfa herb.

~ There is always a possibility that infection may be lurking. To deal with this, use barberry root bark at the beginning of the programme.

♦ The colon, liver and kidneys will all vitally need to undergo cleansing.

~ Liver herbs like wild yam root, barberry root bark, cinnamon sticks, dandelion root and milk thistle seeds will be essential.

~ The immune system should be functioning efficiently; include herbs like pau d'arco bark, Siberian ginseng root and echinacea root.

~ Use endocrine herbs to balance and tone the system (avoiding those that encourage oestrogen production). Use a combination of 3 parts false unicorn root, 2 parts squaw vine herb, 2 parts agnus castus berries, and 1 part each of alfalfa herb, sarsaparilla root, Chinese liquorice rhizome, and red raspberry leaves.

~ For excessive cramps and pain, use equal parts of lobelia herb, pasque flower, black cohosh root and cramp bark.

♦ Lose weight if you need to, because fat stores oestrogen. Take 1 mega GLA and spirulina to facilitate weight loss and help with pains and cramps. Increase fibre in your diet, this also absorbs oestrogen and helps remove it through the bowel.

♦ Use vaginal pessaries (see Chapter Eleven) every third night and douche with herbs at least once a week – these methods will help the body to rid the area of localised infection and, encourage the re-growth of normal tissue.

◆ Hot and cold showers and sitz baths will help to maintain circulation in the womb area; this is vital for the healing process.

◆ For pain, use a hot castor oil pack over the area.

ᨠ For pain herbs try coryadalis tuber and poppy petal tincture.

## EMPHYSEMA, PLEURISY AND PNEUMONIA

These are viral, bacterial lung infections which can be exacerbated or caused by pollution and stress. They all need professional attention, but the general directions for home care are strongly advised.

• Refer to the 'Respiratory System' section in Chapter Nine.

## GASTRIC ULCERS

This is very often the culmination of long-term stomach problems, resulting in excessive acidity which can literally 'burn' the stomach walls, leaving them inflamed and even bleeding. It can also mean that mucus membranes of the gut wall are no longer able to function in a healthy way, so that acid and digestive enzymes come in contact with the wall and erode, disturb and irritate. The result is an ulcer, which is very painful. A condition known as 'leaky gut syndrome' can also develop and produce a knee-jerk reaction which increases barrier protection. This 'armour' produces a knock-on effect of larger-than-normal molecules being absorbed by the gut. This, in turn, creates an immune response and general allergy reaction. Both conditions should be treated in the same way.

✿ Start each morning with a glass of spring water and fresh lemon juice – this eradicates excess hydrochloric acid and removes any lingering food from the night before. It can also encourage the correct production of hydrochloric acid.

✿ Foods should be easily digestible, non-fatty, with no cooked spices, nuts or highly fibrous food.

✿ Include culinary herbs to aid digestion, such as fennel, gentian, caraway, mint, ginger and basil.

✿ Eat apple purée, rice, puréed vegetables and all easily digestible foods (see Chapter Four) while the healing process is taking place.

✿ Eat pineapples and papayas for extra digestive help; include aloe vera juice as a drink to prevent any harm to the stomach walls.

✿ Take 1 tbsp of cider vinegar daily in half a cup of apple juice.

✿ Food intake should be slow, unhurried and calm. Chewing should be thorough and slow. Eating and no talking can be helpful initially.

ᨠ If a major cause of the ulcer is stress and worry, take chamomile flower tea to feed and calm the nervous system. Valerian rhizome will be invaluable in the short term.

❧ Daily meadowsweet herb will help to soothe balance stomach acids and general digestive enzymes.

❧ 3 tsp of slippery elm inner bark powder mashed into a ripe banana should be taken 3 times daily before meals. This regime can replace meals altogether on very bad days and simply more quantity can be consumed if hungry.

❧ Very often the cause of gastric ulcers is nerve-related, so nerve soothers and feeders will be useful. Try equal amounts of chamomile flowers, wood betony herb, skullcap herb and wild lettuce leaves. For short-term usage take valerian rhizome.

◆ Liver and bowel cleanses will be vital. (See Chapter Six.)

❧ To heal the ulcer, use powders of: 3 parts slippery elm inner bark, 2 parts marshmallow root, 2 parts meadowsweet herb and 1 part barberry root bark. These can be mixed with aloe vera gel and eaten as a 'mush' with honey, several times a day. These herbs will coat, heal, allow tissue regrowth and sustain a lubricated seal between incoming food, stomach acids, and the painful ulcer.

◆ Exercise, sing, dance and meditate to relieve any stress.

## GASTRITIS

This literally means inflammation of the stomach. It may be due to a number of causes. Very often it is not so much an infection as a condition brought about by the fierce acidity of the digestive juices (which is usually enough to kill most bacteria). Often, poisons have been swallowed – sometimes in the form of bacteria on food or from improperly prepared or preserved foods. Alcohol, aspirin or even tar from cigarettes are other causes.

✿ Fasting is recommended in this situation to give the stomach as little to work upon – or to revolt against – as possible. It is best to drink water at room temperature (that is, neither hot nor cold).

✿ The first foods should be onion and garlic soup, alternated with slippery elm powder stirred into water or a ripe banana. (Or, try the herbal formula of powdered slippery elm inner bark, marshmallow root, liquorice rhizome and peppermint leaves).

◆ Take acidophilus capsules to help repopulate beneficial bowel flora.

❧ When you are able to keep things down, take echinacea tincture diluted in water.

❧ Take cayenne pepper to rebuild the mucous membrane lining and take daily meadowsweet.

## GERMAN MEASLES – RUBELLA

This is another viral infection, which, if you are lucky, can be very mild. Starting with a sore throat and swollen lymph glands, often accompanied by a reddening of the eyelids, rubella will graduate into a reddish rash of small pink spots starting on the face and spreading down over the body. The itching is difficult for about three days but, after this, things generally improve.

Children with German measles should be kept away from pregnant women.

✿ Follow the diet for mumps and chickenpox.
ᘄ Internally use immuno aids like echinacea, barberry root and garlic clove.
◖ Treatment of the skin is very much the same as for chickenpox.
◖ For swollen glands treat in the same way as mumps.

## GLANDULAR FEVER

This begins with flu-like symptoms – aches, tiredness, runny nose, etc., and occasionally a rash similar to German measles. This is a herpes-like organism called Epstein-Barr virus. The lymph glands in the neck swell and, very occasionally, there are rashes, a sore throat or digestive upset.

A blood test will confirm glandular fever, and this can be useful as it can last months. It should be handled very, very carefully as post-viral fatigue syndrome can easily ensue if the body's energies are not supported and fortified. It has become a common precursor of ME.

✿ Excellent food programmes will be vital: start with juices and Superfood.
✿ Reduce protein intake (meat, eggs, fish, etc.)
• See fever in Chapter Seven and mumps in this chapter.
◖ Perform colon, liver and kidney cleanses and use herbs for these areas (see Chapter Six).
ᘄ Siberian ginseng root will be vital for general long-term adaptogenic support.
ᘄ Immune herbs such as echinacea root, myrrh resin and poke root alongside blood cleansers like burdock root and dandelion root will also be needed.
◖ Include very moderate exercise and massage.

## GOUT

This is really a variation on the theme of arthritis and rheumatism. Uric acid builds up to high levels in the joints, causing inflammation and pain. The condition can be exacerbated by excessive alcohol or acid-forming food intake.

✿ Moving body fluids via the kidneys will help; use home-made barley water for this. (See Chapter Four.)
ᘄ Yarrow herb, milk thistle seed, dandelion root, burdock root and celery seed are all useful herbs.
◖ Cooling and clearing the liver and making sure the bowel is cleansed will be important.
◖ Castor oil packs will relieve pain.
◖ Hot and cold showers will encourage healing and relieve stiffness.

## HAEMORRHOIDS (PILES) AND ANAL FISSURE

Haemorrhoids are ballooning flaps of skin in the rectum and/or anus which are very painful, usually more so when passing a motion, as they are irritated by the pressure. An anal fissure forms when weakened and stretched tissue has split, remaining as a wound that is constantly sore and difficult to heal.

With haemorrhoids (or piles) it's important to consider the state of the whole digestive system, including constipation, diarrhoea, bowel irritability and liver function, which is often found to be faulty in this situation.

♦ Use a mixture of black walnut inner hulls, a little oak bark and some yarrow herb, marshmallow root to soothe, myrrh resin to disinfect, a touch of cayenne pepper in case of bleeding, and some rhubarb as an all-round bowel balancer. Make into an ointment with a base of olive oil and coconut butter with benzoin essential oil and witch hazel essential oil. Use the ointment very frequently, before and after bowel movements and in between if possible. The same herbs can be mixed as powders. Use equal parts, put into capsules and take daily. Neat or diluted witch hazel can help for quick relief.

✪ Drink plenty of water and eat fibre in the form of fruit and vegetables.

❧ Aloe vera juice and meadowsweet herb tea will be two basic herbs to start with.

♦ A slant board treatment will be useful. (See Chapter Five.)

♦ Take cold sitz baths which can help severely prolapsed piles, as can sitting on bags of frozen peas at intervals.

❧ An anal suppository (see Chapter Three) will help heal and support the area. Useful herbs would be barberry bark powder, walnut powder, a pinch of cayenne and witch hazel essential oil.

## HAY FEVER

This is an allergy to pollen which is attracted by the sticky mucus in the body. Symptoms may range from watery, itchy eyes to blocked sinuses and sneezing, a constricted chest, which can cause, bring on or mimic asthma, and general nasal and sinus inflammation. It is an allergy possibly stemming from poor digestive capabilities and a weak immune system, often linked to weak adrenal glands.

✪ Change your diet (see Chapter Four). Start by cutting out wheat, dairy products, tea and coffee. If your diet is already good, you are probably low immunally, or simply have poor digestive abilities, stress, pollution, etc.

✪ Taking local organic honey year-round can provide a 'natural' immunity. 1–2 grains of pollen daily, taken consistently, is the key, especially for the one and a half months prior to your particular pollen season.

♦ Your immune system needs strengthening; refer to Chapter Seven for advice.

♦ Liver and bowel cleanses will be vital to address intestinal and digestive imbalances.

❧ General herbs to address all the above issues would include: 4 parts mullein flowers, 3 parts echinacea root, 3 parts burdock, 2 parts barberry root bark, 2 parts elder flowers 2 parts marshmallow root, 2 parts astragalus root (2 parts St. John's wort flower), 2 parts eyebright herb, 1 part gentian root, 1 part lobelia herb, 1 part cayenne pods and 1 part liquorice rhizome. Many others will work for different reasons.

❧ Plantain herb is a natural anti-histamine and soothes irritated mucus membranes as well as helping with actual infections. It also dissolves mucus and, being so common, like elder flowers, it's an easy plant to identify and collect away from car fumes. Meadowsweet herb would do a similar job, in addition to helping digestive juices to be produced in the correct balance.

◆ Make your own rose petal oil – it helps all allergies.
◆ If your sinuses are very congested, use snuff (see Chapter Eleven) to relieve the pressure.
◆ If your eyes are itchy, use the eye formula suggested in Chapter Eleven under 'Eye Injury and Temporary Blindness'. Refrain from scratching them.
◆ Rub castor oil round the eyes if itchy and swollen.

## HEADACHES, MIGRAINES

These can be of many types and have many causes. Among the most common causes are a toxic bowel, constipation, liver overload, pre-menstrual tension and other hormonal imbalances, high blood pressure and a faulty diet rich in stimulants, chocolates and sweets. Occasional headaches can often be part of a circulatory problem. A simple way of finding out whether they are or not is to test with a hot flannel or ice on the temples (see below for details of these tests). An acid build-up can also produce migraines. Correct diagnosis as to what type of headache you have will be all-important.

∾ If a hot flannel calms the headache, this means the blood vessels are constricted and need dilating. Rosemary herb tea will calm and feed the nervous system, yet dilate the blood vessels; gingko leaf and prickly ash berries will help get oxygen to the brain if this is what is needed.
∾ If ice on the temples relieves the pain, you need to calm and close down your over-dilated blood vessels, then use lime tree flowers and chamomile flowers.
✿ Dietary changes will be vital, particularly omitting dairy products, wheat products, alcohol, tea and coffee. Drink plenty of water.
∾ Herbs for the nervous system will help to relieve stress headaches, while other headaches may come from the liver, diet or the bowel – you may need some further diagnosis here.
∾ Willow bark and meadowsweet herb both contain salicylic acid, which helps to relieve the pain of headaches – make decoctions.
∾ Feverfew herb tea can particularly help migraines.
◆ Liver and colon cleanses will be necessary if the headache originates from toxicity.
◆ If you suffer from sinus headaches you will need to use herbal snuff (see 'Nose Problems') and inhalations of essential oils.

## HEART ATTACK AND STROKE

Many circulatory and heart problems can lead to a heart attack (episode) or stroke. These can be demoralising and scary, and may leave permanent damage or impairment. Yet, a warning can be just the jolt needed to radically change your eating habits and lifestyle to very beneficial effects, as many people have discovered.

High cholesterol levels and fatty and plaque deposits, with resultant severe blockages in the system, can cause heart attacks and strokes. Other causes can be high blood pressure, clotting of blood vessels – thrombosis – and blood stickiness, caused by platelets clumping together and blocking veins. Thus, anyone who has any of these problems should be aware that there are some very useful herbal first aid measures available. I have seen these prevent what could have probably been much more serious situations, time and again.

**These first aid measures can be used in cases of suspected heart attack (episode) or stroke, while waiting for an ambulance.**

- Cayenne tincture should always be the first step. It helps to relieve the heart spasm, partly because it is rich in magnesium, It also stabilises blood pressure quickly. Always have some tincture at hand – in your handbag, car or kitchen cupboard. Put one tsp in a glass of warm water and drink as much as possible immediately.
- Next, take a few drops of lobelia tincture. This will also relax spasms, relieve shock and balance whatever extremes of the nervous system are being displayed. The patient will usually feel a difference in moments.
- If you have it at hand and can remember to use it, place a drop or two of camphor essential oil over the patient's heart and under his nose. Camphor is a vaso-constrictor and increases blood pressure quite quickly. It's a useful item to have at hand for those in a risk category.

**For long-term treatment: (Also see Chapter Nine.)**

- Eat an appropriate diet.
- Long-term heart herbs like hawthorn flowers, leaves and berries can make huge improvements.
- If you smoke, then STOP.
- Good food, exercise and a generally good lifestyle are essential (see angina).
- Doctors often prescribe aspirin for people who've had a stroke because it helps to thin the blood and prevent blood stickiness and clotting. Unfortunately, aspirin can really disrupt your stomach lining and your digestion. You may wish to include meadowsweet herb and white willow bark tea – these are both rich in salicylate – or red clover tea which is rich in blood thinners.
- Hormone Replacement Therapy is often recommended as a protection against heart attacks in older women. In fact, a 19-year study by a department of preventative medicine at the University of California, San Diego found no change in heart attack death rates among menopausal women taking HRT during this time. However, balanced hormone levels are important, including thyroid function, so women should use herbs to balance these – as should men.
- Massage oils made with lavender, frankincense, geranium or ylang ylang (grades 1 or 2) would also be useful and a few drops in the bath would be calming.

## HEART DISEASE (ANGINA PECTORIS)

The pains across the chest experienced in angina are caused by a lack of blood supply to the heart, resulting in a lack of usable oxygen in the heart tissue. Nitroglycerine (an explosive!) is given to angina sufferers – the drugs used are often called 'calcium channel blockers' because, just like many other muscle pains, a heart pain, or angina, is often due to a lack of calcium. This lack of calcium causes an uncomfortable tightening or tensing. Usually when the symptoms are diagnosed as angina pectoris (simply meaning 'pains across the chest') no doctor knows what the specific cause is. Indeed, I have seen this diagnosis given to a variety of conditions, from simple emotional upset to sudden strenuous exercise, high cholesterol or excessive plaque in the arteries. The clogging effects of excess cholesterol, general debris and/or calcium (plaque), causes the arteries and veins leading to and from the heart to become blocked, occasionally only allowing a trickle of blood through at a time. This causes chest pains. Another cause of circulatory blockage can be when pieces of this plaque break off and float round the circulatory system, perhaps finally lodging somewhere where a natural narrowing occurs, blocking off the vessel to a greater or lesser degree. What makes it worse is the formation of fresh blood clots, making the obstruction greater. These could be fatal, causing a heart attack (episode). Angina can be a warning of that ongoing possibility. Stress can also cause a lack of oxygen availability to the heart. (Chronic candida and indigestion can mirror and cause angina pains.)

For lesser problems, the vessels need immediate dilation to allow more blood through. For long-term treatment of the cause, the blockage – whether it be fatty or calcium – must be cleared.

- ✪ Fats to avoid are polyunsaturated margarine, dairy products and meat. Soya margarine would be safe. Virgin olive oil, either low-heated (i.e. not above 90°F) or raw, is also beneficial.
- ◗ Vitamin C and lysine will be vital.
- ✪ Avoid coffee, tea, alcohol and spicy (cooked) foods.
- ✪ You need lots of garlic – at least two fat cloves of garlic for lunch and two for supper. There is no cheaper or more perfect medicine.
- ✪ Lots of leeks, onions and spring onions would be good too.
- ∾ You should also take some source of GLA: evening primrose seed oil or blackcurrant seed oil.
- ∾ If you usually feel cold, add cayenne powder to your regime. Take three capsules three times daily – having started on a much lower dose than this and gradually built up as your body became acclimatised. Continue for three months, then stop if you wish.
- ∾ A herbal formula that will immediately help the heart and will work long-term would be: 2 parts hawthorn berries, 1 part gingko. 1 part motherwort herb and 1 part cayenne pods. They can be used in tincture form if capsules are unsuitable.
- ∾ Herbs to calm and relax would be skullcap herb, black cohosh root, oat straw, passion flower, gotu kola herb, lobelia pods, and, in the short term, valerian rhizome.

∾ A nutritional herbal drink would be equal parts of alfalfa herb, red clover flowers and nettle leaf tea.

♦ Cleanses and hot and cold showers will be vital.

♦ Exercise, but pace yourself. You will need expert help and guidance here, because overdoing it could be dangerous. Taking no exercise at all, however, could be equally dangerous. You need to find the correct medium for your own needs. Start with gentle walking interspersed with frequent rests, making sure that you have someone else with you in case any problems arise. Increase as your heart and chest pains allow. You could eventually walk alone but always let someone know you're out and roughly how long you intend to be. Eventually, cycling and a wider variety of exercise will hopefully be possible.

## HEPATITIS

This is a term given to a form of liver disease which has several different causal agents, currently labelled A, B and C. Less common ones also exist. It takes the form of liver inflammation, usually caused by a viral infection, which leaves the liver enlarged and unable to function properly. Treatment before travel to countries where the diseases are endemic is preferable to vaccination; I have known of many cases where the patient felt the vaccination was responsible for later symptoms, and, occasionally, for the full-blown disease. Conventional medicine will openly admit that vaccination does not necessarily stop one from contracting hepatitis. Symptoms include headaches, facial flushing, inflamed gums, tenderness from inflammation in the liver area, diarrhoea, a yellow coating on the side of the tongue, a profound sense of fatigue and loss of well-being, and possibly migraine headaches. Hepatitis A is transmitted through food, blood, water, body fluid and other sources of infection, and is usually acute and infectious. Hepatitis B is more likely to be transmitted by body fluid and blood. It has an incubation period of three months, and is usually chronic. Hepatitis C is also infectious, present in blood and broken, weeping skin. Current treatment of Hepatitis C involves prolonged doses of interferon which can make the patient feel permanently ill with flu-like symptoms, while simply delaying the regeneration of the liver. Hepatitis is known to increase the likelihood of other liver disease in later life.

Chronic hepatitis is when hepatitis lasts longer than six months. Chills, fever and malaise accompany acute hepatitis. Although liver function tests can be useful, generally no specific treatment is recommended except rest for hepatitis A and B and possibly isolation, depending on the type.

Hepatitis needs individual treatment depending on the type. However, all types will respond to the following treatments:

∾ Bile needs to be de-congested in this situation and the 'fire' and 'heat' of the problem purged and cooled. Many herbs common to the kitchen and garden will help this: dandelion root, turmeric root, mint leaves, oregano leaves and burdock root. Avoid cooked and raw hot spices and alcohol at all cost.

ᴄᴡ Gentian root is a bitter tonic to be taken before meals. It is an ancient European remedy for all digestive and liver/gall-bladder problems. Meadowsweet herb, commonly found in Europe, will also be useful. Siberian ginseng root for tonic support will be vital, so may other tonic herbs depending on the symptoms displayed, e.g. sweating. Advice will be vital.

ᴄᴡ Use milk thistle seed – it is safe even in large doses with practically no side-effects. The silymarin it contains has been found to have protective and regenerative properties, making it effective in chronic and post-acute hepatitis. Milk thistle is known to protect liver cells from injury, toxins, free radicals and viral toxins, and increase the population of liver enzymes. All this encourages a quick recovery from injury, while stimulating regeneration of liver tissue.

♦ Liver and gall-bladder cleanses along with a colon cleanse, will be vital. Use barberry root bark and other liver and bowel cleansers as well.

ᴄᴡ The spleen will need to be assisted to perform better (it can occasionally show slight enlargement with hepatitis C). Use echinacea root or olive leaf and turmeric rhizome to help with the spleen (and liver).

♦ Castor oil packs over the liver will help.

♦ For more natural healing practices, diet and routines for the liver, gall bladder and spleen, refer to Chapter Nine. A bland diet with steamed, stewed food is essential. Hard work will keep this disease to a minimum, so that it neither recurs nor worsens.

## HIGH BLOOD PRESSURE (HYPERTENSION)

This is a well-known and common condition in society nowadays, probably because of our diets and lifestyle. It can be hereditary, or caused by individual habits and stress levels. High blood pressure can be caused by heart and circulatory imbalance, troubled kidneys, sluggish or over-active hormones, a lack of calcium or defective calcium metabolism, obesity, clogged arteries, nervousness and worry. The dangers of persistent high blood pressure are damage to the brain, heart and kidneys. The brain, kidneys, adrenal glands and autonomic nervous system control blood pressure.

♦ Refer to angina for information. See 'Circulatory System' (Chapter Nine) in order to develop a general awareness of diet, natural healing, herbs and cleansing programmes.

✿ Eat sensibly, cut out tea, coffee, salt, alcohol, sugar, chocolate, fats and cigarettes.

✿ Avoid hot cooked spices, except for cayenne capsules, and take large amounts of garlic, with cool herbs like thyme, chives, marjoram, coriander, fennel and cumin.

✿ Search out potassium-rich foods, e.g. bananas, dried fruit, nectarines, melons, potatoes (with skins), broccoli, pumpkins, and potassium broth. (See Chapter Five.)

✿ Good internal oils to use are those rich in Omega 3 and 6. These can be found in the form of linseed oil capsules, GLA capsules and olive oil.

ᴄᴡ Good basic herbs are hawthorn flowers, leaves and berries, lime tree flowers and gingko leaves to support, buffer, elasticate, dilate and clear blockages in the veins and arteries.

❧ If your high blood pressure is known to be emotionally based, then learn to relax and breathe. Consider valerian in the short term, oat straw and skullcap in the long term, in order to feed the nervous system.

❧ If the body is physically tense, use ³/₄ cramp bark accompanied by ¹/₄ lobelia herb.

◆ Exercise and hydrotherapy are vital for increasing circulation.

## HYPOGLYCAEMIA – LOW BLOOD SUGAR

This is currently a very prevalent problem, especially among women and is often at its worst when a woman is pre-menstrual. Men can also suffer, but they are in a minority. Sugar cravings can take the form of outright sugar bingeing with the consumption of unusual amounts of chocolate or more discreet searches for dried fruit around the kitchen. Like diabetes, hypoglycaemia is an imbalance of blood sugar levels. It shows as a deficiency of sugar in the blood due to over-production of the hormone insulin in an attempt to provide much-needed supplies of energy. Excess insulin causes too much sugar to be driven into the cells, resulting in a sudden blood sugar drop. The brain is particularly affected and normal thinking will become difficult as will talking, driving, or 'making sense'. Never leave low blood sugar untreated because when brain function is inhibited and therefore poor, the nervous system will deplete. The need to stop and sleep can be overpowering, should chocolate, coffee, cigarettes or alcohol not be available to prop the situation up! It can also produce impatience and aggression. So what causes this? There are many reasons – for instance, skipped meals and crash diets, unremitting stress, sudden weight loss or the intake of excessive amounts of refined carbohydrates, e.g. crisps, cakes, snacks and sweets; excessive sugar intake, excessive tea, coffee and alcohol intake. In women, causes may include general endocrine imbalances, including pre-menstrual problems, menstrual imbalances, pregnancy, breast-feeding and the menopause. For both sexes pancreatic weakness, vitamin and mineral imbalances can contribute, including vitamin B, magnesium, chromium, manganese, zinc and potassium. Poor liver function, digestive excesses and insufficiencies, adrenal and thyroid function can also be factors. Candida can also be a highly likely cause.

Many people do not know that they are hypoglycaemic but 'swimming' feelings, shakiness, driven hunger, irritability, fatigue, indigestion, headaches, hyperactivity, anxiety, paranoia, sudden energy drops, even blackouts or 'must sleep' times, may all indicate this. The list can be endless – sweating, bad dreams, lack of libido, epilepsy, stomach cramps and general allergies. It may be necessary to find a specialist to make a diagnosis for you. However, very often the problem is constantly covered up and 'supported' by increasing sugar intake when the worst feelings arrive. If left untreated, anaemia, calcium depletion, immune deficiency, cancer, pre-menstrual tension and many other conditions may arise. If too many sweetly flavoured, refined sugar foods and drinks are succumbed to, then protein requirements will increase. If this cycle continues, one often sees a meat/sugar desire becoming stronger and stronger. A desire for sugar can also arise from a deficiency of protein due to the controlling function which protein has on sugar; the metabolism decreases if protein is not provided and consequently the sugar cravings increase. The 'conventional' medical profession rarely diagnoses it, so many people are left untreated or confused. The truth of the matter is often seen when sugar in all its forms, apart from fresh fruit, is removed from the diet. At first this will feel incredibly drastic, but by exchanging sugar for food and herbs which support blood sugar levels when they are very low, the problem will begin to even itself out. For sugar substitutes see Chapter Four. If you treat this condition carefully, you will avoid its possible development into something worse.

- ✪ Follow the diet and herbal advice for diabetes and look at the adrenal glands, as these need support. Pay special attention to the intake of garlic, fibre and water.
- ◖ Take acidophilus capsules.
- ✪ Superfood is wonderful for sustaining blood sugar levels between meals.
- ◕ Take evening primrose oil capsules (mega GLA).
- ◕ Take herbs to stimulate, tone and support all digestive processes: meadowsweet herb, aloe vera leaf gel, gentian root, sorrel leaves and dandelion root.
- ◖ Liver and bowel cleanses are vital.
- ◖ Take gentle exercise; walking and deep breathing are initially the best until your balance and stamina are developed. Exhausting activities like swimming, saunas and so on should be avoided until the body is stronger.

## IMPETIGO

This is a skin infection caused by staphylococci bacteria, which forms clusters of yellowing, crusting patches and small abscesses. This is a contagious disease and needs constant attention regarding hygiene, using separate towels, water, clothes, and so on.

- ✪ The food programme should be of the highest level of vitality – wholefoods, seaweeds, algae, nuts, seeds, beans, fresh organic vegetable juices like carrot and apple. Drink plenty of water.
- ◕ Use immune and adrenal herbs, such as equal parts of echinacea root and Siberian ginseng root, for support internally.
- ◕ Chamomile flowers in quite high doses as a tincture or tea will kill off the infection very quickly and relieve the itching.
- ◖ In the long term or, better still, in the short term, liver, kidney and colon cleanses will be necessary.
- ◖ Externally, use herbal ointments containing walnut husk, neem leaf, plantain leaf and marigold flowers.

## INCONTINENCE OR SLIGHT BLADDER WEAKNESS

A weak nervous system, genetic weakness in the area, those suffering from stroke and paralysis or the very old are most likely to suffer from this condition. Yet a surprising number of apparently healthy middle-aged people are also prone to such problems. Physical obstructions – like a swollen prostate gland in men – can be one common cause. Giving birth causes weakening of the pelvic floor muscles and pre- and post-natal exercises will help this. Hormone disturbances, especially around menopause,

SELF HEAL

can be a factor (special exercises can help enormously, enquire for details). A tumour causing pressure or even being overweight are other possibilities. Chronic constipation is yet another common cause. With help from a practitioner one should find the cause and treat it, at the same time strengthening the sphincter muscle of the bladder and other muscles in the area.

- Carry out a 1 day kidney cleanse.
- If fear, worry and anxiety are the cause, calcium and magnesium-rich foods will help; seaweeds, almonds, barley water, sesame, and herbal teas or formulas to include equal parts of valerian rhizome and chamomile flowers.
- Use equal parts of parsley leaf, rehmannia root, black cohosh root, blue cohosh root, marshmallow root, gravel root, uva ursi leaf, lobelia herb and ginger rhizome.
- Use chamomile and lavender essential oils via massage or in the bath.

## INDIGESTION

This is the inability to digest food properly. It is a 20th century problem and the cause of many allergies and conditions. Among its many causes are tension and stress and unbalanced intestinal flora. When a poor balance of stomach flora is allowed to proliferate to a point where it cannot rebalance itself, constipation and other forms of bowel dysfunction can manifest. The small and large intestine are largely interconnected and are, therefore, unable to function properly on their own. A sluggish or over-active liver, weak spleen and pancreas and over-pressured heart can all disturb the harmonious function of the small intestine, resulting in indigestion.

### Excess Acidity

- Avoid alcohol, fried foods and cooked spices. Also avoid wheat, dairy products and caffeine.
- Very fibrous foods can irritate.
- Foods that require a lot of chewing and digestion, like nuts, should be avoided for a while.
- A one-day fast on slippery elm inner bark powder may help. Mix 3 tsps of powder with water and drink or, if you prefer, you could mash it into a ripe banana.
- A little rice may be tolerated after the one-day fast, with some cabbage juice; keep up the slippery elm. Slowly come back to other foods.
- Avoid acidic foods – except for lemons and apple cider vinegar, unless you have an obvious reaction to them.
- Long-term use of drug antacids will make the problem worse, as drug-induced suppression will eventually lead to increased excess acidity. Drink 3 cups meadowsweet herb and blessed thistle herb tea daily.

### Insufficient Digestive Juices

This is a lack or total absence of hydrochloric acid. Average levels stand at 3% in healthy people. Very often, lack of hydrochloric acid can denote a lack of ability to

194

absorb vitamin B12, and a deficiency of another digestive enzyme – pepsin. A great many cancer patients (including those with stomach cancer) are found to be deficient in hydrochloric acid and pepsin, so too children, especially those with allergies like childhood candida, asthma and eczema.

✿ Avoid tea, coffee, fried food, alcohol, cooked spices or an excess of raw ones, salt and smoking.

✿ Hydrochloric acid and pepsin production can be balanced by using apple cider vinegar. Take between one and three tbsp daily in apple juice and /or honey and water.

✿ Eat pineapples and papaya for extra digestive help; the bromelain in the pineapple is good at breaking down half-digested food matter and the papain in papaya digests proteins and starches, soothing the stomach as it does so.

∾ Resurrect beneficial stomach flora with acidophilus capsules and garlic.

∾ Meadowsweet stimulates the parietal cells in the stomach to produce hydrochloric acid and pepsinogen, if necessary. Take this herb daily as a tea or a tincture.

∾ Include digestive herbs as frequently as possible. Try using equal parts of cinnamon sticks, angelica root, fennel seed, Chinese liquorice rhizome, wormwood herb and gentian root. Blessed thistle herb is useful, as it stimulates all digestive juices as well as encouraging correct acid production.

∾ Increase your general immunity if necessary through occasional use of echinacea root, elderberry or thuja or olive leaves.

## INSOMNIA AND DISTURBED PATTERNS OF SLEEP

✿ Follow a healthy diet, totally removing all dietary stimulants like coffee, tea and sugar.

∾ Take 3 parts valerian rhizome in the short term, with 2 parts passion flower and 1 part lobelia herb. These will alleviate sleep disturbance whether it has short-term or long-term causes. Long-term use of herbs such as 2 parts skullcap herb, 2 parts vervain leaf and 1 part lobelia herb will be needed to support and regenerate the nervous system.

◆ Practise barefoot walking on grass, sand and pebbles to ground and disperse any static electricity.

◆ Do breathing exercises and meditation.

◆ Take saunas, hot and cold showers and practise skin brushing.

◆ It is important to remember that we need stimulation in order to sleep. Therefore go running or dancing, take a long hike or swim in the sea and then learn to relax. Sunbathe for short periods of time or take catnaps.

◆ Cleanses will be of key importance in helping balance the body and restore correct metabolism.

## IRREGULAR AND DYSFUNCTIONAL PERIODS – MENORRHAGIA

Early periods are those occurring eight or nine days prior to the expected twenty-five to twenty-nine day cycle. Much variance outside the normal cycle will cause the body to feel tired and depleted. If your period is constantly early, you may feel consistently anxious. An early period can be caused by insufficient progesterone, shortening the second phase (the phase after ovulation). It is also possible that ovulation occurs early, in which case a little oestrogen will help extend and complete the first phase. Very occasionally, ovulation doesn't take place at all, in which case the general health of the entire body will need to be attended to, as other irregularities can occur (osteoporosis for instance). Periods which are consistently late may be due to hormonal imbalance, congestion and stagnation, anaemia or bowel and liver conditions.

☼ A dietary overhaul will be needed. Avoid tea, coffee, food containing synthetic hormones and any other foods that cause allergies.

ꝏ Insufficient oestrogen – Use 3 parts false unicorn root, 2 parts red clover flowers, 2 parts black cohosh root, 2 parts hops, 1 part sage herb and 1 part liquorice rhizome.

ꝏ Insufficient progesterone – Use 2 parts agnus castus berries and 1 part sarsaparilla root.

ꝏ If there is congestion, use equal amounts of warming, relaxing and moving herbs like ginger rhizome, cayenne pepper, pennyroyal leaf, black cohosh root, cramp bark and lobelia herb.

ꝏ Lack of ovulation or general hormonal imbalance can be dealt with through cleanses (especially liver and bowel) and a good mixed herbal formula taken regularly. Dr. Christopher's female formula would be ideal in this situation: Use equal parts of blessed thistle herb, cayenne pod, cramp bark, false unicorn root, ginger rhizome, barberry root bark, red raspberry leaves, squaw vine herb, uva ursi leaf and agnus castus berries.

♦ Colon and liver cleanses will be necessary (see Chapter Six).
♦ Use vaginal pessaries (see Chapter Three).
♦ Take hot and cold showers.
♦ Exercise regularly.

IRRITABLE BOWEL SYNDROME

This is the most common bowel complaint seen by doctors. The bowel has irregular muscular contractions which cause food and toxins to become trapped and stored, leading to bloating, constipation, diarrhoea and excessive mucus production, all of which will cause pain. This is often a precursor to other complaints. In general, follow directions for diverticulitis and colitis.

☼ You will need to radically change your diet – see Chapter Four, and repopulate colon bacteria – take acidophilus.

ꝏ A bowel cleanse with appropriate herbs to suit the individual will be vital. A liver cleanse would also be advised. Consider using equal parts of slippery elm inner bark, marshmallow root and meadowsweet herb if diarrhoea predominates.

♦ Gentle massage with essential oils of chamomile and ylang ylang is helpful.

- Use a hot castor oil pack with chamomile and ylang ylang essential oil – place on the abdomen; reheat and replace till the pain has subsided.
- Take plenty of exercise.

## JAUNDICE

This is a yellowing of the skin and eyes caused by discoloration from a build-up of waste products in the bloodstream, normally dealt with by the liver. This can be caused by a blockage in the bile duct, an infection or liver disease.

- Take carrot juice, wheat germ, lots of steamed broccoli, artichokes, cabbage and rice and plenty of garlic and turmeric.
- Temporarily, at least, use other sources of protein instead of meat or dairy products.
- You will need to do a liver cleanse and eventually a bowel cleanse.
- Daily burdock root, dandelion root, red clover flowers and nettle leaf tea will all help, try rotating these. Dandelion is one of the best day-to-day treatments for cooling and strengthening the liver. Both the roots and leaves can be used.
- Use equal amounts of barberry root bark, milk thistle seed, dandelion root, burdock root, yellow dock root, gentian root and turmeric rhizome as a tincture daily.
- If the immune system is weak use echinacea root or olive leaves.
- Chicory enemas and castor oil packs over the liver accompanied by hot and then cold showers directly over the area may help and reduce the bile.

## KIDNEY STONES

The incidence of these has risen dramatically over the last 100 years due to a huge increase in the consumption of animal fats and proteins. Stones can be found in the kidneys, bladder and ureter and can vary in size tremendously. They are generally composed of calcium oxalate. Normally the body controls the pH level of urine and any deleterious components remain suspended in solution. However, with imbalanced pH levels or with lowered immunity these mechanisms fail, the compounds crystallise and the crystals start clumping together. The pain of stones, which radiates from the upper back down to the groin, is excruciating. Other symptoms include fever or a chill, or blood in the urine. The composition of the stones can vary e.g. they may contain cystine (an amino acid). If diagnosis shows what type of stone/gravel composition you have, then a more exact diet can be tailored to your particular needs; but this is not easy to detect nor do hospitals have the time or technology to do it very often, so general guidelines usually have to do.

Often people are unaware of stones until they have passed one, which is an incredibly excruciating experience. However, it is likely there will be more, so this is the time to start treating them.

- Avoid tea, coffee, chocolate, peanuts, rhubarb, Swiss chard, spinach, tomatoes, strawberries and beetroot and any other foods containing oxalic acid.
- Avoid eggs and fish in particular as they are very high in oxalic acid levels, but also stop eating animal fats and protein because they will interfere with oxalate absorption.

197

✿ Avoid salt, alcohol, refined foods, fried foods and sugars.

✿ Foods rich in natural silicon will help maintain a stone-free urinary system. Silicon is found in the skins of organically grown grains, fruits and vegetables, particularly oats, radishes and garlic, in unpolluted seaweeds and in bee pollen. Foods rich in vitamin A will also help: melon, pumpkin, yams and carrots.

✿ Drink plenty of water to ensure a constant flushing of the entire urinary system. Choose low or no mineral content water. Distilled water is free from any minerals and so flushes through at a faster rate. A good substitute for distilled water is spring water. Sometimes add quite large quantities of fresh lemon juice as this will ease the pain.

✿ Make and drink barley water three times daily – see Chapter Four for the recipe.

~ Occasionally a problem in which the urine flows backwards when the bladder is not emptying sufficiently can cause stone formation (or, indeed, urinary infections). Diuretic herbs like dandelion root and leaf will largely solve this.

~ To start dissolving the stones and ease their journey through the body, use equal amounts of herbs like gravel root and hydrangea root, combined with demulcents like marshmallow root or corn silk; they help prevent inflammation and bleeding. You can soak the herbs in apple juice overnight and simmer them. Drink the liquid throughout the day – at least 30ml at half-hourly intervals. Continue for a few days. Even the hardest calculi will eventually turn into softer balls with no hard edges, which can then be more easily passed to support the whole body.

~ If your immune system is low take olive leaf or echinacea root and other immune herbs. Take Siberian ginseng root longer term.

● Take baths and massage with geranium, juniper, chamomile and sweet fennel essential oil.

● A kidney cleanse will be vital (see Chapter Six).

● A sedate lifestyle with little or no exercise encourages the accumulation of calcium in the bloodstream. Exercise will redirect it into the bones.

**A stone stuck anywhere at awkward entrances and bends in the kidneys, urethra or bladder is extremely painful. Most people contact their GP or arrange to be taken to casualty immediately if the pain is unbearable, but, while waiting for professional help to arrive:**

~ Try drinking a diuretic fluid, such as dandelion root coffee, or, if you have none, drink lots of water.

● A compress of lobelia herb (see compresses in Chapter Three) when placed over the kidney area and some drops of lobelia herb tincture taken internally is soothing. Make the compress as hot as you can (a wet, hot rag with lobelia tincturepoured onto it is quick), then put a hot water bottle over it.

● A cold compress on the forehead will ease any nausea or fever.

LIVER SPOTS

These are brown blotches which often occur on the backs of hands, face and neck generally in later life. They are sometimes referred to as age spots. They are an indication of a strained liver, so it is necessary to clear and regulate the liver and gall bladder. Excessive exposure to the sun can exacerbate their appearance. Liver 'coat hangers' or liver 'inflated spots' are the same, only three-dimensional, and can be a nuisance as they catch on clothing.

- ✿ Increase intake of vitamins B, C and E and appropriate foods to help the liver function better – see Body Systems, Chapter Nine.
- ∾ Colon and liver cleanses will be necessary along with the herbs associated with them – see Chapter Six.
- ◆ Treat topically with a mix of equal amounts of lemon juice and castor oil nightly.
- ◆ Stay out of direct sunlight while treating this condition, wear sunscreen.

## Low Blood Pressure (Hypotension)

This can be hereditary, you can have naturally low blood pressure. Vegans and vegetarians certainly have naturally lower blood pressure than flesh and dairy eaters. A vegetarian's normal blood pressure is 110/70 compared to an average meat eater's blood pressure of 120/80. For an accurate indication of blood pressure health, note how the person feels. Is he or she tired, lethargic and regularly yawning? If you suspect or know that your blood pressure is very low, get professional help in examining your diet, exercise, adrenals and thyroid function, also your bowel, lymph and other systems for signs of imbalance. Seriously consider the possibility of anaemia.

- • See anaemia and poor circulation, this chapter.

## Lung or Sinus Infection, Bacterial or Viral

The quality and quantity of mucus production is directly linked to the well-being of the lungs. If the lungs maintain a light, moist protective coating of mucus, this can be considered healthy. If the lungs are over-congested with mucus and the air passages are generally inflamed this will attract infection. Exercise can remove some of the excess build-up. Lack of exercise can make the situation worse, leading to a severely hindered and ineffective lung capacity. As a lot of lung problems manifest themselves in the autumn with the onset of damp and cooler weather, special attention should be paid at this time. Some lung problems are a result of poor digestion, and low stomach and bowel flora through lack of enzymes.

- ✿ Adopt a mucus-free diet, especially avoiding milk, yoghurt, cheese and eggs.
- ✿ Take no alcohol, tea or coffee.
- ✿ Avoid gluten-rich grains like wheat, or refined grains like wheat pasta.
- ✿ Avoid sugar, meat or fried foods.
- ✿ If you already have what you feel to be a healthy diet, then excess mucus is probably an indication of general low health, a cold body and a weakened immune system. This will need to be generally sustained and strengthened with tonic and supportive herbs and foods. Natural food choices should predominantly be those which grow regionally and seasonally.

✿ Eat onions, leeks, spring onions, garlic, turnips, fresh lemons, limes, ginger, cinnamon, cloves, cabbage, cabbage juice, rice and maize.

✿ Make and drink barley water (see Chapter Four).

❧ The immune system may be low and in need of motivation and support, therefore use echinacea root and Siberian ginseng root.

❧ Dr. Vogel, the respected herbalist, says that weak lungs need plenty of calcium, an easily available source of which is daily nettle leaf tea, made from young nettles (preferably picked in the spring, and not later than July).

♦ Practise breathing exercises.

**If the mucus is yellow, brown or green, you need to cool the body down:**

✿ Use plenty of lemons, limes and garlic, alongside a little ginger, cinnamon and cloves.

♦ Essential oils of lime and lemon with a little eucalyptus in a base oil could be massaged on the chest and back morning and night.

**If you have white or transparent mucus then you may feel more cold and shivery and need extra heat and energy:**

✿ Use fewer fresh fruits and raw vegetables. Take plenty of horseradish sauce, baked onions and grated ginger in dishes and drink ginger tea.

♦ Massage with marjoram, rosemary and black pepper essential oils. Or use them in the bath.

**For any kind of mucus and blocked nose, sinus and/or chest:**

✿ Use the Ayurvedic method – chew 12 raw peppercorns.

❧ Plantain leaves, elder flowers and berries, edible lichens, nettle leaves, yarrow herb and pine needles can all be made into teas.

❧ Take some garlic syrup and elder flower and elderberry syrup.

❧ Lobelia herb is a prime lung herb. A tremendous anti-spasmodic and expectorant, it is very useful for asthmatics who can learn to use it instead of Ventolin for calming and assisting breathing and also for bringing up excessive phlegm. A few drops at a time is generally adequate.

♦ Make sure your bowels are working properly; any bowel disorders will affect the proper working of the lungs.

♦ Exercise helps the lungs. Horse-riding encourages the diaphragm to push strongly up and down, particularly when galloping. Go cycling, swimming, running and dancing. Strong emotions like apprehension and fear can be physically dissipated with these simple pleasures.

♦ Take hot and cold showers. Direct the jet onto the chest and back, from the shoulders to the waist and directly on the lungs. If you are frail or weak, make sure this treatment is done under expert supervision. But, given the go-ahead and adequate help, it is a great lung strengthener, and can help turn a chronic condition right around.

♦ Inhale a variety of eucalyptus, lime, pine, lemon, fennel or cubeb essential oils. If you find yourself coughing, take a break and try again in a few moments. The inhalation oils can also be added to the bath or sprinkle the essential oils onto handkerchiefs, pillows, sheets and nightwear. When lying down, the whole body becomes more clogged and congested and these essential oils can work well at this time.

- Massage your chest. Your lungs practically touch your collarbone ʾso make movements extending up to your shoulders and down to the bottom of your rib cage; and don't forget that both your back and front house your lungs.
- Reflexology. You don't need to be an expert – just rub and stroke your feet. This is best done just before you go to bed.
- If problems are severe then, just before you go to bed, use garlic paste (see Chapter Three). During this treatment the body will bring the garlic very effectively into the lungs, helping relieve any congestion, mucus or infection. (The Vaseline is vital to prevent the skin burning; therefore ensure you use plenty).

## MEASLES

This is a viral respiratory tract infection that is highly contagious. It takes fourteen days from initial exposure to incubate and the child (or adult) will be infectious on the seventh day of exposure until ten days after the appearance of the rash. It affects the eyes and skin as well and is spread by coughing and sneezing.

The first signs are usually a cold or runny nose, followed by a fever. However, when one of my daughters developed it (she was not vaccinated), she went straight into a slight fever and rash which was found in the mouth as Koplik's spots (white ones on the cheek lining) and brownish-red spots on the body. The whole episode was over in three days, although doctors cite ten days as the normal duration of the illness. At times the reddish-brown spots can also be found behind the ears and on the face and neck where they often originate, before finally spreading to the body.

The fever generally increases as the rash develops; fluids only should be taken during this stage.

- Take a few drops of lobelia herb every hour to ease the pain and add drops of lobelia herb to bath water.
- Drink herbal teas like yarrow herb, red raspberry leaf, red clover flowers, mullein flowers and nettle leaves; carrot juice or potassium broth and Superfood.
- Use immune-enhancing herbs and those that will help calm the fever and encourage the correct function of elimination channels – see Chickenpox.
- Grapefruit seed extract and olive oil has been shown to neutralise the virus. Echinacea will also be useful to increase the body's immune response.

## MULTIPLE SCLEROSIS, MUSCULAR DYSTROPHY AND MYASTHENIA GRAVIS

These diseases involve the slow destruction of the sheath covering the nerve endings – the myelin sheath – which then becomes replaced by scar tissue. We do not know what causes them, but some speculate on a virus which encourages the immune system to kill myelin-producing cells by overzealous killer T-cells – an auto-immune reaction. Muscular weakness, pins and needles, coordination impairment and vertigo all complicate movement and produce intense pain. These conditions can be genetically inherited and all require professional help. Immune abnormalities are often the reason behind neurological breakdowns. Whether under viral, bacterial or parasitic attack, the immune system must be supported. Likewise the hormone system.

✿ Good food, rich in B vitamins and other nerve foods must predominate. Include wholefoods, plenty of water but absolutely no dairy products or wheat. Herbalist Richard Schulze makes the point that nerve foods like spirulina and non-active yeasts enter the bloodstream and are used very quickly, with little digestion required. Superfood would be ideal.

ॐ Take evening primrose oil capsules (mega GLA) and linseed oil capsules.

ॐ Take supportive and immune herbs like Siberian ginseng root and pfaffia root, but do not ingest echinacea root.

ॐ Take nerve tonics to include lobelia. Also hormone regulatory herbs (see Chapter Nine).

ॐ The herbalist Richard Schulze uses a formula designed to build, stimulate and awaken. It contains 3 parts oat straw, 3 parts skullcap herb, 3 parts St. John's wort flower, 2 parts lavender flowers, 2 parts celery seed, 2 parts kola nut, 1 part coffee beans and 1 part lobelia herb. The coffee in this formula is in simulative, therapeutic quantities and should be organic: ordinarily it must not be consumed. You can substitute prickly ash bark if you prefer, or use it as well as the coffee, in which case, halve the amount of coffee beans used. Take small amounts initially, as it will not suit everyone. (A few doses will let you know.)

• Take hot and cold showers, along with other hydrotherapy and massage.

◆ Liver, kidney and colon cleanses are absolutely vital (see Chapter Six).

MUMPS

This is a viral infection, the result of toxic mucus accumulation in the body. It takes two or three weeks to incubate and is usually caught from other children which means that your child's immune and glandular system is a little low or clogged. The infectious time is one day before the glands swell until three days after they have gone down; they can be swollen for three to seven days. The face will look swollen due to the fact that the glands around the tonsils and the salivary glands are highly inflamed, causing difficulty in swallowing: this is probably the most uncomfortable symptom.

✿ Organic vegetable juices, such as carrot, would be best at this stage, also frequent gargling is helpful (see mouth gargle in Chapter Eleven).

✿ Drink plenty of water, followed by lemon juice and water when the throat pain is over; fresh vegetable and fruit juices during the swollen phase and then graduate to salads, raw foods, rice and lots of garlic.

ॐ You may also like to use the herbal B & B ear formula in Chapter Eleven.

ॐ Internally, a formula which aids the immune system, clears the liver, cleans the blood and clears the lymph will be needed: 3 parts echinacea root, 2 parts red clover flower, 2 parts poke root, 2 parts mullein flowers, 2 parts cleavers herb and 1 part lobelia herb. Separate mullein flower tea would be excellent.

◆ A neck oil applied over the affected glands can be comforting: try a mixture of 4mls lavender, 2mls eucalyptus and 2mls tea tree in 250mls base oil (olive oil is fine); apply warmed through and hold over the glands with a muslin cloth – add some mullein flower tincture to this hot compress as it is an excellent lymph decongestant.

## Muscle Cramps

Severe cramps can occur at any time, but they most commonly occur at night. They mainly involve the legs (especially the calf muscles) and feet. Muscle cramps often affect children and adolescents in the form of growing pains. Women also suffer from menstrual cramps. Pregnant women and the elderly also commonly suffer from cramps. They can be caused by many things including calcium, magnesium, iron and vitamin E deficiency, anaemia, dehydration or poor circulation. For some people, cramps indicate a liver or gall-bladder problem, so seek out a professional diagnosis if the cramps continue.

✿ Eat foods rich in calcium, magnesium, iron (see Chapter Four), vitamin B, especially B6, and vitamin E.

✿ Take Floradix (a multi-vitamin and mineral supplement) for anaemia along with other herbs and foods rich in iron. For further information see anaemia.

∾ Use equal parts of lobelia herb, cramp bark and pasque flower tincture. This will quickly relax the individual and reduce the spasms.

∾ Include herbs that are rich in calcium and magnesium: black cohosh root, boneset herb, cramp bark, nettle leaves and red raspberry leaves; add valerian rhizome for the first three nights to induce sleep. Agnus castus berries are also a relaxant and can beneficially balance the hormone system.

◆ Moderate or increased exercise will help, increasing circulation and oxygenation of muscles.

◆ Using a hot water bottle for womb and other cramps can help, with hot and cold showers over the limbs affected.

## Nose Problems

Along with an increase in asthma and catarrhal build-ups as an allergic response to our diets and environmental pollution, blocked noses are also on the increase, often causing long-term and deep-rooted infections. External pollutants like benzine from car exhausts, chlorine gases from swimming, paints, etc. can lead to mucus production becoming extreme. Blocked nasal passages are often inevitable. Also look to weakened digestive systems caused by lack of enzymes and gut flora imbalances.

✿ Ensure a junk food-free, mucus-free diet, i.e. no carbonated drinks, sugar, wheat, dairy products – see Chapter Four on food.

✿ Eat onions, chives and garlic, all of which are rich in sulphur.

○ Horseradish, raw cayenne and black pepper will also help.

○ No tea, coffee (or decaffeinated versions), chocolate, carbonated drinks, sweets, cakes. Drink plenty of water.

○ Drink juices and eat light foods – rice, steamed vegetables.

◒ Herbs that help the immune system in general and directly cope with pollen, traffic and household irritations are:--mullein flowers, pfaffia herb, gentian root, plantain herb, barberry root bark, cayenne pods, echinacea root, lobelia pods, eyebright flowers, juniper berries, burdock root and liquorice rhizome.

◒ Other herbs that help maintain the positive function of the lungs and nasal polyps (helping to clear excess mucus and, in turn, to empower the ability for oxygen replenishment) are: chickweed herb, eucalyptus leaves, liquorice rhizome, horehound herb, elecampane herb. Use in equal parts. In the short term, small amounts of coltsfoot herb.

◆ Determine what kind of weakened digestive system you have, and treat appropriately – refer to 'The Digestive System' in Chapter Nine.

◒ Lymph herbs may help to decongest a very clogged system; use 3 parts mullein flowers, 2 parts poke root, 2 parts cleavers herb and 1 part lobelia herb.

◒ Use herbal snuff: a mixture of powdered herbs in equal amounts: American ephedra herb, barberry root bark, bayberry bark, lobelia seed pod, cayenne pod, horseradish root and mustard seed. Put a tiny amount on the back of the hand and sniff, in turn, into each nostril. Hold as long as possible, then blow your nose. Repeat procedure twice daily. This is also useful for nasal polyps.

◆ Essential oil inhalers: Use one, more, or all of the following: peppermint, eucalyptus, pine and camphor. Breathe in deeply until the nose feels clearer.

◒ An ointment can be made of the inhalant herbs (or bought ready-made) and used over the chest, back and nasal passages, particularly at night time, to help with the extra clogging that occurs during this static time.

◒ Dr. Christopher's B & B ear drops (see Chapter Eleven) can be useful, because a release in the ears can often help release the nasal passages.

## OEDEMA (WATER RETENTION)

Retaining excess water in the body is a problem that women in particular are prone to, especially pre-menstrually. However, both men and women can be susceptible. Particular 'holding' areas are the fingers, under the eyes and (due to gravity) the ankles and feet. Water retention may be part of the many symptoms of a faulty or congested liver. It can also be connected to the hormone system, the heart and the kidneys. When the liver becomes overburdened with toxins, it cannot keep up with its work and so passes on the job to the kidneys which, in turn, may overload and stagnate. The same applies to an overburdened circulatory or lymph system. Constipation, diabetes and thyroid problems can also cause oedema, therefore individual treatment will be necessary.

○ Avoid refined salt, unless you are told specifically not to by a practitioner. Avoid foods that exacerbate the problem, like dairy products and wheat products.

✿ Include plenty of leeks, parsley, celery seeds and sticks, and cucumber. For fruits choose apples, pears, melons, peaches, pineapples and bilberries.

✿ Eat plenty of dark green vegetables, chlorella and algae which are rich in B vitamins, particularly B6. Drink Superfood.

∾ Herbs that remove excess water are easy to find, the safest being dandelion root. Use in teas or tinctures. In addition, when in season, the leaf can go into fresh salads.

◆ A colon cleanse will help balance the water level in the body and relieve the oedema.

◆ A liver cleanse will be useful along with a kidney cleanse; this combination will make the kidneys work much more efficiently.

◆ Massage the affected areas with juniper oil or add it to your bath water.

OSTEOPOROSIS

This is a decrease in bone mass. It affects 1 in 3 women by the age of 70. However, younger people can be affected as a result of the body being unable to absorb and utilise nutrients properly (or during pregnancy, especially if you become pregnant frequently). The menopause can also affect magnesium and calcium levels, due to a reduction in oestrogen, so pay attention to calcium and magnesium needs from the age of forty. This will prepare and strengthen you in readiness for the menopause, and also support kidney function. A large meat intake will also inhibit calcium absorption. Meat also contains large amounts of phosphorus which ruins the calcium/phosphorus balance by inhibiting calcium levels. Any prolonged cortisone treatment will also take its toll; cortisone inhibits bone formation and decreases absorption of calcium in the stomach. Those with rheumatoid arthritis are often treated with steroids and may suffer from osteoporosis later on.

Early warning signs include broken nails, leg cramps, joint pain and restless behaviour. More advanced cases will exhibit loss of spinal movement and a decrease in height.

**Test for Osteoporosis.**

The McCue Cuba Clinical Machine is able to measure bone density and structure without the use of radiation or a body scan. The test cost is minimal and involves placing your bare foot on a plate that is connected to a computer for data processing. Diagnosis is printed out in two minutes. (See 'Resources' at the end of this chapter).

✿ Eat and drink foods rich in calcium and magnesium foods (refer to Chapter Four). In addition, Aqua-Mag is a wonderful natural product available from Springfield Pharmacy.

✿ Cut out coffee and tea in particular.

✿ Drink Superfood on waking and at bedtime.

∾ Drink nettle leaf tea as a bedtime drink as bone mass is decreased the most while one sleeps. Pau d'arco bark also contains high levels of calcium, and assists any immune or inflammatory problems.

- Kidney cleanses will help this function, and oestrogen output will remain balanced.
- Herbs to help maintain hormone levels at menopause include dong quai root, agnus castus berries, blue and black cohosh root, wild yam tuber, hops strobile, fennel seed – and many more
- HRT (Hormone Replacement Therapy): has been proven to increase the likelihood of osteoporosis by causing other mineral deficiencies which, in turn, cause hormone deficiencies. Natural progesterone is an alternative option (though not used by the authoress in her clinic); contact Dr. Shamim Daya (see 'Resources' section at the end of this chapter).

## OVARIAN CYSTS, UTERINE FIBROIDS, CERVICAL POLYPS AND CYSTS

An ovarian cyst develops when an ovarian follicle fails to release an egg as it should. Instead it fills with a clear fluid and becomes sac-like and slightly firm. Cysts are, some say, a defence system against serious toxicity or more malignant problems; 89% of them are benign. Some even suggest they are more like localised mini livers. There is a similar view about uterine fibroids (benign tumours) which grow inside or outside the uterus wall. Very often they remain small but they can grow. At this point they will often become painful and even bleed. If very large, doctors will want to remove them (occasionally they also remove the womb, but this is becoming more unusual). Ranking as the most common female reproductive tumour, fibroids affect one fifth of all women. Note that they are almost never malignant (cancerous). Most fibroids grow inside a capsule, which acts as a barrier between the uterine wall and the fibroid itself. As they are heavily oestrogen dependent, the intake of oestrogen, as with ovarian cysts, must be kept to a minimum.

Cervical cysts and polyps are completely harmless. They are found inside the uterus but can protrude and bleed and are best dealt with quickly. They are comparatively simple and effective to treat, and the bleeding can be stopped with herbs and natural healing.

Polycystic ovaries indicate a hormonal imbalance and are often connected to infertility.

- Decrease all oestrogenic food and drink intake. This will include, among others, coffee, tea, chocolate, dairy products and hormone-fed meat.
- If you are overweight, lose weight, as oestrogen is stored in fatty tissue. Weight loss is enhanced by taking GLA and spirulina or Superfood.
- Adopt a good food and cleansing programme – see general suggestions for endometriosis.
- Take one evening primrose oil capsule (mega GLA) daily.
- Colon, kidney and liver cleanses will be vital as this condition indicates sluggishness and congestion.
- Use herbs to balance the endocrine system and especially ones that tend to be more progestogenic in action e.g. agnus castus berries and sarsaparilla root, but a rounded formula is fine.

- Use vaginal pessaries (see Chapter Three).
- Pain or cramping can be alleviated with equal amounts of lobelia pods, pasque flower and cramp bark tincture, and also castor oil packs.
- Have sitz baths and hot and cold showers to encourage blood supply/flow. (See Chapter Five.)
- Exercise to encourage blood supply.

## OVER-ACTIVE THYROID – HYPERTHYROIDISM

This is when the thyroid gland over-produces thyroid hormones according to a blood test, which in turn overactivates the body's metabolism. The general symptoms include irritability, heat, increased perspiration, insomnia, fatigue; less frequent and increased flow of menstruation; rapid digestion and bowel movements and mal-absorption. Goitre can also develop. (For under-active thyroid, see page 219.)

- Ground and support the body with 'earthy' foods like barley, rice, millet, quinoa and all the root vegetables, particularly the sweeter ones like carrot, parsnip and sweet potato. Also eat plenty of cabbage, Brussels sprouts, cauliflower, kale, mustard greens and watercress to suppress excess thyroid hormone production.
- Try eating six small meals rather than three large meals a day.
- Avoid dairy products and all stimulants including tea, coffee, alcohol etc.
- Avoid seaweeds, particularly bladderwrack and kelp, as they contain iodine which will over-provoke the thyroid.
- The nervous system needs to be treated with sedatives to calm and feed it. Use chamomile flowers, skullcap herb and even valerian rhizome as a short-term measure. More specific treatments may be needed according to the individual picture.
- Immune and adrenal debility is often the cause (or an added problem), so echinacea root and Siberian ginseng root are useful.
- Hormonal tonic herbs: agnus castus berries for both women and men or saw palmetto berries for men (or both for both sexes) with fenugreek seed and a little Chinese liquorice rhizome.
- The liver, colon and the entire endocrine system will need individual assistance and support for overall balance. (See Thyroid, Chapter Nine.)

## PAINFUL PERIODS – DYSMENORRHOEA

Dysmenorrhoea can be initiated by an inadequate calcium and magnesium supply which is needed to flex and squeeze the womb wall muscles in order for menstruation to begin. The womb can also be burdened with old toxic and stagnant discharge as a result of poor monthly flow due to poor circulation and/or because of inadequate womb peristalsis. The resulting congestion can cause tremendous pain. Often, once a womb has expanded to hold a baby and gone through the huge peristaltic waves needed for childbirth, this problem diminishes. Some women can experience dysmenorrhoea for the first time after childbirth, however, due to the huge drop in magnesium and calcium levels associated with pregnancy and breast-feeding. These levels need to be replenished. Occasionally, a uterus is positioned in a way that makes menstruation difficult. This can be looked into should all else fail, but the uterus is normally individually aligned and will change alignment throughout one's life. Older women (30-35 years old) may suddenly develop an aching abdomen, legs and thighs which may be caused by a congestive build-up. Symptoms include sweating, fever, nausea, fainting and intense physical pain caused by muscle spasms. Fibroids, endometriosis, hypothroidism and other problems should also be considered and then professionally explored if simple treatments are failing to alleviate the problems.

○ You must increase calcium and magnesium intake: include seaweeds like wakame and hijiki, both from the kelp family, to ensure that your physical and nutritional needs in general are met.

○ Make sure that your iron and folic acid intake is adequate, as an insufficiency can cause leg cramps and twitching.

◐ Herbs to increase calcium and magnesium include pau d'arco bark, oat straw, nettle leaves and Irish moss.

◐ Useful herbs for spasm, pain relief and hormone balance include: 3 parts agnus castus berries, 3 parts false unicorn root, 3 parts squaw vine root, 3 parts dong quai root, 3 parts cramp bark, 2 parts blue cohosh root, 2 parts black cohosh root, 2 parts nettle leaves, 2 parts sarsaparilla herb, 2 parts blessed thistle herb and 1 part lobelia herb.

◐ If you suspect congestion and stagnation in the uterus, use dong quai root and cayenne pepper capsules for general circulation.

◆ Liver, kidney and bowel cleanses will be vital.

◐ Use general hormone balancers like agnus castus berries and sarsaparilla herb, false unicorn root and blessed thistle herb.

◆ Practise deep breathing at all times, but spend a concentrated 20 minutes doing belly breathing in a warm bath to really let go and relax.

◆ Relax in a warm bath with a few drops of rosemary essential oil.

◆ Gentle daily exercise should include yoga.

◆ Exercise regularly to increase circulation and decrease congestion.

◆ Use a slant board (Chapter Five) or put your feet up as high as you can against a wall.

◆ Put a muslin cloth which has been soaked in chamomile essential oil and sunflower oil over the abdomen underneath a hot water bottle for extra relief.

## PALPITATIONS

This is the erratic or fast beating of the heart. It is not necessarily dangerous but it can be disturbing, especially if it is partially caused by (or is in conjunction with) anxiety, stress, anger or other emotional outbursts. Checking your blood pressure will give you an insight into the effect these palpitations are having. Likewise, the outcome may suggest possible treatment. The condition can also be a symptom of food allergy or candida.

✪ Refer to angina suggestions for dietary guidance.

✪ Make sure your digestion is good and, if you're not sure, take a tsp of cider vinegar three times daily.

ༀ If there is undue stress and nervousness, add valerian root and skullcap herb for a limited period. Stop the valerian after three weeks but keep using the skullcap for at least three months. Lobelia herb would also be ideal for any panic moments – take a few drops at a time.

ༀ Hawthorn berries would be an ideal herb to use every day as a general heart and circulatory balancer.

ༀ If you often feel cold, take cayenne capsules.

♦ Massage with lavender, ylang ylang (grade 1 or 2), peppermint and rosemary essential oil. Or use them in the bath.

## PANCREATITIS

This can be associated with alcoholism, trauma or infection of the biliary tract. This latter is the duct shared with the gall-bladder and this often causes the problem, especially if the duct is blocked with gallstones. However this is by no means always the case. Inflammation of the pancreas due to the potent digestive enzymes created by the pancreas itself can cause it to attack its own pancreatic tissue.

✪ Drink vegetable juices, but avoid fruit juices due to high sugar content.

✪ Drink plenty of water because dehydration can often be the root cause of this condition.

✪ Eat lots of garlic.

ༀ Eat powdered digestive herbs – slippery elm inner bark, meadowsweet herb, fennel seed and liquorice rhizome.

ༀ Long-term herbs for the pancreas will include cedar berries, fenugreek seed and liquorice rhizome.

♦ Perform liver, kidney and colon cleanses. (See Chapter Six.)

♦ Use castor oil packs directly over the pancreas. (See Chapter Three.)

♦ Take hot and cold showers, especially over the pancreas.

♦ Look at advice for diabetes for extra tips.

## PARKINSON'S AND ALZHEIMER'S DISEASE

Parkinson's is a degenerative disease in which neurotransmitter messages no longer function properly and motor functions gradually decrease. Alzheimer's disease is a chronic dementia causing great distress for those around the patient. It is sadly on the increase. The patient will become forgetful, disorientated, have mood swings, and become less and less able to walk, eat and function normally. Some practitioners feel that the mercury from dental fillings will drastically increase the risk of Alzheimer's disease. Aluminium from cooking pots and utensils is also suspected to be involved. Another theory is that the brain attacks itself in an over-active and misguided immune response. Mercury, aluminium, pesticides and other modern processing agents added to food are also felt to contribute. I have reason to believe that the bowel and liver have a huge effect on all the above diseases and, when these organs and systems are cleared, I have seen fundamental changes take place.

- ✿ Refer to Chapter Four and adopt a good diet, free of foods that will harm the nervous system e.g. stimulants like coffee, tea and sugar. Malnutrition is felt to be a large factor in both Parkinson's and Alzheimer's disease.
- ✿ Nerve foods like soaked oats, non-active yeast and spirulina will be important.
- ✿ Eat antioxidant foods (see Chapter Four).
- ❧ Nerve sedatives will help to promote sleep: valerian rhizome in the short term and skullcap herb in the longer term.
- ❧ Nerve relaxants and tonics must become a daily ritual. Use equal amounts of: gotu kola nut, vervain herb, wood betony herb, lemon balm, lobelia herb and St. John's wort flower.
- ❧ Time and again it has been shown that treating the 'shakes' experienced by Parkinson's sufferers with herbal stimulants is effective. In effect the body needs waking up and rebuilding. Refer to 'The Nervous System' in Chapter Nine.
- ◆ Intensive cleanses for the kidneys, liver and the colon with the use of juices and organic food will be vital, as clearing the liver and colon helps the brain function more effectively. Many health workers feel that liver toxicity underpins both these conditions.
- ◆ Relaxation methods, together with significant exercise, should be pursued.
- ◆ Use deep body work, reflexology and massage.
- ◆ Persistent hydrotherapy can be helpful according to the individual and the carer's time and abilities.

## PELVIC INFLAMMATORY DISEASE (P.I.D.) – SALPINGITIS

This is inflammation of the pelvic organs due to infection from the uterus which can sometimes be linked to, or follow on from, endometriosis. It may also develop independently. The uterus, ovaries or fallopian tubes become congested, with water retention and pus-like secretions. The pain, which can be treated easily if the condition is caught quickly, can become intense and bleeding can occur. I've had patients who have endured it for years in severe and almost constant pain, sometimes caused in part by abscesses. Some people feel that it can be caused by initial infections like chlamydia, gonorrhoea and other bacterial infections. Appendicitis, extra-uterine pregnancy, IUDs (inter-uterine devices), fallopian tube twisting, abortion, gynaecological procedures and the use of tampons, can be other causes.

- • Look at the general routine recommended for endometriosis for extra information on diet and lifestyle.
- ❧ Use immune herbs like pau d'arco bark, garlic clove, echinacea root, barberry root bark and pine needle tinctures internally.
- ❧ For pain and cramping, use equal parts of cramp bark, pasque flower, lobelia herb and valerian rhizome.

∿ To balance the system, take endocrine herbs and uterine tonics such as false unicorn root, agnus castus berries, squaw vine herb and wild yam root.
♦ The bowel and liver will be vitally in need of cleansing. (See Chapter Six.)
♦ Make sure the kidneys are well flushed – drink fresh lemon water (this also cleans the bloodstream) and dandelion root coffee. Take lymph system herbs like cleavers herb and marigold flowers, and consider a kidney cleanse.

## PHELONEPHRITIS (PYLETIS), NEPHRITIS AND GLOMERULONEPHRITIS

These systemic infections are very often accompanied by fever, so correct fever treatment is important. I've known dangerously high fevers rage, in particular with nephritis, and permanent damage to eyesight and other areas may follow if it is not carefully treated with the help of a practitioner. All these conditions need professional help, but prolonged use of antibiotics invariably makes the situation much worse and they should be avoided after any initial use. The general recommendation is to rest and relieve the kidneys as much as possible.

✿ No salt, animal protein, dairy products, tea, coffee or alcohol should be taken.
✿ Assess and correct individual nutritional deficiencies.
✿ Use lots of garlic when you are cooking.
✿ Plenty of barley water will help, as will non-roasted dandelion tea.
✿ Avoid sugar, as it encourages bacterial growths. Vegetable and fruit juices, raw foods, steamed vegetables, fruits and spring water are needed here.
∿ Use general guidelines and herbs for cystitis, along with the use of uva ursi leaves and buchu leaves made as a tea; however, more personal, professional treatment is advised.
♦ Kidney cleanses will be vital. (See Chapter Six.)

## POOR CIRCULATION AND CHILBLAINS

Cold hands and feet are quite common. They are really worth working on, rather than leaving them to simply make your life miserable and allowing them to turn into something more troublesome.

✿ Eat horseradish, the hot English mustards and root ginger frequently.
✿ Refer to dietary advice for angina.
∿ Take the following herbs in equal amounts: cayenne pepper pods, prickly ash berries and hawthorn flowers, berries and leaves.
♦ Stop or cut down on smoking.
♦ Exercise frequently.
♦ Take hot and cold showers.
♦ Use a hot ointment or massage oil containing mustard, chilli, juniper, pine, cubeb and rosemary essential oils.

## PRE-MENSTRUAL TENSION (OR PRE-MENSTRUAL SYNDROME)

The range of symptoms experienced pre-menstrually is quite alarming: headaches, stomach bloating, breast tenderness, cysts, mastitis, general water retention, cramps, acne, joint aches and pains, depression, irrational anger, over-sensitivity, lethargy, extreme tiredness, sugar and chocolate cravings and nausea. There are many more!

Pre-menstrual tension can often be caused by a congested liver. If the liver is not breaking down excess hormones effectively, transitional stress hormones can linger, making the person irritable, angry or depressed. It is for these reasons that the liver is often associated with anger. The liver can also contain an excess of hormones that it is supposed to be able to deal with, but which it is unable to for a variety of reasons. In this case, the heat caused by this excess must be purged; dandelion and milk thistle will greatly help here. The health of the liver has a strong connection to the female gynaecological system. A congested, immobile liver often results in pre-menstrual tension and period pains, while a deficiency of cholesterol made in the liver leads to underproduction of progesterone which is vital for women at this time of the month.

The whole endocrine system needs looking at, especially the oestrogen and progesterone balance, along with levels of prolactin, thyroid and adrenal hormones. Constipation or diarrhoea will greatly affect PMS, therefore look for bowel problems.

✿ Do not eat red meat; all red meat is rich in excessive oestrogen. Eat no meat at all if it is not organically reared, if possible.

✿ Include foods containing sulphur, like garlic and onions.

✿ Decrease intake of cabbage family foods for one week before your period.

✿ Follow a wholesome diet with particular attention to 'liver' foods (see Chapter Nine).

✿ Eat plenty of fresh fruits, whole-grains, olive oil and lemon juice.

✿ No fats (with the exception of olive oil, which is wonderful to use), tea, coffee, alcohol, sugar or chocolate should be taken.

❧ Take evening primrose oil capsules, or other sources of GLA.

◗ A liver cleanse and use of liver herbs should be a primary step, followed by colon and kidney cleanses.

❧ Take daily dandelion root and nettle leaf tea with fresh dandelion leaves in salads to meet iron, magnesium and calcium needs. The dandelion can also be put with other kidney herbs like uva ursi and corn silk made up as a tea in order to alleviate any water retention problems.

❧ General hormone balancing herbs will be useful throughout the month. Combine equal amounts of the following herbs to make a formula: agnus castus berries, sarsaparilla root, black cohosh root, milk thistle seeds, blessed thistle herb, liquorice rhizome, false unicorn root, wild yam root and squaw vine herb. Take 1 tsp 3 times daily.

❧ Replace the above herbs 10 days prior to menstruation with herbs that will need to be individually chosen and tailored to your own particular chemistry. However, a general formula to help with pain, the liver, water retention and the hormones themselves would be 3 parts agnus castus berries, 3 parts pasque flower, 3 parts black cohosh root, 3 parts wild yam root, 2 parts milk thistle seed, 2 parts fennel seed, 2 parts pulsatilla herb, 1 part lobelia herb, 1 part pennyroyal herb, 1 part red raspberry leaf and 1 part buchu leaf.

◆ Exercise consistently but lightly. Avoid taxing physical exercise and do more walking, dancing, yoga, meditation and breathing exercises.
◆ Try special abdominal/pelvic exercises and perhaps lie on a slant board.
◆ Take long relaxing baths and get early nights to conserve energy.
◆ Hot and cold showers during the month will help, but avoid them just prior to and during menstruation.

## PROSTATE ENLARGEMENT

This can be a common problem for men in later life. They experience pain on urination and the constant urge to urinate can produce fitful nights and become quite exhausting. One cause of this can be a bacterial infection invading the prostate. However, the herbalist James Green tells us it mostly affects men between 40 and 59 years old and this suggests a hormonal imbalance or gland stagnation. Sometimes a dull ache will be felt in the lower stomach area: this is the prostate pressing into the urethra. Occasionally blood in the semen and in the urine is noticeable. Treating the condition quickly is important. If it is left untreated, the retained urine, which is unable to be expelled, can eventually cause cystitis or prostitis as it flows back into the bloodstream, while the pressure on the bladder and kidneys can become very dangerous. The prostate gland is occasionally removed if the problem has been allowed to develop too far without proper attention. If left untreated, the whole prostate could become cancerous.

✪ Consume plenty of zinc-rich foods, as this normalises testosterone production. Use sea vegetables, organically grown pumpkin seeds, pumpkins themselves, sunflower seeds, garlic, capsicums, mushrooms, bilberries and soya beans.
✪ Steer absolutely clear of coffee, tea, alcohol, sugar and refined foods.
✪ Eat plenty of grains, fresh vegetables and fruit.
✪ Drink lots of barley water and water with lemon juice.
♋ Do not buy cheap zinc tablets. Zinc can boost the immune defences, but excessive intake in the form of zinc tablets can undermine and impede the immune system. Herbs which are rich in zinc include skullcap, Siberian ginseng, nettle and chickweed, all of which can be taken for their general tonic properties.
◆ James Green also suggests herbal enemas – this is well worth a try and you can use the herbs mentioned below.
♋ A herbal formula that will generally help to balance the hormones and strengthen the kidney and bladder in the long term would be: 3 parts saw palmetto berries, and 1 part each of damiana herb, dandelion root, rehmannia root, chickweed herb, marsh-mallow root, lobelia herb, ginkgo leaf, astragalus herb, burdock root, parsley leaves and uva ursi leaves. Saw palmetto berries will also help to relax the nervous system.
♋ To ease inflammation use tincture or teas of: gravel root, hydrangea root, corn silks and marshmallow root in equal amounts.
♋ For infection, use garlic cloves and echinacea root.
◆ Some medical practitioners feel that the cause of the enlargement is an accumulation of testosterone in the prostate itself. Using up the testosterone is

possibly an answer, so continue sport, sexual activity and work with continued zeal, if you can. If the prostate feels hot and unbearably inflamed and urination is a nightmare, use a clay poultice over the area at night time. Use equal parts of the following: bentonite clay, slippery elm inner bark, barberry root bark, lavender herb powder with enough castor oil to turn it all into a paste.

- ◆ Take regular exercise to increase circulation and oxygen to the area.
- ◆ Hot and cold showers will also increase circulation and oxygen to the area.

## PSORIASIS

No-one knows quite how or why this disease appears. However, some now believe that it occurs when skin cells are produced about ten times faster than usual. Many practitioners suspect that the thinning of the small intestine walls can allow poisons to enter into the circulatory and lymph system. The theories of the cause also include auto-immune conditions; digestive incapability, food allergies, constipation, candida and immunisation. In severe cases, the thickened white, red and silvery scaly skin (sometimes with yellowish pustules) can be very dry and itchy and constantly flake off – though, of course, it can be less severe. It can be all over the body, including the scalp, but is most commonly found on the arms, legs, elbows and knees.

- ✿ One-day, three-day and five-day fasts should be done as directed by a practitioner, using fruits and vegetables appropriate to individual needs. Water intake will be vital at all times.
- ✿ Make sure that your hydrochloric acid levels are sufficient and increase essential fatty acid intake via GLA and olive oil.
- ✿ Eat lots of apples, grapes, carrots and garlic.
- ✿ Seaweed should be used both internally and externally, especially if the skin is hot, red and producing pus.
- ✿ For hot skin, cooling foods will help: raw fruits and vegetables, bilberries, celery, grapefruit, spinach, melon, cucumber and apples are all good.
- ✿ For cold skin and low body heat, warming foods will help: raw ginger, chilli, horseradish, garlic and onion.
- ✿ Drink fresh lemon juice in distilled water – it will naturally cleanse and clear.
- ✿ Garlic will be one of the prime foods because of its immune qualities and its sulphur content, cleaning and clearing the skin.
- ∾ Oregon grape inhibits the growth of skin cells, so bathe the affected areas with a solution of it and also take internally.
- ∾ Use equal parts of nettle leaves, echinacea root, lavender herb, burdock root, gentian root, cleavers herb, skullcap herb, red clover flowers, barberry root bark, liquorice root, sarsaparilla root, dandelion root, poke root, plantain leaves and yellow dock root as general liver, digestive and blood cleansers and to provide immune support.
- ∾ Drink three cups of burdock root tea daily.
- ∾ Use 3 parts skullcap herb and 1 part lobelia herb to nourish the nervous system.
- ◆ Clean and detoxify the eliminative channels – liver, kidney and colon. (See Chapter Six.)

🜆 Aloe vera gel is absolutely brilliant at soothing and cooling. It has in-built anti-microbial abilities and is easy to apply from freshly cut leaves if these are available.

🜆 A seaweed and clay skin treatment is cooling, cleansing and restorative. Mash bentonite clay powder with dulse and other crumbled seaweeds, add enough virgin olive oil to make a paste. Apply liberally and then bandage. If the psoriasis is on the scalp, apply a cotton bath cap and treat during the evening, washing off before bedtime.

🜆 For less severe psoriasis, use plantain herb and chickweed leaf along with other herbs as an ointment.

🜆 A dusting powder can help alleviate itching, use equal amounts of the following powders: lavender herb, chickweed herb, neem leaf, yarrow herb, chamomile flowers and plantain leaf.

🜆 Avoid all commonly found shampoos and stick to those which are gentle and designed for such conditions or those containing low doses of appropriate essential oils with enriching, soothing and pH balanced soaps. However, avoid any shampooing when not completely necessary and do not use soap on the body.

🜆 Skin brush; however, do not skin brush on inflamed scaling areas, only on healthy skin.

🜆 Sweating may give relief, so have saunas, but interspersed with frequent cold showers, starting on the top of the head.

🜆 Exercise is essential.

🜆 Use clothing and bed linen made from natural fibres.

🜆 Try to make sure no undue stresses and strains exist.

• Read section on eczema for extra tips.

## RINGWORM

This is a surprisingly common skin disease. It is a fungus that causes ring-shaped marks on the skin. Sometimes, the middle of the ring heals, but not the outer ring. A common site is the scalp but sometimes it occurs around the nails. This is the so-called 'true ringworm', but 'dhobi itch' is also a form of ringworm. So called after the heat and wet of tropical monsoon regions where it originated, this affects the area of the groin.

✪ Avoid sugar and yeasts until it has cleared up.

꩜ Drink pau d'arco bark decoction.

🜆 Use a few of the following: marigold flowers, lavender herb, neem leaf, walnut inner hull or other anti-fungal herbs as powders for dusting affected areas like the scalp, groin and nails.

🜆 Keep the areas clean and dry at all times. Cleanses will help clear the skin and individual organs.

## SCIATICA

Although classified as a neurological disease, it is usually caused by poisons collecting in the kinks and pockets of the sigmoid section of the bowel up to the descending colon and over to the rectal area. The poisons collect in the upper leg area and, in turn, irritate the sciatic nerve, eventually dislocating the sacroiliac bone. The resulting inflammation and pain around the nerves is excruciating. Eventually, muscle wasting will add to the problem.

- A colon cleanse will be a vital first step.
- Adjustment by a chiropractic (or osteopath) can help.
- Massage will ease the pain.
- Hot and cold showers over the area will help.
- Take exercise.

## SHINGLES – HERPES ZOSTER

Shingles is a close relative of chickenpox and can be triggered in adults by contact with children who have chickenpox, so if you are run down and feel low, take care. The virus, once it has set in, can remain for some time if it is not treated.

- Adopt a good diet – see Chapter Four on food. Include plenty of garlic and water.
- Eat liver cleansers like dandelion leaves, artichokes, asparagus, olives and olive oil.
- Ensure that you eat plenty of foods rich in magnesium, calcium and B vitamins (refer to Chapter Four).
- Consume plenty of Superfood.
- Take mega GLA capsules daily (evening primrose seed oil).
- Take nerve restorative and tonic herbs like Siberian ginseng root, astragalus herb, skullcap herb, vervain leaf, wood betony herb, lobelia herb all in the long term and valerian rhizome in the short term.
- Liver, colon and kidney cleanses prevent recurrences.
- Immune herbs like echinacea root and elderberries will greatly help.
- Use neem leaves, chickweed herb and lavender flowers in powder form to dust over the itchy areas.
- Nourish the nervous system and immune system on general natural healing level, relaxing and resting as much as possible (see Body Systems, Chapter Nine).

## SINUSITIS

This is an inflammation of the nasal sinuses, mainly affecting the area around the eyes and either side of the nose. It can also affect the other systems in this area, with excess mucus production building up due to allergies or viral or bacterial infection. If you have small sinuses they will clog up more quickly. Symptoms include headaches, earache and facial pain.

- Adopt a mucus-free diet, especially cutting out wheat and dairy products. Investigate any food allergies you may have and support these to balance digestive enzyme action, etc.
- Take acidophilus capsules.

- You need to take small but consistent amounts of lobelia herb in order to purge the lungs of old tissue, mucus and other foreign materials. But be careful, as taking too much will cause vomiting.
- General respiratory herbs will help as a daily formula like horehound herb, wild cherry bark and elecampagne herb. Also take immune herbs to help with infection. Use equal parts of garlic clove, echinacea herb, mullein flowers and Siberian ginseng root.
- Take steam inhalations of essentials like chamomile and lavender. Afterwards take a cold shower and eat twelve raw black peppercorns; you will feel cleansed and soothed.
- Put two drops of eucalyptus or lavender essential oil, into the bath. Inhale the water into each nostril and similarly blow out of each nostril. It really clears the nose and can help first thing in the morning when the mucus and blocking is usually at its worst.
- Use herbal snuff (see Nose Problems). Sometimes the problem is so severe and deep-rooted that repeated use of the snuff will be necessary.
- Dr. Christopher's B & B herbal ear drops may be necessary (Chapter Eleven). Indeed, it may be worth using these even if you do not have earache.
- Avoid decongestants and surgery.

## STROKE

This is a very common neurological disorder. It occurs because of a blockage or rupture in a brain blood vessel. It can affect movement and speech. High-risk people include smokers and those with diabetes, obesity, an excessive alcohol intake, high blood pressure and high cholesterol. Strokes can be genetic, but can also be directly linked to lifestyle. A change in diet is probably the most important first step in treating them.

Refer to 'The Circulatory System' in Chapter Nine.

- Lobelia herb is most effective when used immediately after the stroke and continued for several days afterwards. Five drops at the base of the tongue every hour for an adult will be very beneficial.
- Cayenne pods and prickly ash bark or berries will help circulation and long-term use of skullcap herb to nourish the nervous system will also be beneficial.
- Other choices of herbs include ginger rhizome, rosemary leaves, gingko leaves and gotu kola nut. These are all especially helpful for the brain.
- Take hot and cold showers.
- Skin brushing will also be beneficial.
- Other natural healing procedures will help, e.g. massage and all cleanses.

## THROAT PROBLEMS – LARYNGITIS, TONSILLITIS AND PHARYNGITIS

Problems can arise here from the lungs, sinuses, mouth, ears or even the stomach and bowel. The glands may simply be swollen due to toxic overload from the bowel or allergic reactions in the stomach. The lungs and/or the whole ear, throat and nose network may be congested.

- Treat laryngitis, tonsillitis and pharyngitis in basically the same way, paying close attention to the cause, as well as easing the symptoms.
- Read the sections on mumps and glandular fever, swollen glands and mouth gargle, then combine recommendations as appropriate.

## THROMBOSIS, PHLEBITIS, THROMBOPHLEBITIS

Phlebitis is inflammation of veins, while thrombosis is a blood clot. The condition can be deep or superficial; phlebitis is the more common and is often caused by pregnancy, standing for long periods of time, a lack of exercise or smoking. Deep thrombosis is more serious because the veins affected are deep within the muscle. With thrombosis, blood clots can break off and travel around the circulatory system. Circulation and oxygen are impeded by the ensuing blockage and surrounding organs served by blood vessels may be damaged, depending on where the blockage is. Thrombosis can be a very serious problem which may potentially cause death. Occurrence of clots or ruptures in the brain are often referred to as stroke, while in the chest they are known as pulmonary thromboses (asthma can be an additional factor here). Deep vein thrombosis often comes with no symptoms and can surprise all concerned; diagnosis can be difficult.

The aim is to clear the vessels, reduce the stickiness of blood platelets which are clumping together and to strengthen the vascular walls through the use of calcium and rutin.

- Refer to dietary and herbal advice for angina and circulatory system. You must ensure that you have good circulation, therefore look at the relevant sections. Seek professional advice.
- Take exercise and generally engage in sensible activities. For the bedridden, this can be a serious problem, so massage will be vital.
- If you smoke – STOP.
- If the inflammation or phlebitis itself is visible, use an external poultice made with equal parts of tincture of oak bark, horse chestnut and comfrey leaf plus a few drops of lavender essential oil in a little St. John's wort flower oil. It should be used ice cold, so make the mixture strong, then put it in the freezer. Apply twice daily for ten minutes. Depending on the cause of the phlebitis, individual essential oils could be chosen.
- Take regular hydrotherapy and use a slant board.

## TINNITUS AND MENIÈRE'S SYNDROME

Tinnitus is a fairly common condition, causing ringing or buzzing in the ears. which may be accompanied by dizziness, nausea and balance problems. It may develop due to an infection, an obstruction, an accident or excessively noisy environments.

218

Symptoms of Menière's syndrome include variable loss of hearing, loss of balance, dizziness, nausea and vomiting. It is an inner ear problem affecting one or both ears. Many believe it is rooted in the nervous system while others believe it is a metabolic imbalance related to hypoglycaemia. Others suggest that poor circulation and inadequate blood flow to the brain are to blame. Both conditions are initially treated in exactly the same way. According to the speed of recovery, treatment is either short-term or longer term up to nine months.

- ✿ Maintain or develop a good diet with no dairy or wheat products; eat wholesome, nerve feeding foods in small but regular meals. Avoid tea and coffee.
- ✿ Superfood will be invaluable for keeping good blood sugar levels and supplying plenty of B vitamins.
- ✿ The ears are associated with the kidneys, so supportive kidney foods will also help.
- ✿ Drink lots of barley water.
- ♦ Colon, kidney and liver cleanses are vital for long-term treatment.
- ∾ Use equal parts of the following nerve herbs to support and nourish: skullcap herb, lobelia herb, vervain herb and passion flower.
- ∾ Use Dr. Christopher's B & B herbal ear formula (see Chapter Eleven) which is based on nervines, lymphatics, immune stimulants and antispasmodics. Use the ear drops nightly, then choose other herbs from the recommended list above to use as a regular teas and tinctures.
- ♦ Hot and cold showers will stimulate the whole head, and the neck in particular.

## UNDER-ACTIVE THYROID – HYPOTHYROIDISM

This is caused by insufficient thyroid hormones, and leads to general sluggishness, a sensitivity to the cold and general low body temperature. It can cause, in particular, cold hands and feet, slow heart rate, poor and slow digestion and a loss of appetite with weight gain; painful menstruation and other hormonal problems, sometimes including infertility; constipation, general low immunity; dry skin and hair, thinning eyebrows and overall fatigue. Goitre may also occur.

- ✿ If there is weight gain still eat three very balanced but light meals a day; rice, steamed vegetables, fruit and vegetables. Juicing fruits or vegetables is excellent as part of this food programme, especially those rich in digestive enzymes.
- ✿ Avoid cabbage, Brussels sprouts, kale, broccoli, watercress, turnip, cauliflower and mustard greens as they suppress thyroid hormone production.
- ✿ Gently increase seaweed intake as part of your food programme. Bladderwrack and kelp are especially beneficial incorporated into cooking.
- ♦ Use 3 parts Siberian ginseng root, 2 parts skullcap herb and 1 part lobelia herb to support the nerves and adrenal glands. Nerve stimulants like celery seed and oat straw will be vital. Take male and female hormones like agnus castus berries and saw palmetto berries. Heart, circulatory and digestive herbs will be needed. Do not use herbs that sedate the nervous system like valerian root. Use bladderwrack

seaweed as a tincture or capsule to balance the thyroid. If the immune system is low take echinacea root periodically (see Chapter Nine).

◆ Take hot and cold showers twice a day directing the water over the thyroid.
◆ Massage, using light strokes.

## UNUSUALLY STRONG MENSTRUAL FLOW

Occasionally, and always when it's least expected or wanted, one's period can flood. Should the flood be of short duration, there is no problem; but if it continues for days on end, or repeats itself each month, hormone imbalances and/or spinal, hip displacement must be considered and professional help sought. Sometimes menorrhagia occurs because there has been no ovulation; then the increased thickening of the uterus wall can cause congestive infection.

- General tips in Chapter Eight (Menstruation) must be followed. Professional advice should be sought if the problem persists.
- ✿ An increase in iodine through your diet is important (Take kelp tablets or eat extra seaweed.)
- ✿ Consume plenty of Superfood.
- ✿ Keep the diet simple yet supportive with just whole-grains, vegetables and fruit.
- ∾ It is useful to have astringent herbs to staunch the flow. A classic choice would be red raspberry – an astringent rich in iron and calcium. Other herbs would include lady's mantle herb, geranium herb or yarrow leaf. Yarrow is available for picking from spring to late autumn; use it to make a tea.
- ∾ To balance the hormones, there are many herb choices to use but an individual choice of plants will probably be necessary. Start with false unicorn root and squaw vine root.
- Don't exercise heavily until the flow has decreased and keep any water contact gentle and warm.

## URETHRITIS

This is infection of the urethra and needs similar treatment to cystitis, but extra mucilaginous and soothing herbs are usually needed, e.g. increase your intake of marshmallow root.

- ✿ Keep your diet simple yet supportive with whole-grains, vegetables and fruits initially.
- ✿ Drink plenty of barley water, and water in general.

## VAGINAL INFECTIONS – LEUCORRHOEA, TRICHOMONIASIS, VAGINITIS, ETC.

Friendly to invaders, the warmth and moisture of the vagina provide the perfect breeding ground for all kinds of undesirables. Tampons, vaginal deodorants, nylon tights, sexual lubricants, dirty hands and many other factors can tip the balance, causing an infection of some kind, especially if the immune system is a little low. Add to this a poor diet, stress, little exercise and a congested bowel or sluggish liver, and you have the ideal circumstances for the growth of yeasts, micro-organisms, protozoa and so on. Orthodox medicine generally deals with these problems with the use of sulphur drugs and antibiotics, which do work to a certain extent. They also leave the cause uninvestigated, thereby leaving the possibility of recurrence wide open. Whether it is the white discharge of leucorrhoea, the irritation of candida and other yeast infections or the tenacious bacteria-based trichomoniasis and gardnerella, there are basic rules to bear in mind. Be alert to vaginal itching, red swellings, discharge and odours.

✿ Avoid all tea, coffee, cola, juices, alcohol, squashes, sugar and chocolate – yeasts thrive on these.

✿ Refined foods and fats should be omitted from the diet, along with farmed meats and fish: pesticides and synthetic hormones will not help.

✿ Refer to Chapter Four and eat well. Eat lots of garlic and drink copious amount of water.

✿ Take lemon juice and apple cider vinegar daily, you can dilute these in water.

◆ Take acidophilus; make rejuvelac (see Chapter Four).

◆ Bowel, liver and kidney cleanses will be vital, over a period of time.

∾ Use equal amounts of endocrine balancing herbs: agnus castus berries, squaw vine herb and blessed thistle herb.

∾ Use some or all of these plants in equal parts: antibacterial or antimicrobial herbs internally like myrrh resin, echinacea root, barberry root bark or thuja leaves and lymphatics like poke root, cleavers leaves and mullein flower.

◆ Any blood-stained discharge should be reported to a doctor immediately.

◆ Wear cotton or silk underwear. Nylon tights will retain moisture and produce the environment that infections love; over-the-knee socks and stockings are better, or wear a suspender belt. If wearing trousers, use natural fibres like cotton, silk or wool.

◆ Use cotton-based sanitary towels. Avoid tampons.

◆ Discontinue internal lovemaking until the episode is over.

∾ Use vaginal pessaries (see Chapter Three).

∾ Consider vaginal douches using oak bark and other herbs.

◆ Make your own garlic vaginal suppositories by wrapping a whole clove of garlic (peeled) in two pieces of muslin with a pull-out string. Use during the day so that, if you experience any burning sensation, you can remove it: the delicate tissue of the vagina must not be damaged. Garlic is lethal to yeasts and stubborn bacteria like trichomonas and gardnerella. For further information on garlic see Chapters Four and Seven.

◆ Take only warm baths and always finish with a cold shower. You must cool the area to discourage bacterial and fungal growth. Add 5 drops of lavender essential oil and 1 drop of tea tree essential oil to your bath.

◆ Sitz baths will encourage circulation to the area (see Chapter Five).

◆ After the bath, use a herbal vaginal dusting powder or gel (see Chapter Eleven).

## VARICOSE VEINS AND ULCERS

Veins have the job of assisting the arteries with the job of circulating the blood. If the tiny valves of the inner walls of the veins do not work properly, then blood accumulates and causes stretching and bulging. Varicose veins look lumpy and bluish and can ache and feel sore. They may be the result of constipation, thrombophlebitis, liver disorders, calcium and magnesium deficiency, an hereditary history, working in jobs that require a lot of standing, habitually sitting with crossed legs, wearing tight clothing, being pregnant or having borne children, along with poor diet and smoking.

- ✿ Refer to angina, haemorrhoids and thrombophlebitis for dietary advice on circulatory well-being, and the circulatory system in Chapter Nine for general advice.
- ❧ Take linseed oil capsules (Omega 3).
- ❧ Take natural lecithin, preferably in capsules.
- ❧ As a preventative measure, drink 2 cups daily of a herbal tea made up of equal parts of nettle leaves and gingko leaves.
- ❧ Take three cayenne capsules three times daily.
- ❧ Take a mixture of equal parts lime tree flowers (vessel strengthener), prickly ash bark (to stimulate circulation), hawthorn berries and leaves (essential for heart and vascular support) and dandelion root (for water balance).
- ♦ Maintain good exercise routines.
- ♦ Use cold sitz baths over the legs and follow warm baths with powerful cold showers.
- ♦ Explore and maintain skin brushing.
- ♦ Keep your feet up above heart level when at rest.
- ♦ Make a massage rub with equal amounts of oak bark tincture, chestnut tincture and castor oil. Add 4mls each of witch hazel and cypress essential oil to 250ml of the base oil.

## WARTS AND VERRUCAS

Warts are small growths found anywhere on the body including the genitalia. They are caused by a virus and are highly contagious. Warts on the feet are often known as verrucas or plantar warts.

- ✿ Include plenty of fresh garlic in your diet.
- ✿ Avoid coffee, tea, cakes, and junk food.
- ❧ Use general immune and specific anti-viral herbs like echinacea root, pau d'arco bark, thuja leaves and elderberry. Vary as tinctures, teas and syrups.
- ❧ Repeatedly apply the white juice of dandelions and ground spurge onto the affected area.
- ❧ Viral verrucas and warts need to be treated specifically to keep ahead of the virus. Use a threesome of targeted essential oils. Use one a week – start with lemon, then tea tree, then bergamot, keep this up for 3 to 6 weeks.

## WORMS AND AMOEBIC INFESTATIONS

Parasites that live in the intestines are becoming more prevalent due to the poor health of factory-produced meats. They are opportunistic creatures and thrive in our modern day immunally-low bodies which have been bombarded with antibiotics and drugs of all kinds. Parasitic threadworm is, and always has been, very common; probably one in five children will have them at some time, but adults also get infestations. More and more children are becoming infested with parasites, particularly after MMR and other vaccinations due to their overwhelming impact on the immune system. Travelling can also lay one open to all kinds of unusual parasites, and parasitic diarrhoea is a common occurrence. Intestinal parasites like giardia, ascaria, hookworm and amoeba are now becoming very common too. They were once associated with visiting foreign climates but they are becoming increasingly more common in Britain, whereas tapeworms have always occurred here, particularly from cooked meat. The problem is that a lot of parasites are only active in hot temperatures, so baths, electric blankets and saunas will encourage their proliferation. (Testing for them in a British pathology laboratory is usually disappointing because they hibernate in the cold and few laboratories appear to take this presently into consideration. People are often 'tested' for infestations but the stools are not kept hot, which is vital. Thus the organisms die or hibernate. This means that the results will prove negative.) Colonics can give you a good feedback on parasitic activity.

✿ Eat lots of raw garlic, freshly capsulated for children if necessary.
✿ Avoid clogging, sticky mucus-forming food as this time, in particular wheat and diary products.
❧ There are many herbs that can be chosen to treat parasites and it will vary accordingly, but wormwood leaves, walnut fruits and olive leaves with barberry root bark, cascara sagrada root and other vital bowel laxatives and liver aids will work. Alongside this, take freshly crushed cloves to kill the eggs.
♦ Follow the programme in Chapter Six, accompanied by the three-stage colon cleanse.
♦ Colon cleansing and colonics will be vital. Warm to hot water can be used in the colonic, enticing out the parasites with its heat. Colonics are not necessary for children with threadworm, but will be invaluable for those with parasites.

## CANCER AND OTHER 'INCURABLE' OR SO-CALLED 'TERMINAL' CHRONIC DISEASES

Cancer requires a very broad, individual approach. The whole person will need to be carefully considered on all levels, physically, mentally and emotionally. Many people should be involved with this, not simply one practitioner or just the hospital, but rather a team of practitioners and therapists and a network of friends and carers.

FOR THE VERY SICK

When there is no time to lose and conventional medicine has pronounced someone 'terminally ill', a minimal 30-day natural healing and cleansing programme can be undertaken, under the guidance of a qualified practitioner, hospital consultants and the patient's own GP and a team of 2 or 3 assistants/carers. Guidance on this routine will be very specific with many individual considerations.

Herbs to support the body in general will be vital, those called 'adaptogens' (see Chapter Seven) will be specifically required. Siberian ginseng taken as a tincture (1 tsp 3 or 4 times daily) is a very good choice, astragalus is another. Adaptogens make sure that the body can cope with any incoming stress, helping the body to 'adapt' when it is asked to do things rather than 'crash'. It will help keep a person's weight stable, rather than allowing it to fall off as it often does with cancer. If you experience weight loss, drinking 3 cups a day of fenugreek seed tea will be very helpful.

Herbs used for cancer are called neoplastics. This means that they have a 'blocking' or 'inhibiting' effect on the new growth, the neoplasm. A simple and famous neoplastic is garlic, while others include mistletoe berries, poke root, burdock root and red clover flowers.

Herbs that clean the bloodstream will also be vital for cancer and other chronic diseases, as they support the body through its process of releasing toxins shed from cancerous growths. A blood nourisher and general stimulator, vital for all chronic diseases, is cayenne. Use very hot cayenne – it is vital. Herbs with liver balancing or neoplastic abilities combined, like burdock root, red clover flowers, yellow dock root, cleavers leaves and dandelion root, should be used.

Other foods and herbs will be required to support and nourish the nervous system. (See Chapter Nine.)

Immuno enhancers and lymphatic cleansers like echinacea root, grapefruit seed, neem leaf, barberry root bark, turmeric root, poke root, mullein flowers and lobelia seeds will be vital. When dealing with lymph cancers DO NOT use echinacea as this plant encourages white cell production. Instead use choices like pau d'arco bark, but there are many others.

All eliminative channels (to include the kidney, liver and bowel) will need to be cleansed and balanced. For this you will need plants like buplerum herb, milk thistle seed, cascara sagrada bark and corn silk. Specific cleansing routines will be essential – see Chapter Six.

Some individual areas will need assessment – for instance, breast cancers will need a raising in progesterone-rich herbs to counteract the oestrogen surge which can often cause the cancer. Herbs rich in oestrogen like red clover flowers and hops strobile will need to be avoided.

The digestive system is a key factor in cases of cancer. This must work efficiently. Many cancer patients have low hydrochloride levels. Therefore, use meadowsweet herb and other digestives like gentian root. Food programmes, however individualised, will need to be based around plenty of freshly-juiced vegetables and fruits – based on 72% carrot, with the rest taken from the cabbage family vegetables (avoiding beetroot and beet tops and avoiding cabbage if certain thyroid conditions exist). In addition, take Superfood-type nutritional drinks and raw food in general, especially garlic. Precautions are necessary to ensure that plenty of raw food and juices are eaten and drunk without causing an excess of cold and therefore creating excess mucus, coldness and tiredness and a less efficient spleen. Listen to your body, if you overdo anything it will let you know.

Vaginal and anal suppositories (see Chapter Three), poultices, compresses and castor oil packs will be vital to deal with the manifestations of the cancers and other diseases, e.g. tumours and cysts. This 'drawing out' and healing routine will either pull the toxins up and out to the surface or help flush them through the blood and lymph systems and finally the bowel. Flower remedies and essential oils will be part of the routine just as the herbs in their forms are.

Other requirements will be exercise, acupuncture, massage, reflexology and lymph drainage and hydrotherapy routines, some of which are very specific to chronic diseases. Of course emotional support and/or therapy with plenty of laughter to encourage the healing process will be vital.

## BOOK LIST

*Cure for All Cancers* by Hilda Clark (New Century)
*Herbal Healing for Women* by Rosemary Gladstar (Simon & Schuster)
*Male Herbal* by James Green (Crossing Press)
*Women's Guide to Herbal Medicine* by Carol Rogers (Hamish Hamilton)
*Encyclopedia of Herbs* by Andrew Chevaillier (Dorling Kindersley)

## RESOURCES

Measuring Bone Density: McCue PLC, PO Box 84, Winchester, SO121 2RO
**Acidophilus:** Biocare, Lakeside, 180 Lifford Lane, Kings Norton, Birmingham, B30 3NT. Tel: 0121 433 3879
**Nature's Biotics:** Springfield Pharmacy, Mr. J N Patel, 124 Sheen Road, Richmond, Surrey TW9 1UR. Tel: 0181 940 2304

# ELEVEN

# First Aid

Knowing how to give first aid in emergencies can and does save lives.

Herbal remedies have their limitations, and the help of modern medicine should be enlisted for any serious injury or illness. In fact, trauma medicine and trauma surgery are the best kinds of so-called 'conventional' medicine; make sure you call for their help if necessary. Take a first aid course to gain basic skills which can help until professional help arrives.

While following the golden rule, 'Do Not Harm', you must also accept the principle of the calculated risk in first aid. Even if there is some risk, it is right to apply a treatment that will benefit the majority of casualties. You must not, however, use a doubtful treatment just for the sake of doing something.

## EMERGENCIES

### Bee Stings

Bee stings are painful and can cause fever and headache, allergic reactions (due to the body's release of histamine), swelling, redness and rash. With bee stings, the poison bag may still be attached to the sting; remove this with tweezers, without damaging the poison bag, then apply freshly crushed plantain leaf, lavender essential oil or crushed garlic directly onto the sting.

A cold chamomile compress made with diluted essential oil could be equally well applied. One neat drop of chamomile essential oil can be applied directly to the sting and this may be repeated every few hours (or when irritation occurs) for 2 or 3 days. St. John's wort flower oil or tincture is also helpful as is echinacea root tincture used topically.

### Bites and Stings – Serious

Calm the patient. Then immerse the affected area in a bowl of cold water containing ice cubes and a teaspoon of baking powder. This slows the circulation and helps prevent the poison spreading. Alternatively, apply fresh raw onion over the area or cover with wheatgerm oil, put an ice bag on top and apply calendula ointment. This should be done before anything else. Give Dr. Bach Rescue Remedy (a flower remedy available from specialist shops and pharmacies, including Boots), arnica (a homeopathic remedy), or a few drops of lobelia herb tincture. Allergic reactions need to be treated with cortisone and/or adrenaline for which you must seek urgent medical help: administer coffee in the short term. If the patient loses consciousness, apply a few drops of lobelia tincture to the lips. This very often brings them back.

Don't scratch or squeeze the wound, as this can encourage infection. Use lavender, tea tree or rosemary essential oil, or lemon juice. Also apply echinacea root tincture topically. When in natural surroundings, look for plantain leaves and either rub on fresh or prepare as an extra strong tea (i.e. boiled for 10 minutes) and apply to the wound on cotton wool.

## BLEEDING

Dr. Christopher, as well as a number of other popular herbalists, recommends the treating of the wound with cayenne pepper in order to stop bleeding both internally and externally. Other herbs with predominantly styptic qualities are plantain leaves, yarrow herb, cranesbill root, slippery elm inner bark, oak bark and ground ivy. All these herbs are best used in powder form. Find out the cause of the bleeding and seek appropriate further treatment.

## BURNS

Burns can be divided into four groups:

First degree – affecting the epidermis.
Second degree – involving the dermis (blistering falls into this category).
Third degree – includes the epidermis, dermis and underlying tissues.
Fourth degree – down to and including bone.

With third and fourth degree burns, the pain may be less because there is often a loss of sensation due to nerve damage.

### First and Second Degree Burns

Initially some St. John's wort flower oil poured over the burn will ease the nerve pain. Make or buy 'burn paste' (see 'Other Items' in this chapter) and pack the wound with this. The paste will gradually be absorbed during the healing process and should be 'topped up' when necessary – but do not remove the previous application. The paste will form a soft cast-like bandage, but initially a light bandage or covering will be required on top. The use of burn paste does not require the cleansing of the burned area to clinical standards; there have been no reports of infection with this treatment. It eventually falls off just like a scab that has healed.

## EYE INJURY AND TEMPORARY BLINDNESS

An Ayurvedic remedy for eye injuries is simple: lemon juice squeezed and put in with an eye bath. Plantain leaves, eyebright herb and chamomile flowers are also very useful for treating eye injuries, either on their own or combined – make as a tea first and wash your eyes with the fluid using an eye bath.

## Temporary Blindness Caused by Chemicals or Acids

Flood the eyes with cold water or milk in order to wash away and minimise the effect of the irritant. Follow by carefully placing a tiny amount of cayenne pepper in the eyes; only a very small amount should be used, so as not to cause further pain to the eye. Cayenne pepper, as well as being a high-quality healer, is intended as an irritant, causing the eyes to water freely, for tears contain a number of healing factors which can begin to effect repair. The discomfort experienced by using cayenne in the eye is short-lived. (Mid-stream urine or breast milk can be used to flush out the eye in an emergency.)

## Gashes and Lacerations – Deep Wounds

Use a few drops of lobelia herb and cayenne pod tincture orally and then pack with 'deep wound' paste. (see 'Other Items' at the end of this chapter for recipe). Renew paste on a daily basis.

## Heat Stroke and Sun Stroke

The onset of this is usually slow and is heralded by a confused feeling, headache, drowsiness, a raised temperature, discomfort in the kidney area and a lower urine output than expected. The skin appears flushed, hot and dry. This type of temperature needs to be brought down quickly. Feed plenty of liquids, ideally involving infusions from plants with a high sodium content e.g. seaweed, kelp, lichens or liquorice rhizome. If mineral salt has to be added, use minimal quantities only.

## Insect Repellents

Elder leaves and flowers can be bruised and made into a concoction. Applied to the skin it will act as a repellent, but can also be used as a poultice after the event (i.e. if bitten by insects). Lemon grass or citronella also make excellent insect repellents.

## Shock and Fainting

Use lobelia herb tincture; a few drops on the tongue will help in any shock situation, from grief to a car accident. It also helps revive patients suffering blackouts. The tincture only needs to be rubbed onto the lips in situations where swallowing or access is limited. Dr. Bach 'Rescue Remedy' will also work well in this situation.

## Sleeplessness with Extremely Shocked or Exhausted Nerves

Use valerian root capsules. Use tincture or capsules (an average adult dose) three hours before bedtime and then more just prior to retiring to ensure good sleep. More can be taken if waking in the night is a problem but a 2-hour interval should have elapsed since the bedtime dose. This treatment can be used for a week or more but real nerve-building is also required; for this use skullcap herb, chamomile flowers, lime flowers and lobelia herb long-term.

## Snake Bites

Lavender has a long history of use against the venom produced by the European adder; however, lavender essential oil and echinacea root tincture applied externally together are more effective. Echinacea root should also be administered by mouth as a tincture in frequent doses. (Echinacea root has been used for centuries for rattlesnake bites in Canada and America). Just a few drops of lobelia herb tincture applied both topically and internally will help prevent the body going into anaphylactic shock. Do not suck the bite – any injury in the mouth would become contaminated; filled teeth can also harbour the venom and may cause the jaw to swell to an enormous size. You can buy anti-venom treatments from the chemist. The shape of the snake's eyes can give a rough indication as to its type: i.e. round – non-poisonous, elongated – poisonous.

## Wasp Stings

For wasp stings, which are alkaline, it is best to neutralise the sting with cider vinegar or lemon juice first. Then treat with applications of lavender and chamomile essential oil for 2 or 3 days.

## Unconsciousness

Apply a few drops of lobelia herb tincture and Dr. Bach Rescue Remedy to the lips and wrists. If the patient does not regain consciousness within three minutes; call for an ambulance.

# NON-EMERGENCIES

This is a brief outline of some of the more frequent everyday problems you may encounter, with suggestions on how relief may be obtained by herbal and other methods.

## Blisters

Apply 1 drop of lavender and chamomile essential oil neat. Apply gently and rub in thoroughly. Or use lavender spray, followed by finely-powdered myrrh and cover with padded Band-Aid.

## Bruises

Apply hot and cold packs to increase the circulation. Follow this with applications of comfrey leaf ointment, to which calendula, hyssop or plantain leaf could be added. These herbs can equally well be made into a poultice. Tincture of arnica flower and marigold flower, applied directly to the bruise several times a day, can be equally soothing. (Do not ingest arnica in any form as this is poisonous if used internally.) St. John's wort oil would also be a good alternative.

## CHILBLAINS

Chilblains are caused by poor circulation. I have heard many a tale of traditional remedies – including cayenne pepper in the socks and onions in the stockings – and they all seem to work. But ultimately you need to work on the problem internally, which means investigating the reasons for your poor circulation. (See Chapter Nine.)

## DIARRHOEA, STOMACH ULCERS, BOWEL PAIN, ETC.

Mix slippery elm bark or arrowroot with cold water into a drinkable gruel. This is excellent as a convalescence food too.

## INFECTION

Use echinacea root because when it is ingested the white blood cell count will increase dramatically upon each dose. The best course of treatment is to take it for ten days, have four days off, and then, if necessary, continue with another ten-day course. In the first few days you can take half-hourly doses of ten drops and this can be reduced as you feel better. Echinacea root can also be very effective when put directly on to an infected cut. If you do not have any echinacea, use something like garlic and turmeric (both of which are readily available from local shops, or you may already have some in the kitchen). These can be very effective when made into a paste, added to mashed potato and applied directly to a wound. You should also eat some! Chamomile flower tea will also help because of its anti-microbial qualities.

## TOOTHACHE

Make an immediate appointment to see the dentist.

Meanwhile, chew a clove for a while and then spit it out, or put a little clove oil on a cotton bud and gently apply to the affected area. Take echinacea root tea or tincture, in case an abscess has begun to form. Constantly gargle with herbal mouthwash containing oak bark, myrrh resin and St. John's wort flowers. (See 'Other Items' later on in this chapter).

## SPRAINS AND STRAINS

Use a cold compress soaked in a strong decoction made from all or some of the following herbs: ginger rhizome, thyme, lavender herb, marigold flowers, St. John's wort flowers, plantain leaf and chamomile flowers. This will reduce swelling. Alternatively, soak the affected area in a hot decoction made from chamomile flowers, comfrey leaf, rosemary herb and wormwood herb. Alternate this with cold soaks and treat with trauma oil (see formula under 'Other Items' later in this chapter).

## CONTENTS OF A FIRST AID KIT

### MATERIALS

- 6 triangular bandages
- A selection of bandages: at least 4 elasticated, 4 crepe, tubular bandages with applicator, and gauze of various sizes
- Cling film
- Cotton wool: pads can be made using cotton wool and open weave or gauze bandages
- Dental mirror
- Dextrose tablets
- Eye bath and small mixing container
- First Aid Manual
- Foil blanket (or a wool blanket if there is room) or a polythene survival bag
- Grain alcohol
- Hot and cold packs – available from chemists
- Magnifying glass
- Notepad and pencil
- Plasters and butterfly stitches
- Plastic gloves or disposable gloves (to wear when dressing wounds and handling waste)
- Pointed and flat tweezers
- Safety pins and clips for securing bandages
- Scalpel
- Scissors
- Selection of sterile dressings
- Tape
- Torch
- Venom remover (if travelling abroad)
- Whistle
- Wooden spatula

Bandaging primarily protects and supports, but it can also be used to apply pressure, thus arresting bleeding. It can support a fracture, help with pain control and give psychological benefits. The actual technique of bandaging is a vast subject and has been more than adequately covered in first aid manuals and the Barefoot Doctor's Manual (see 'Resources' section at the end of this chapter).

### HERBAL FIRST AID ITEMS

All items must be labelled clearly. All other items (except tincture) should be in plastic containers.

- 10ml cayenne pepper tincture – bleeding, shock and cold.
- 50ml echinacea root tincture – topical and internal use for bites, cuts and so on.

- 10ml lobelia tincture – shock.
- Dr. Bach Rescue Remedy – shock.
- 10ml St. John's wort flower tincture – for toothache, bruises, cuts and trauma in general.
- Codeine – this should be used, as we do not have legal access to painkilling opium.
- 30ml coffee tincture – for alcohol poisoning and other situations where a nerve stimulant is necessary. Prickly ash will also work in a similar way.
- Colon capsules – both strong and mild.
- For diarrhoea – slippery elm bark powder or use bentonite clay for serious diarrhoea.
- Fresh juniper berries – for those unable to urinate.
- 30 or 50ml formula of 5 parts hawthorn leaf and 1 part cayenne pepper tincture – heart attack tonic.
- 30 or 50ml formula of 1 part valerian rhizome and 1 part lobelia herb – nerve sedative.
- 50ml formula of 30ml agnus castus berries and 20ml cramp bark tincture – pre-menstrual symptoms, cramps and so on.

## LOBELIA AND CAYENNE

### Two Major Components of a First Aid Kit

### Lobelia (Lobelia inflata)

Lobelia is one of the most useful systemic relaxants available to us. It has a general depressant action on the central and autonomic nervous systems and on neuro-muscular action. Lobelia contains alkaloids called pyridine and piperidine – these act to stimulate and then to block autonomic nervous activity. It is very useful in a first aid situation for shock and trauma. It may be used in many conditions and in combination with other herbs to further its effectiveness.

It is specifically used for bronchial asthma and bronchitis. Lobelia is a powerful respiratory stimulant, whilst the chemical isolobelinine found in lobelia is an emetic and respiratory stimulant, which will stimulate catarrhal secretion and expectoration whilst relaxing the muscles of the respiratory system. The overall action is a truly holistic combination of stimulation and relaxation! It can be used for any internal or external situation, 'drops' in most cases being sufficient. (It is a Section 12 herb.)

### Cayenne Pepper (Capsicum minimum)

Cayenne pepper is unsurpassed in its effect on the circulatory system. Cayenne is a herb which everyone should have in tincture or powder form, in the kitchen, the bathroom and in the car. As a prime first aid measure it will prevent fainting or loss of consciousness, as it keeps the blood supply constant; yet it will not allow damaged arteries to lose dangerous quantities of blood, as it also assists in blood clotting in certain circumstances. Cayenne pepper stops bleeding immediately and its high level of vitamins A and C also cleans and disinfects.

Again, it may be used internally and externally (though caution should be observed when causing pain to open wounds in shocked/fragile patients).

## OTHER ITEMS

**Burn paste (also for sprains and wounds):** made from 1 part slippery elm bark, 2 parts comfrey leaves and flowers, 1 part lobelia herb powder, $^1/_4$ part lavender leaves and flowers powder and $^1/_4$ part bentonite clay. Carry the ingredients separately and mix when needed in a base of (equal parts) honey, wheatgerm oil and aloe vera gel. Spread evenly over area and leave on, simply adding more to it as required.

**Digestive and travel tincture:** ginger rhizome, sweet fennel seed and peppermint herb. Combine in equal parts. Take drops as needed.

**Mallow and walnut ointment (Dr. Christopher's bone, flesh and cartilage formula):** powdered herbs of: 6 parts oak bark, 3 parts gravel root, 3 parts mullein herb, 3 parts marshmallow root, 3 parts walnut bark and leaves, 2 parts wormwood herb, 1 part lobelia herb, 1 part skullcap herb and 1 part comfrey leaf. See 'Ointment Making', Chapter Three.

It is useful for regeneration of tendons, ligaments, bone and flesh, as designed and used by Dr. Christopher.

**Dr. Christopher's B & B ear formula:** made from equal parts of garlic bulb and mullein flower oil, blue cohosh root, black cohosh root, blue vervain herb, skullcap herb, lobelia herb.

With an eye dropper, insert 8–12 drops of the oil into each ear at night. Warm the dropper full of the intended drops on a radiator (leave on a saucer). Then plug ear with cotton wool. Keep the plug in overnight. If you prefer, go into the procedure gradually, building up to every, or every other night. Flush the ears out with equal amount of warm water and cider vinegar the morning after each treatement. If you continue the treatment for longer than five or six weeks with no beneficial results, go to your GP or to an outpatients' clinic at a hospital and get a nurse to syringe your ears out.

**Dr. Christopher's anti-miscarriage formula:** 3 parts false unicorn root and 1 part lobelia root. Get plenty of bed rest and drink tea made from these herbs at regular intervals: drink $^1/_2$ cup of tea, or take 10 drops of tincture, at hourly intervals, until the bleeding stops. Follow with a half dose (every 2 hours) for the next 24 hours. Seek medical advice.

**Dr. Schulze's deep tissue oil:** made from equal parts of: wintergreen, menthol crystals, arnica herb, St. John's wort flower oil, chilli oil and marigold flowers in a base of olive oil.

**Marigold and comfrey ointment (general healing salve):** equal parts (50g each) of marigold flowers, comfrey root, lobelia flowers, plantain herb, thyme leaves, lavender flowers and turmeric root. Useful as a first aid measure for cuts and grazes. See ointment making, Chapter Three.

**Trauma oil or ointment:** this contains arnica flower oil, St. John's wort flower and marigold flower oil. Mix equal parts of each in a base of organic virgin cold-pressed olive oil.

**Plantain and barberry ointment (eczema ointment):** equal parts (50g each) black walnut inner hull, barberry root, chickweed herb, plantain leaf, marigold flower and lavender essential oil. Useful in the treatment of eczema and similar skin conditions. See 'Ointment Making', Chapter Three.

**Healing and antiseptic ointment:** use barberry root, marigold flowers and thyme. Mix equal parts in an olive oil and beeswax base – see 'Ointment Making', Chapter Three.

**Herbal cast or deep wound paste:** equal parts of: comfrey root, marshmallow root, slippery elm bark and turmeric rhizome powders. Make into workable paste with olive oil and lavender essential oil. Pack into the wound and bandage. Do not worry about cleaning out the paste, it will grow into and become the new tissue – simply add more if any comes away when bathing. See 'Ointment Making', Chapter Three.

**Herbal snuff:** powdered: barberry root bark, mustard seeds, horseradish root, garlic bulb and cayenne pepper. Combine equal quantities of these herb powders (for further details see 'Nose Problems' in Chapter Ten).

**Insect repellent:** 1 part thyme leaf, 2 parts lemon grass, 1 part lavender herb and 1 part peppermint leaf mixed with wheatgerm oil.

**Lavender spray for burns and bites:** 250ml distilled water and 4-5ml lavender essential oil.

**Mouth gargle:** use for a sore throat, inflamed mouth, painful tonsils or abscesses. Gargle three times daily with a mixture of 500ml spring water, 200ml oak bark tincture, 200ml barberry root bark tincture and 200ml myrrh tincture or neem leaf tincture. Choose two or three of the following essential oils and add two or three drops of each: cinnamon, sweet fennel, sage, thyme, angelica, tea tree, myrrh and rosemary. Only a qualified herbalist should make up this formula due to the essential oil content to be used orally. Store in a dark cupboard.

**Pain and headache:** a tincture of white and black willow bark, wild lettuce juice, feverfew herb, meadowsweet leaf and flower, St. John's wort flower and lavender flower: take 1tsp hourly. Corydalis can also be aded for extra pain relief.

**Swollen glands:** use 3 parts mullein leaf and 1 part lobelia herb in tea, tincture or powder form during or after the first bout of swollen glands; take 1tsp three times daily.

If the throat, in particular, is painful, use tinctures of: 4 parts echinacea root, 2 parts red clover flowers, 2 parts sage leaf, 2 parts barberry root bark, 2 parts myrrh resin and 1 part Siberian ginseng root as a tincture, take 1tsp three times daily for ten days.

# ENGLISH TO LATIN TRANSLATION AND PARTS OF THE HERB TO USE

| Common Name | Part | Genus species |
|---|---|---|
| Agnus Castus | herb | *Vitex agnus castus* |
| Agrimony | herb | *Agrimonia eupatoria* |
| Aloe | leaf, gel | *Aloe ferrox / spicata* |
| Angelica | root | *Angelica archangelica* |
| Apple | pectin | *Malus communis* |
| Artichoke | globe bud | *Cynara scolymus* |
| Astragalus | herb | *Astragalus membranious / complanatus* |
| Balm of Gilead | bud / resin | *Commiphera opobalsamum / Populus balsamifera* |
| Barberry | root bark | *Berberis vulgaris* |
| Black Pepper | seeds | *Piper nigrum* |
| Black Walnut | inner hull | *Juglans nigra* |
| Black Cohosh | root | *Cimicifuga racemosa* |
| Bladderwrack | herb | *Fucus vesculosis* |
| Blessed Thistle | herb | *Cnicus benedictus* |
| Blue Cohosh | root | *Caulophyllum thalictroides* |
| Boneset | herb | *Eupatorium perfoliatum* |
| Boswellia | root | *Boswellia serrata* |
| Buchu | leaf | *Agathosma betulina* |
| Buplerum | herb | *Bupleurum scorzonerifolium* |
| Burdock | seed, root, | *Arctium lappa* |
| Butternut | inner hull | *Junglans cinerea* |
| Cascara Sagrada | aged bark | *Rhamnus purshiana* |
| Catnip | herb | *Nepeta cataria* |
| Cayenne | fruit | *Capsicum annum / minimum* |
| Celery | seed | *Apium graveolens* |
| Chamomile (Roman) | flowers | *Anthemis nobilis* |
| Chamomile (German) | flowers | *Chamomilla recutita* |

| | | |
|---|---|---|
| Chickweed | herb | *Stellaria media* |
| Cleavers | herb | *Galium aparine* |
| Clove | bud oil | *Syzygium aromaticum* |
| Coltsfoot | leaf | *Tussilago farfara* |
| Comfrey | leaf | *Symphytum officinale* |
| Corn | silk | *Zea mays* |
| Corydalis | tuber | *Corydalis bulbosa* |
| Crampbark | bark | *Viburnum opulus* |
| Cranesbill (American) | root | *Geranium maculatum* |
| Damiana | leaf, herb | *Turnera aphrodisiaca, diffusa* |
| Dandelion | root, leaf | *Taraxacum officinale* |
| Devils Claw | root | *Harpagophytum procumbens* |
| Dong Quai | root | *Angelica sinensis (Asia)* |
| Echinacea | root, flower, leaf | *Echinacea angustifolia, purpurea* |
| Elecampane | root | *Inula helenium* |
| Elder | berry, flower, leaf | *Sambucus nigra* |
| Eucalyptus | oil, leaf | *Eucalyptus globulus* |
| Eyebright | herb | *Euphrasia officinalis* |
| False Unicorn | root | *Chamaelirium luteum* |
| Fennel | seed | *Foeniculum vulgare* |
| Fenugreek | seed | *Trigonella foenum-græcum* |
| Feverfew | herb | *Tanacetum parthenium* |
| Figwort | root | *Scrophularia nodosa* |
| Flax | seed, oil | *Linum usitatissimum* |
| Gentian | root | *Gentiana lutea* |
| Ginger | rhizome | *Zingiber officinale* |
| Ginkgo | leaf | *Ginkgo biloba* |
| Ginseng USA | root | *Panax quinquefolium (notoginseng)* |
| Ginseng Chinese | root | *Panax ginseng (sp. Rhen Shen)* |
| Golden Seal | root | *Hydrastis canadensis* |
| Gotu Kola | root | *Hydrocotyl asiatica* |
| Gravel Root | root | *Eupatorium purpureum* |
| Hawthorn | berry, flower, leaf | *Crataegus oxycantha* |
| Hibiscus | flowers | *Hibiscus abelmoschus* |
| Holy Thistle | herb | *Cardus benedictus* |
| Hops | flower (strobile) | *Humulus lupulus* |
| Horehound | herb | *Ballota nigra* |
| Horseradish | root | *Armoracia rusticana* |
| Horsetail | herb | *Equisetum arvense* |
| Hydrangea | root | *Hydrangea arborescens* |
| Juniper | berries | *Juniperis communis* |
| Kola | nut | *Cola acuminata / vera* |
| Ladies Mantle | herb | *Alchemilla vulgaris* |
| Lavender | flower, oil | *Lavandula vera / officinalis* |

| | | |
|---|---|---|
| Liquorice | root | *Glycyrrhiza glabra / uralensis* |
| Lemon Balm | leaf | *Melissa officinalis* |
| Lime Blossom | flowers | *Tilia europea* |
| Lobelia | herb, seed, pod | *Lobelia inflata* |
| Marigold | flower | *Calendula officinalis* |
| Marshmallow | root | *Althea officinales* |
| Meadowsweet | leaf, flower | *Filipendula ulmaria* |
| Milk Thistle | seed | *Silybum marianum* |
| Mistletoe | leaf, berry | *iscum album* |
| Mahonia | root, root bark, berries | *Mahonia aquifolium* |
| Motherwort | herb | *Leonurus cardiaca* |
| Mugwort | whole plant | *Artemisia vulgaris* |
| Mullein | leaf | *Verbascum thapsus* |
| Mustard | seed | *Brassica alba / nigra* |
| Myrrh | resin | *Commiphora myrrha / molmol* |
| Neem Tree (Nim) | seeds, leaf | *Azadirachta indica* |
| Nettles | leaf | *Urtica dioica* |
| Oak | bark, gall, twig | *Quercus alba* |
| Olive | leaf | *Olea europea* |
| Oregon grape | root bark | *Berberis aquifolium* |
| Parsley | root, leaf | *Petroselinum crispum* |
| Pasque Flower | herb | *Anemone pulsatilla* |
| Passion Flower | leaves | *Passiflora incarnata* |
| Pau d'arco | inner bark | *Tabebuia impetigenosa* |
| Pennyroyal | leaf | *Mentha pulegium* |
| Peppermint, Spearmint | leaf, oil | *Mentha piperita / spicata* |
| Pfaffia | root | *Pfaffia paniculata* |
| Pine | resin, needles | *Pinus species* |
| Plantain | leaf, juice | *Plantago major* |
| Poke | root | *Phytolacca americana / decandra* |
| Prickly Ash | berry | *Zanthoxylum bungeanum / americanum* |
| Psyllium | husks | *Plantago ovata* |
| Pumpkin | seeds | *Cucurbita pepo* |
| Red Clover | blossoms | *Trifolium pratense* |
| Red Raspberry | leaf | *Rubus idoeus* |
| Rehmannia | root | *Rehmannia glutinosa* |
| Rhubarb | root | *Rheum palmatum / rhaponticum* |
| Rosemary | herb | *Rosmarinus officinalis* |
| Sage | leaf | *Salvia officinalis* |
| Sphagnum Moss | herb | *Sphagnum cymbilifolium* |
| Sarsaparilla | root | *Smilax officinale / ornate* |
| Saw Palmetto | berry | *Serenoa serrulata* |

| Senna | leaf, pod, root | *Cassia angustifolia* |
|---|---|---|
| Schizandra | berries | *Schizandra chinensis* |
| Siberian Ginseng | root | *Eleutherococcus senticosus* |
| Skullcap | herb | *Scutellaria lateriflora* |
| Slippery Elm | inner bark | *Ulmus fulva* |
| Squaw Vine | herb | *Mitchella repens* |
| St. John's Wort | flower | *Hypericum perforatum* |
| Tea Tree | oil | *Melaleuca alternifolia* |
| Thuja | leaf, seed, | *Thuja occidentalis* |
| Thyme | leaves | *Thymus vulgaris* |
| Turmeric | rhizome | *Curcuma longa* |
| Usnea | whole plant | *Usnea longissima* |
| Uva Ursi (Bearberry) | leaf | *Arctostaphylos uva-ursi* |
| Valerian | rhizome | *Valeriana officinalis* |
| Vervain | leaf, tops | *Verbena officinalis* |
| Wild Cherry | bark | *Prunus serotina* |
| Wild Lettuce | leaf | *Lactuca virosa* |
| Wild Oats | herb | *Avena sativa* |
| Wild Yam | root | *Dioscorea villosa* |
| Willow | bark | *Salix alba* |
| Wood Betony | herb | *Stachys betonica* |
| Wormwood | herb | *Artemisia absinthium* |
| Yarrow | herb | *Achillea millefolium* |
| Yellow Dock | root | *Rumex crispus* |

# APPENDIX 2

# LATIN TO ENGLISH TRANSLATION

| Genus species | Common Name |
| --- | --- |
| *Achillea millefolium* | Yarrow |
| *Agathosma betulina* | Buchu |
| *Agrimonia eupatoria* | Agrimony |
| *Alchemilla vulgaris* | Ladies Mantle |
| *Aloe ferrox / spicata* | Aloe |
| *Althea officinales* | Marshmallow |
| *Anemone pulsatilla* | Pasque flower |
| *Angelica archangelica* | Angelica |
| *Angelica sinensis (Asia)* | Dong Quai |
| *Anthemis nobilis* | Chamomile (Roman) |
| *Apium graveolens* | Celery |
| *Arctium lappa* | Burdock |
| *Arctostaphylos uva-ursi* | Uva Ursi (Bearberry) |
| *Armoracia rusticana* | Horseradish |
| *Artemisia absinthium* | Wormwood |
| *Artemisia vulgaris* | Mugwort |
| *Astragalus membranious /complanatus* | Astragalus |
| *Avena sativa* | Wild Oats |
| *Azadirachta indica* | Neem Tree (Nim) |
| *Ballota nigra* | Horehound |
| *Berberis aquifolium* | Oregon grape |
| *Berberis vulgaris* | Barberry |
| *Boswellia serrata* | Boswellia |
| *Brassica alba / nigra* | Mustard |
| *Bupleurum scorzonerifolium* | Buplerum |
| *Calendula officinalis* | Marigold |
| *Capsicum annum / minimum* | Cayenne |
| *Cardus benedictus* | Holy Thistle |
| *Cassia angustifolia* | Senna |
| *Caulophyllum thalictroides* | Blue Cohosh |
| *Chamaelirium luteum* | False Unicorn |

| | |
|---|---|
| *Chamomilla recutita* | Chamomile (German) |
| *Cimicifuga racemosa* | Black Cohosh |
| *Cnicus benedictus* | Blessed Thistle |
| *Cola acuminata / vera* | Kola |
| *Corydalis* | Corydalis |
| *Commiphera opobalsamum / Populus balsamifera* | Balm of Gilead |
| *Commiphora myrrha / molmol* | Myrrh |
| *Crataegus oxycantha* | Hawthorn |
| *Cucurbita pepo* | Pumpkin |
| *Curcuma longa* | Turmeric |
| *Cynara scolymus* | Artichoke |
| *Dioscorea villosa* | Wild Yam |
| *Echinacea angustifolia, purpurea* | Echinacea |
| *Eleutherococcus senticosus* | Siberian Ginseng |
| *Equisetum arvense* | Horsetail |
| *Eucalyptus globulus* | Eucalyptus |
| *Eupatorium perfoliatum* | Boneset |
| *Eupatorium purpureum* | Gravel Root |
| *Euphrasia officinalis* | Eyebright |
| *Filipendula ulmaria* | Meadowsweet |
| *Foeniculum vulgare* | Fennel |
| *Fucus vesculosis* | Bladderwrack |
| *Galium aparine* | Cleavers |
| *Gentiana lutea* | Gentian |
| *Geranium maculatum* | Cranesbill (American) |
| *Ginkgo biloba* | Ginkgo |
| *Glycyrrhiza glabra* | Liquorice |
| *Harpagophytum procumbens* | Devils Claw |
| *Hibiscus abelmoschus* | Hibiscus |
| *Humulus lupulus* | Hops |
| *Hydrangea arborescens* | Hydrangea |
| *Hydrastis canadensis* | Golden Seal |
| *Hydrocotyl asiatica* | Gotu Kola |
| *Hypericum perforatum* | St. John's Wort |
| *Inula helenium* | Elecampane |
| *Juglans nigra* | Black Walnut |
| *Junglans cinerea* | Butternut |
| *Juniperis communis* | Juniper |
| *Lactuca virosa* | Wild Lettuce |
| *Lavandula vera / officinalis* | Lavender |
| *Leonurus cardiaca* | Motherwort |
| *Linum usitatissimum* | Flax |
| *Lobelia inflata* | Lobelia |
| *Mahonia aquifolium* | Mahonia |

240

| | |
|---|---|
| *Malus communis* | Apple |
| *Melaleuca alternifolia* | Tea Tree |
| *Melissa officinalis* | Lemon Balm |
| *Mentha piperita / spicata* | Peppermint, Spearmint |
| *Mentha pulegium* | Pennyroyal |
| *Mitchella repens* | Squaw Vine |
| *Nepeta cataria* | Catnip |
| *Olea europea* | Olive |
| *Panax ginseng (sp. Rhen Shen)* | Ginseng (male) Chinese |
| *Panax quinquefolium (notoginseng)* | Ginseng (female) USA |
| *Passiflora incarnata* | Passion Flower |
| *Petroselinum crispum* | Parsley |
| *Pfaffia paniculata* | Pfaffia |
| *Phytolacca americana / decandra* | Poke |
| *Pinus species* | Pine |
| *Piper nigrum* | Black Pepper |
| *Plantago major* | Plantain |
| *Plantago ovata* | Psyllium |
| *Prunus serotina* | Wild Cherry |
| *Quercus alba* | Oak |
| *Rehmannia glutinosa* | Rehmannia |
| *Rhamnus purshiana* | Cascara Sagrada |
| *Rheum palmatum / Rheum rhaponticum* | Rhubarb |
| *Rosmarinus officinalis* | Rosemary |
| *Rubus idoeus* | Red Raspberry |
| *Rumex crispus* | Yellow Dock |
| *Salix alba* | Willow |
| *Salvia officinalis* | Sage |
| *Sambucus nigra* | Elder |
| *Schizandra chinensis* | Schizandra |
| *Scrophularia nodosa* | Figwort |
| *Scutellaria lateriflora* | Skullcap |
| *Serenoa serrulata* | Saw Palmetto |
| *Silybum marianum* | Milk Thistle |
| *Smilax officinale / ornate* | Sarsaparilla |
| *Sphagnum cymbilifolium* | Sphagnum Moss |
| *Stachys betonica* | Wood Betony |
| *Stellaria media* | Chickweed |
| *Symphytum officinale* | Comfrey |
| *Syzygium aromaticum* | Clove |
| *Tabebuia impetigenosa* | Pau d'arco |
| *Tanacetum parthenium* | Feverfew |
| *Taraxacum officinale* | Dandelion |
| *Thuja occidentalis* | Thuja |

| | |
|---|---|
| *Thymus vulgaris* | Thyme |
| *Tilia europea* | Lime Blossom |
| *Trifolium pratense* | Red Clover |
| *Trigonella foenum-græum* | Fenugreek |
| *Turnera aphrodisiaca, diffusa* | Damiana |
| *Tussilago farfara* | Coltsfoot |
| *Ulmus fulva* | Slippery Elm |
| *Urtica dioica* | Nettles |
| *Usnea longissima* | Usnea |
| *Valeriana officinalis* | Valerian |
| *Verbascum thapsus* | Mullein |
| *Verbena officinalis* | Vervain |
| *Viburnum opulus* | Crampbark |
| *Viscum album* | Mistletoe |
| *Vitex agnus castus* | Agnus Castus |
| *Zanthoxylum bungeanum / americanum* | Prickly Ash |
| *Zea mays* | Corn |
| *Zingiber officinale* | Ginger |

# APPENDIX 3

# HOW TO MAKE A HERBAL PROFILE

Making a herbal profile of your own can be a worthwhile and enjoyable experience. It will ultimately give you a deep understanding of 12 or so herbs which surround your home and with which you will be able to treat many commonly experienced diseases or preferably how to help resist their manifestation in the first place. Some ideal choices in Britain would be oak, apple, yarrow, plantain, nettles, hawthorn, red clover, dandelion, burdock. Only choose the very common ones or you will defeat the main purpose of the herbal profile.

A ring binder, with clear plastic A4 covers to protect pictures and writing alike, will be useful. Either photograph, paint, draw (using colour) or freshly press the herb. You can buy a flower press or make your own from MDF board, rigid poles and wing-nuts with card and blotting paper. This will be ideal for keeping at home, but too bulky to take out into the field, except by car.

If you want to make your own large, but more portable flower press, construct it to the Herbarium size of approx. 480mm x 285mm (17" x 11"), and make it with 30mm (1¼") squares using 15mm (¾") slatted wood. To create layers, you will require quantities of sugar paper or blotting paper with kitchen roll and card. To tighten your press you will need to use fixed Velcro luggage straps (something like a horse girth with clasps, capable of expanding to any width is ideal). Small or large numbers of plant specimens may have to be accommodated at another time in the press, so this ability to open, close, tighten and loosen is vital.

When you first pick your plant, thank it, then shake off any excess water or dew. When dry, place carefully and with consideration as to its arrangement, on white kitchen paper, underneath which you have placed several layers of blotting paper, thick card and the base of the press. If leaves are overlapping each other, carefully spread them out, and if there are really too many, carefully pluck some out. Spread any flower petals out carefully so that they don't get crushed and distorted. After this, put kitchen paper on top, then blotting paper, more card and finally the lid of the press. Until you become more dexterous, get another pair of hands to help you with all of this, the result will be better. Finally tighten the press, but only gently – only as the water starts to leave the plants can you gradually tighten it more. Every day you should change the kitchen paper until the very wet stage is over. Also tighten your straps or wing-nuts a little more each time. The time taken to reach the dry plant stage will vary according to the climate you are in and the lushness or density of the plant you are using. Once it is really dry and there is no longer any more water content, there will be far less risk of colour fading.

To mount your plant pressings, use a white background and glue. Label, using both the Latin and the common name. If you can, list the kind of area and soil you found your plant growing in.

Take at least one year over your herbal profile – though two are often needed and the pleasure doubled! It is important that you experience each season with the plants or trees of your choice. It can be fun to photograph the plant one season and paint it the next, or photograph the berries or flowers, and paint the whole plant.

When writing a description of the plants, you may wish to use botanical language but only do so if it means something to you. For instance 'palmate' is a botanical term for the visual description of a plant with leaves that resemble the hand – i.e. with a palm and fingers coming from it. Otherwise, simply describe the plant in language that means something to everybody including yourself. Note the exact sensory details as seen, felt and experienced by you, e.g. 'the beautiful blue grey bark is also smooth, shiny and smelling faintly musky/sweet in summer, but hardly smelling at all in winter...' Make sure you describe everything – the roots, stem, bark, height, breadth, colour, shape, size, leaf shape and size, flowers blossom, seeds, fruit, needles, smells and taste. Keep the information easy to read, adding sub-headings like 'Flowering Time'. This helps both the writer and the reader.

Dealing descriptively in this much detail involves spending many hours of intimate time with each plant. This could involve sleeping against your chosen tree, or peering at it through a magnifying glass. Both approaches will be needed. Watching plants with this much sensitivity gives you pleasure and joy, with a sense of bonding to nature. Writing down the actions and medicinal uses will be additionally helpful. You will gain much from knowing the action of a plant in relationship to a particular body system as well as the actual diseases it treats.

Folklore information will bring a sense of historical use into your quest, while modern scientific research will give you even more invaluable information.

## RESOURCES

Flower Presses available from:
Fred Aldous, PO Box 135, 37 Lever Street, Manchester M60 1UX. Tel: 0161 236 2477

# An Example of a Healing Programme Timetable

|  | Food Ideas | Natural Healing | Drinks To Be Consumed | Herbal Additions |
|---|---|---|---|---|
| On Rising | N/A | Hydrotherapy & Skin Brushing | Lemon Juice & Water | Tincture 40 drops |
| Breakfast Time | Liver Drink | N/A | Herbal Tea | N/A |
| Mid Morning | Superfood | Belly Breathing 5 minutes | Water | Tincture 40 drops |
| Lunch Time | Salad and Rice | N/A | Herbal Tea | N/A |
| Mid Afternoon | N/A | Belly Breathing | Water | Tincture 40 drops |
| Supper Time | Dahl and Rice with Salad | N/A | Herbal Tea | N/A |
| Before Bed | N/A | Massage / Meditation | Water | Tincture 40 drops |

FOR YOU TO COPY AND USE IF YOU WISH:

|  | Food Ideas | Natural Healing | Drinks To Be Consumed | Herbal Additions |
|---|---|---|---|---|
| On Rising |  |  |  |  |
| Breakfast Time |  |  |  |  |
| Mid Morning |  |  |  |  |
| Lunch Time |  |  |  |  |
| Mid Afternoon |  |  |  |  |
| Supper Time |  |  |  |  |
| Before Bed |  |  |  |  |

# GLOSSARY

**Acid-Alkaline** – This is the pH scale of the residue ash which forms when a given food is oxidized.

**Acupuncture** – The Chinese practice of inserting fine needles into the body at specific points, to energise, unblock or re-route subtle energies, also known as chi.

**Agribusiness** – Generic term referring to the business of agriculture and its associated politics.

**Alkaline** – see above.

**Allicin** – The active component of garlic.

**Antispasmodic** – A herb that limits, corrects or prevents excessive involuntary muscular contractions.

**Antioxidants** – These substances found commonly in high-chlorophyll plants, especially those high in flavonoids, protect the cells from free-radical damage.

**Aphrodisiac** – Any herb that increases sexual desire and potency. Some herbs are shared, some are gender specific.

**Ayurveda** – The healing modality of ancient East India, based on the comprehension of constitutional typing into three basic Dashas (or dispositions); Pitta (Fire), Vala (Air), and Kapha (Moisture).

**Carminative** – A herb that expels gas from the gastro-intestinal tract through excitation of internal peristalsis.

**CFCs** – abbreviation of chloro-fluorocarbon, any of various usually gaseous substances, commonly used in refrigeration, thought to be harmful to the ozone layer.

**Detoxification** – This is the general term indicating a systematic cleansing of the body/mind in total or specific systems.

**Endocrine System** – Glands which govern and regulate body comprising pituitary, thyroid, parathyroid, thymus, adrenal, liver, pancreas, testes and ovary.

**Enzymes** – Substances secreted in the body, and present in live foods, that aid digestion.

**Faecal** – Pertaining to the physical material of the stool.

**Fibroids** – These are non-malignant growths that form from muscle and connective tissue.

**Flavonoids:** Flavonoids are generally capable of free-radical scavenging as they are classified as anti-oxidant.

**High Density Lipo-Proteins** – These are the high ratio protein to fat proteins that carry cholesterol from tissue to the liver. Low density lipo-proteins are considered to be more harmful.

**H I V** – The retro virus considered to be the precursor to AIDS.

**Immunity** – The capacity and function of the body to fend off foreign bodies (fungi, virus, bacteria), and/or disarm and eject them.

**Lymphatic System** – This is the system of glands that secrets white blood cells.

**Maceration** – A medicinal oil that has been made by infusing a base oil with a herb or a number of herbs over a period of time. A typical maceration would be of St John's wort in a vase of olive oil and is used for cuts and bruises.

**Micro-flora** – Tiny plant cells.

**Mucilaginous** – Having the quality of mucus, that is viscous; thick and sticky. Internally used to soothe raw membranes.

**Mucus** – Is the quality of thickness and stickiness in plant and flesh foods. Something described as mucus is said to be binding.

**Oestrogen** – This is the female hormone whose production in the body is lessened during menopause.

**Olfactory organ** – The nose and its glands.

**Organo-phosphates** – Chemical fertilisers.

**Oxygenators** – Substances that bring oxygen into the system.

**Phagocytosis** – A mechanism of three phases, chemotaxis, adherents and ingestion. After it ingests a particle a phagocyte unleashes chemicals that kill any microbes and digest the remains.

**Probiotics** – Substances that increase the presence of 'friendly' bacteria in the intestines.

**Progesterone** – The female hormone of the second phase of the menstrual cycle that prepares for and supports pregnancy.

**Polysaccharides** – A large number of sugars linked together where energy is stored in living tissue.

**Rubefacient** – A category of herb defined by its capacity to draw blood to the surface of the body causing redness by stimulating capillary action. e.g. cayenne.

**Steroids** – In the body essential fatty acids are converted into hormone-like substances called polysaccharides; steroids block their production in order to relieve clotting and pain.

**Stimulant** – Any herb that increases energy and function in the body.

**T-Cells** – Also called T-lymphocytes, these are immune cells that play several roles in the body's defences. T-cells are so called because they mature in the thymus.

**Uterine** – Pertaining to the uterus.

**Vibration** – In the esoteric sciences, all beings are considered to have an energetic quality, also known as their vibration.

**Virus** – Any of a group of minute infective and disease-producing agents consisting of a core of nucleic acid (DNA or RNA) enclosed in a protein shell. Viruses are acellular and able to function and reproduce only if they can invade a living cell to use the cell's system to replicate themselves. In the process they may disrupt or alter the host cell's own DNA.

**Vitamin** – Any of a number of unrelated organic compounds, essential in small quantities for the normal functioning of the body.

# REFERENCES

*Advanced Treatise in Herbology* by Dr. Edward Shook
*Bartram's Encyclopedia of Herbal Medicine* by Thomas Bartram
*Book of Sound Therapy* by Olivea Dewhurst-Maddock
*Botanical Safety Handbook* by Michael McGuffin
*Confessions of a Medical Heretic* by Robert Mendlesohn
*Forest Gardening* by Robert A de Hart
*Healing with Wholefoods* by Paul Pritchard
*Herbal Home Healthcare* by Dr. J Christopher (formerly *Childhood Diseases*)
*Herbal Pharmacopoeia 1996* by BHMA
*Eat Right For Your Type* by Peter D'Adamo with Caroline Whitney
*Light Eating for Survival* by Marcia Mudhuri
*New Holistic Herbal* by David Hoffman
*Nutritional Herbology* by Mark Pederson
*Parasites, An Epidemic in Disguise* by Stanley Weinberger
*Rejuvenation through Elimination* by Dr. J Christopher
*School of Natural Healing* by Dr. J Christopher
*Staying Healthy with Nutrition* by Earnest Haus
*Textbook of Advanced Herbology* by Terry Willard
*Textbook of Modern Herbology* by Terry Willard
*The Manual of Conventional Medicine for Alternative Practitioners* by Stephen Gascoigne
*Water Can Undermine Your Health* by N.W. Walker

# USEFUL ADDRESSES

## PRACTITIONERS

For a list of herbal practitioners, specific schools and their associations will need to be contacted. The umbrella organisation the E.H.P.A. houses the full names and addresses as required (see under Associations). For practitioners trained in the Materia Medica and practices of this book enquire: Selfheal School for Natural Healers and Herbalists, The Cabins, Station Warehouse, Station Road, Pulham Market, Norfolk IP21 4XF. Tel: 01379 608 007. Fax & Tel: 01379 608 201

*Nutritional Medicine and Consultations or accessing nutritional needs.*

### Professor Linda Fellows Phd. M.RED.A
*Radionics practitioner and Herbal Pharmacist. Consultations both in person and by post.*
3 Broadfield Court, Broadfield Road, Folkestone, Kent, CT20 2JT Tel: 01303 226 674

### Dr. Shamim Daya
*G.P. and Nutritionalist.*
57 Harley Street, London, W1N 1DD Tel: 0171 580 7537

### Dr. Marilyn Glenville
*Nutritionist who specializes in hormone problems.*
37 High Street, New Town, Uckfield, East Sussex, TN22 5DL

## ECOLOGICAL ASSOCIATIONS

### Friends of the Earth
26-28 Underwood Street, London N1 7JQ. Tel: 0171 490 1555

### GreenPeace
30-31 Islington Green, London, N1 8BR. Tel: 0171 865 8100

### Plantlife – Registered Charity to Save British Wild Plants
The Wild Plant Conservation Charity, The Natural History Museum, Cromwell Road, London SW7 5BD. Tel: 0171 938 9123

**Rainforest Action Fund**
103 Whitehall Road, Colchester, Essex, CO2 8HA

## HERBAL AND OTHER ASSOCIATIONS

**B.H.M.A**
*To defend the right of the public to choose herbal remedies and to be able to obtain freely. To encourage a wider knowledge and recognition of the value of herbal medicine working with the MCA (Medicine Control Agency) to protect, maintain and promote high standards of quality and safety of herbal remedies.*
Secretary: Ray Hill
Sun House, Church Street, Stroud, Glos, GL5 1JL
Fax: 01453 751 402 Tel: 01453 751 389

**E.H.P.A.**
*Aims to foster unity within the herbal profession and to promote the availability of professional herbal treatment and to raise standards of training and practice within the profession. Works closely with Europe and the M.C.A. Aims eventually to have a common register of qualified practitioners.*
Chairman: Michael McIntyre
Midsummer Cottage and Clinic, Nether-Westcote, Kingham, Oxfordshire OX7 6SD. Tel: 01993 830 419 Fax: 01993 830 957
Secretary: Peter Jackson. Tel and Fax: 01223 212 744
Website: http://www.users.globalnet.UK/~ehpal

**Guild of Naturopathic Iridologists**
*(Holistic Health College)*
Contact: Angela & Peter Bradbury
94 Grosvenor Road, London SW1 3LF. Tel: 0171 834 3579

**Herb Society**
**For magazine and information on national and local meetings and general information about herbs**
Deddington Hill Farm, Warmington, Banbury, Oxon OX17 IXB
Tel: 0129 569 2900 Fax: 0129 692 905

## COLLEGES, SCHOOLS AND ASSOCIATIONS OF HERBAL MEDICINE

**College of Ayurveda**
Milton Keynes. Tel: 01908 664 518

**Danish Association of Phytotherapy**
Denmark. Tel: 0045 33 936162

**Irish Association of Medical Herbalists**
Dublin. 00353 1 8368965

**I.R.C.H.**
Swansea. Tel: 01792 655 886

**N.I.M.H.**
Exeter, Devon. Tel: 01886 821 026

**R.C.H.M.**
London. Tel: 0171 483 3568

**Register of East West College of Certified Herbalists**
East Sussex TN7 4ET. Tel: 01342 822 312

**Selfheal School for Natural Healers and Herbalists**
**Master Herbalist Association**
The Cabins, Station Warehouse, Station Road, Pulham Market, Norfolk IP21 4XF.
Tel: 01379 608 007. Fax & Tel: 01379 608 201

**Tara College of Tibetan Medicine**
Edinburgh EH5 3DL. Tel: 0131 447 1945

**Swedish Association of Medical Herbalists**
Sweden. Tel: 0046 46 121909

## SUPPLIERS

**Archturus Health Care Ltd**
*Enema kits, supplements and other general health care items*
Strathenry House, Leslie, Fife KY6 3HY Scotland

**Baldwin & Company**
*Herbs, storage bottles, jars and other containers*
171-173 Walworth Road, London, SE17 1RW. Tel: 0171 703 5550

**Bio-Care**
*Quality supplements by post*
180 Lifford Lane, Kings Norton, Birmingham B30 3NT. Tel: 0121 433 3727

**Bristol Bottle Company**
*Storage bottles and jars and other containers*
Unit 1, Ashmead Trading Estate, Ashmead Road, Keynsham, Avon, BS18 1TZ

**Dr. Richard Schulze, American Botanical Pharmacy,**
*Herbal products*
California, USA. Tel & Fax: 001 310 576 6525

**East West Herb Shop**
*Chinese herb suppliers who will supply Western herb tinctures only upon request.*
3 Neals Yard, Covent Garden, London, WC2H 9DP. Tel: 0171 379 1312

## Essential Foods
*A mail order company supplying minerals, celtic salt, Valdina cane sugar and much more. A full catalogue is available on request.*
Essential Foods, PO Box 36, Richmond, Surrey, TW9 3RP. Tel: 0870 606 2755

## Hambelden Herbs
*Organic Herbs by mail order.*
Court Farm, Milverton, Somerset TA4 1NF. Tel: 01823 401 205

## Herbs, Hands, Healing
*Herbal Formulae, organic herbs, Superfood and Herbal Tea Socks*
The Cabins, Station Warehouse, Station Road, Pulham Market, Norfolk IP21 4XF
Tel 01379 608 082, Tel & Fax 01379 608 201

## Neal's Yard Remedies
*Herbal Remedies*
Tel: 0171 379 7222 *Ask for local shops*

## Potters Herbal Supplies
Leyland, Mill Lane, Wigan, Lancashire, WN1 2SB. Tel: 01842 3461

## Springfield Pharmacy
Mr. J N Patel, 124 Sheen Road, Richmond, Surrey TW9 1UR. Tel: 0181 940 2304

## Sunshine Health Shop
Herbal Remedies and Natural Supplements
25 Church Street, Stroud, Gloucester, GL5 1JL

## Wholistic Research Company
*Suppliers of enema kits, water distillers, juicers and much more in a huge catalogue*
Bright Haven, Robins Lane, Lolworth, Cambridge, CB3 8HH Tel: 01954 781 074

# U.S.A. HERBS

## Blessed Herbs (Organic)
109 Barre Plains Road, Oakham, MA01063

## Pacific Botanicals (Organic)
4350 Fish Hatchery Road, Grants Pass, OR 97527

# MISCELLANEOUS

## Cambridge University Botanic Garden
Cory Lodge, Bateman Street, Cambridge, CB2 1JS. Tel: 01223 336 265

## Chiltern Seeds
*for an excellent seed catalogue*
Ulverston, Cumbria LA12 7PB. Tel: 01229 581 137

### Poyntz Field Herb Nursery

*Grower of Siberian ginseng and other herbs, seed and young plants available mail order*
Duncan Ross, Pontyz Field, Herb Nursery, Black Isle, by Dingwell, Ross and Cromalty, Scotland, IV7 8LX

### Diagnostech Ltd.

*For general tests like adrenal, hormone, melatonin and a variety of other tests*
Diagnostech ltd. York Chambers, Yorkshire, Swansea SA1 3NJ
*They will be able to refer you to a practitioner who either works with them or has the tests available on site.*

### Higher Nature Ltd.

The Nutrition Centre, Burwash Common, East Sussex, TN19 7OX. Tel: 01435 882 880

### Royal Botanic Gardens at Kew

47 Kew Green, Richmond, Surrey, TW9 3AB. Tel: 0181 332 5000

### Royal Horticultural Society's Garden

Wisley, Surrey. Tel: 01483 224 234

### Tao of Books

*A fine source for books on alternative medicine and related topics in Europe who produce a fairly comprehensive catalogue and supply mail order. Also available are special lists for Herbalism and Natural Healing books only – extremely comprehensive, covering worldwide titles.*
The Tao of Books, Station Warehouse, Station Road, Pulham Market, Norfolk, IP21 4XF Tel: 01379 676 000

### Nutritional Video

Food Therapy by Dr Shamim Daya:
Food Therapy Ltd, PO Box 434, Richmond, Surrey, TW9 3RN
Tel: 07000 388 388

# INDEX

Note: Numbers in bold indicate pages with substantial references. Where **f**, **r** or **ill** follows a number, a **formula**, **recipe** or **illustration** (respectively) is found in the page range shown.

cysts, 114, 181, 211
  breast, 163–4
  cervical, 206–7
  ovarian, 206–7

dairy products, 44–5, 88, 114
Danazol, 182
dancing, 60, 82
dandelions, **9**, 49, 66, 69, 80, 82, 110, 122,
  133, 135, 138, 144, 145, 205, 212
dandruff, 174
death, cancer, 129
death rate, 141–2
decaffeination, 46
decoctions, 20, **21–2**, 24
deep breathing, *see* breathing
deep wound paste, 234**f**
dehydration, 132, 177, 203
dementia, 209
dengue fever, 86
dental care, 127
deodorants, 153
depressants, *see* anti-depressants
depression (*see also* anti-depressants), 37, 38,
  57, 63, 67, 81, 82, 96, 108, 113, 120,
  121, 122, 123, 134, 140, 141, 142, 149,
  166, 168, 171, **174–5**, 182, 212
dermatitis, 175
detoxification, **63–83**, 134
diabetes, 63, 68, 133, **175–7**, 204, 217
diaphragm, 92
diarrhoea, 11, 13, 36, 38, 96, 103, 105, 127,
  129, 140, 140, 146, 166, 168, 169,
  **177–8**, 182, 190, 196, 212, 230
diet (*see also* nutrition; individual entries for
  conditions and illnesses), xi–xii, 2, 18,
  **30–32**
digestion, 36, **39**, 47, 49, **51–52**, 136, 138,
  139, 165, 168, 184, **194–5**,
  herbs, 135
digestive system, **126–32ill**
digestive and travel tincture, 233**f**
diphtheria, 86, 96
discharges, vaginal, 221
diuretics, 38, 64, 108, 132, **133**
diverticuli, 128
diverticulitis, **178–9**

diverticulosis, 130**ill**
dizziness, 89, 135, 139, 219
douches, 27, 118
Dr. Christopher's anti-miscarriage formula,
  233**f**
Dr. Christopher's B & B ear formula, 233**f**
Dr. Christopher's bone, flesh and cartilage
  formula, 233**f**
drinks, 46–8
Dr. Schulze's deep tissue oil, 233**f**
drugs, 34, 68, 72–3, 128, 142, 168, 172
  addiction, 94
  withdrawal, 150
duodenum, 126**ill** 134, 138
  ulcers, 179–80
dysentery, 86
dysmenorrhoea, 207–8

ear problems, 180, 216, 218–9,
echinacea, **94–6**, 98, 113, 117, 123, 124, 138,
  140, 153, 154, 184, 224, 230, 231
ecobiotics, 90
eczema, 28, 38, 104, 152, **180–81**, 195
  ointment, 234**f**
effleurage, 58
eggs, **45–6**, 114
ejaculation, involuntary, 112
elder, 10
elderberries, 97
elderflower and elderberry compote syrup,
  22**r**
Eleuthero, 94
emergencies, first aid, 226–9
emetics, 232
emotions, 31, 79, 80, 81, 82, 83, 89, 91–2,
  109, 113, 118, 121, 134, 141, 142, 146,
  148, 152, 161, 171, 208, 212
emphysema, 183
endocrine system (*see also* hormones), 47,
  110, 111, 112, 137, 138, 140, 141, 174,
  212
endometrial cancer, 108
endometriosis, 113, **181–3**, 208, 210
enemas, 65, **75–6f**, 98–9
energy, 80, 81, 82, 95, 108, 119, 134, 138,
  140, 192
Engervita, 53, 117

enzymes, 43, 54, 134, 138
epilepsy, 148, 150, 192
Epstein-Barr virus, 185
esophagus, *see* oesophagus
essential oils, 5, 8, 27–8, **97–8**, 113, 123,
    132, 137, 147, 152, 153
eucalyptus, 6–7, 8, 13, 97
excretion, by skin, 152
exercise, 2, **60**, 64, 82, 156
exfoliation, facial, 57
exhaustion, *see* fatigue
eye problems, 96, 113, 135, **227–8**
eyes, xii, 68
eyesight, 211

faecal matter, *see* faeces
faeces, 71, 72, 76, 74, **128**, 129, 131, 158,
    178
fainting, 232, 228
fallopian tubes, 181, 210
famine, 8
farming, 7, 8, 88
fasting, **64–5**, 67, 78, 184, 214
fat, 42, 44, 65, 80, 81, 108, 113, 134, 138,
    142, 159, 189
fatigue, 63, 68, 81, 104, 110, 113, 116, 122,
    140, 141, 166, 167, 171, 185, 192, 199,
    207, 212, 219
fatty acids, 46, 134, 139, 142, 144, 149, 152,
    154
fatty deposits, 188
fennel, 36, 72, 97
fenugreek, 36, 139
fermentation, 52
fermented foods, 51–3
fertility, 34, 61, 47, 107, 137
    treatment, 114
fevers, 13, 26, 38, 82, **98–99**, 106, 167, 168,
    208, 211
fibre, 50, 65, 71, 128, 131, 170
fibrocystic lumps, 164
fibroids, 114, 208
    breasts, 163–4
    uterine, 206–7
first aid, 226–34
first aid kit, 231
fish, 46

flatulence, 36
flat worms, *see* worms
flavonoids, 18, 82
flavours, 39–41
flax, 72, 142
flora, 52, 72, 76, 87, 90, 128, 131, 135, 144,
    166
flowers, 18
flu, 13, 36, 124
fluke worms, *see* worms
foetuses, 116–7, 139
folic acid, 116, 117, 142, 158, 208
food chain, 87, 89
food colourings, 103
food flavouring, 143
food poisoning, 87–8
food production, 3, 34
foot massage, 58
forest gardening, 7
forgetfulness, 163, 209
    *see also* brain; memory
fragrances, 98, 117, 118
free radicals, 41, 44, 63, 124, 143
friction massage, 58
fruit delight, 103**r**
fruit, xi, 35, **49**, 143
    juices, **49–50**, 134
fungal infections, 165, 174, 162, 166
fungi, 71, 97, 129, 215

gall-bladder, 12, 40, 41, 68, 90, 96, 130**ill**,
    131, **133–6**, 138, 203
    cleansing, 77, 134–5
gallstones, 46, 130**ill**, 209
gamma linoleic acid (GLA), 113
gardening, 8
gardnerella, 221
gargles, 98, 234**f**
garlic, 23, 25**f**, 35, **36–7**, 69, 71, 76, **96**, 97,
    124, 134, 139, 143, 144, 145, 160, 176,
    178, 189, 201, 221, 222, 223, 224
gashes, first aid, 228
gastric ulcers, 130**ill**, **183–4**
gastritis, 130**ill**, 184
gastro-intestinal problems, 82
gelatine, 23
genito-urinary problems, 133